Practical Pediatric and Adolescent Gynecology

Practical Pediatric and Adolescent Gynecology

Edited by

Paula J. Adams Hillard MD

Professor, Department of Obstetrics and Gynecology
Stanford University School of Medicine
Stanford, CA
USA

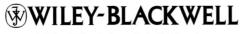

A John Wiley & Sons, Ltd., Publication

This edition first published 2013 © 2013 by John Wiley and Sons, Ltd.

Wiley-Blackwell is an imprint of John Wiley & Sons, formed by the merger of Wiley's global Scientific, Technical and Medical business with Blackwell Publishing.

Registered office: John Wiley & Sons, Ltd, The Atrium, Southern Gate, Chichester, West Sussex, PO19 8SQ, UK

Editorial offices: 9600 Garsington Road, Oxford, OX4 2DQ, UK
The Atrium, Southern Gate, Chichester, West Sussex, PO19 8SQ, UK
111 River Street, Hoboken, NJ 07030-5774, USA

For details of our global editorial offices, for customer services and for information about how to apply for permission to reuse the copyright material in this book please see our website at www.wiley.com/wiley-blackwell

Library of Congress Cataloging-in-Publication Data

Practical pediatric and adolescent gynecology / edited by Paula J. Adams Hillard.
        p. ; cm. – (Gynecology in practice)
    Includes bibliographical references and index.
    ISBN 978-0-470-67387-4 (hardback : alk. paper)
    I. Hillard, Paula Adams. II. [DNLM: 1. Genital Diseases, Female.   2. Adolescent.
3. Child.   4. Gynecological Examination–methods.   5. Infant. WS 360]

    618.92'098–dc23

                                2012037093

A catalogue record for this book is available from the British Library.

Wiley also publishes its books in a variety of electronic formats. Some content that appears in print may not be available in electronic books.

Cover image: (man and woman) © iStockphoto.com/John_Woodcock; (people silhouette) © iStockphoto.com/Kristina
Cover design by Sarah Dickinson

Set in 9/11.5 pt Sabon by Toppan Best-set Premedia Limited
Printed and bound in Singapore by Markono Print Media Pte Ltd

1 2013

Contents

Preface

I'm assuming that you're a "clinician" – a term that I use to mean someone who provides clinical care for individuals – and in the case that you're reading this book, for young girls and adolescent young women. You may be a family physician, a family nurse practitioner, a general gynecologist, a pediatrician, an obstetrician-gynecologist, an internist, a specialist in adolescent medicine, a physician's assistant, a registered nurse, a certified nurse midwife, or a clinician of another stripe/persuasion/training. I specifically don't intend for the audience to be physicians only, as I know that many other varieties of clinicians provide care for girls and teens. I welcome your interest in caring for young girls and adolescents. You may regularly provide care for teens, but want to know more about their gynecologic care, as do many of my colleagues in adolescent medicine. You may provide gynecologic care for adults, but want to learn more about the gynecologic conditions that affect young girls that you see much less frequently, as is the case with my colleagues who are general obstetrician-gynecologists.

I want to remind those who do not regularly provide pediatric care for teens that there are really two parties to keep in mind with the pediatric age group: the designated patient and her parent (usually her mother or other female adult guardian). The challenges of providing the necessary confidential care to our adolescent patients, who live within the context of their family, are many. It's not an easy line for a clinician to walk, and thus several chapters in this text address issues such as the initial consultation visit with an adolescent, confidentiality, and even legal issues for the care of adolescents.

I would strongly encourage you to review those chapters in the section on Adolescent Health as a place to start reading, if you intend to provide gynecologic care for adolescents. This section addresses common issues for all adolescents, even those who don't present with a specific gynecologic problem. For example, Chapter 20 on Adolescent sexuality provides important background on adolescent development. Chapter 19 provides essential legal information on the provision of adolescent healthcare. Another section that will be helpful is Appendix 1, Essential Information, which includes a number of tables that will be relevant to an understanding of adolescent health. Tables on adolescent development, normal menstrual parameters, sexual history taking, psychosocial assessment using the HEEADSSS tool, and indications for a pelvic examination provide a wealth of information summarized in easy to reference tables.

Similarly, providing care for a young girl, particularly one with vulvovaginal symptoms, will be facilitated by pre-reading this Essential Information prior to going to the chapter on a specific symptom or condition.

But after you've read these initial chapters and reviewed the Essential Information, then in all likelihood, you will be reviewing the book with concerns about a specific patient with a specific gynecologic problem. I would first direct you to the appropriate section of the book by age – prepubertal or adolescent. Within the age groupings, each section is further organized by either the presenting sign or symptom or by the specific gynecologic conditionthat occurs in that group. For example, if you are looking for what conditions may cause vaginal discharge in a prepubertal girl, you would look in Section 1 for prepubertal conditions, and then in Part 2 under symptoms and signs. You will then find information about the various conditions that can cause discharge. Alternatively, if you have an adolescent patient whom you have diagnosed as having a specific condition, such as a vulvovaginal yeast infection, and you want to read further about the management of this particular condition, you would look in Section 3 for adolescents, and then under Part 4, gynecologic conditions in adolescent girls.

Finally Appendix 2 includes useful web resources for adolescents, for parents, and for clinicians.

Overall, I hope that the organization of the book will make it both a useful text that will provide background information to allow you to better provide care to teens and young girls, as well as a handy reference that will answer specific questions about girls with specific gynecologic symptoms, signs, or conditions.

The preparation of this book has been quite a project, involving the hard work and dedication of many medical colleagues. My friends and colleagues who have so generously contributed their knowledge to the content of this book have, collectively, many, many years of clinical experience. They are the true experts on each topic, and they have taught me a great deal. I extend my heartfelt thanks to each of them. In addition, the many individuals at Wiley-Blackwell have contributed their professionalism, feedback, guidance, skills, and expert management from the very beginning of the project with the conception of an idea for a book, through the long gestation period of communications with contributors,

editing, and finally the birth of the book through the work of the production staff. They have my gratitude and thanks. Of course I also thank my husband who has seen my free time consumed by this project, yet who has supported me faithfully and lovingly in so many ways. Finally, but perhaps most importantly, I thank my patients and their parents. They continue to teach me daily.

I welcome any thoughts, suggestions, and feedback on this book. We share the goals of providing excellent, knowledgeable medical care that the young girls and developing young women whom we see in our clinical practices deserve. As clinicians, we are privileged to help guide them toward a healthier future.

Paula J. Adams Hillard

Contributors

Elizabeth Alderman MD
Professor of Clinical Pediatrics;
Director, Post-doctoral Fellowship Adolescent
  Medicine
Albert Einstein College of Medicine
Children's Hospital at Montefiore
Bronx, NY, USA

Lisa Allen MD, FRCSC
Associate Professor, Department of Obstetrics and
  Gynecology
University of Toronto;
Section Head Pediatric Gynecology
Hospital for Sick Children
Toronto, ON, Canada

Janice Bacon MD
Lexington Medical Center
Women's Health & Diagnostic Center
West Columbia, SC, USA

Corinne Bazella MD
Assistant Professor of Obstetrics and Gynecology
Case Western Reserve University School of
  Medicine
Cleveland, OH, USA

Kirsten Bechtel MD
Yale New-Haven Children's Hospital
Section of Pediatric Emergency Medicine
New Haven, CT, USA

Uri Belkind MD, MS
Post-doctoral Fellow
Division of Adolescent Medicine
Albert Einstein College of Medicine
Children's Hospital at Montefiore
Bronx, NY, USA

Jennifer L. Bercaw-Pratt MD
Division of Pediatric and Adolescent Gynecology
Department of Obstetrics and Gynecology
Baylor College of Medicine
Houston, TX, USA

Frank M. Biro MD
Rauh Professor of Pediatrics
University of Cincinnati College of Medicine;
Director, Division of Adolescent Medicine
Cincinnati Children's Hospital Medical Center
Cincinnati, OH, USA

Margaret J. Blythe MD
Professor of Pediatrics and Adjunct Professor of
  Gynecology
Adolescent Medicine
Indiana University School of Medicine
Indianapolis, IN, USA

Paula Braverman MD
Professor of Pediatrics
University of Cincinnati College of Medicine;
Division of Adolescent Medicine
Cincinnati Children's Hospital Medical Center
Cincinnati, OH, USA

Lesley L. Breech MD
Associate Professor of Obstetrics and Gynecology,
  Surgery, and Pediatrics
Department of Surgery
Division of Pediatric and Adolescent Gynecology
University of Cincinnati College of Medicine
Cincinnati, OH, USA

Jane E.D. Broecker MD
Assistant Professor of Obstetrics and Gynecology
Ohio University Heritage College of Osteopathic
  Medicine
Athens, OH, USA

Gale R. Burstein MD, MPH
Associate Professor of Clinical Pediatrics
The State University of New York at Buffalo School
    of Medicine and Biomedical Sciences;
Commissioner of Health
Erie County Department of Health
Buffalo, NY, USA

Christopher V. Chambers MD
Department of Family & Community Medicine
    Thomas Jefferson University
Philadelphia, PA, USA

Susan M. Coupey MD
Professor of Pediatrics
Chief, Division of Adolescent Medicine
Albert Einstein College of Medicine
Children's Hospital at Montefiore
Bronx, NY, USA

Stephanie Crewe MD, MHS
Assistant Professor
Division of Adolescent Medicine
Virginia Commonwealth University Medical Center
Richmond, VA, USA

Helen R. Deitch MD
Wellspan Medical Group
York Hospital
Wellspan Women's Specialty Services
York, PA, USA

Dianne Deplewski MD
Assistant Professor of Pediatrics
Director, Pediatric Endocrinology Fellowship
    Program
The University of Chicago Pritzker School of
    Medicine
Section of Pediatric Endocrinology
Chicago, IL, USA

Jennifer E. Dietrich MD, MSc
Associate Professor
Department of Obstetrics and Gynecology;
Division of Pediatric and Adolescent Gynecology
Baylor College of Medicine
Houston, TX, USA

Amy D. DiVasta MD, MMSc
Staff Physician
Divisions of Adolescent and Young Adult Medicine
    and Pediatric and Adolescent Gynecology
Boston Children's Hospital;
Assistant Professor of Pediatrics
Harvard Medical School
Boston, MA, USA

Michael Dobbs MD
Clinical Fellow, Adolescent Medicine
Cincinnati Children's Hospital Medical Center
Division of Adolescent Medicine
Cincinnati, OH, USA

Colleen Bryzik Dodich MD
Assistant Professor, Pediatrics
Oakland University-William Beaumont School of
    Medicine
Beverly Hills Pediatrics, Private Practice
Bingham Farms, MI, USA

Kaiyti Duffy MPH
University of Illinois at Chicago College of
    Medicine
Chicago, IL, USA

James R. Ebert MD, MBA, MPH
Associate Professor of Pediatrics and Community
    Health
Wright State University
Boonshoft School of Medicine
Dayton, OH, USA

Beth L. Emerson MD
Yale School of Medicine
Department of Pediatrics
Section of Pediatric Emergency Medicine
Yale New-Haven Children's Hospital
New Haven, CT, USA

Abigail English JD
Director
Center for Adolescent Health & the Law
Chapel Hill, NC, USA

Elizabeth B. Erbaugh PhD
Visiting Assistant Professor
Department of Sociology;
Research Associate
Institute for Research on Social Issues
Indiana University-Purdue University Indianapolis
Indianapolis, IN, USA

Mariel A. Focseneanu MD
Department of Obstetrics and Gynecology
Division of Pediatric and Adolescent Gynecology
Washington University School of Medicine in St.
    Louis;
Barnes Jewish Hospital
St. Louis, MO, USA

Michelle Forcier MD, MPH
Associate Professor of Pediatrics
Division of Adolescent Medicine
Hasbro Children's Hospital;
Department of Pediatrics
Warren Alpert Medical School of Brown University
Providence, RI, USA

J. Dennis Fortenberry MD, MS
Professor of Pediatrics
Indiana University School of Medicine
Indianapolis, IN, USA

Donna Futterman MD
Director, Adolescent AIDS Program
Professor of Clinical Pediatrics
Montefiore Medical Center
Albert Einstein College of Medicine
Bronx, NY, USA

Melissa Gilliam MD, MPH
Professor, The University of Chicago
Department of Obstetrics and Gynecology
Section of Family Planning and Contraceptive
    Research
Chicago, IL, USA

Emily M. Godfrey MD, MPH
Associate Professor of Family Medicine
Department of Family Medicine
University of Washington
Seattle, WA, USA

Melanie A. Gold DO
Clinical Professor of Pediatrics
Department of Pediatrics
Division of Adolescent Medicine
University of Pittsburgh School of Medicine
Pittsburgh, PA, USA

Neville H. Golden MD
Chief, Division of Adolescent Medicine
The Marron and Mary Elizabeth Kendrick Professor
    in Pediatrics
Department of Pediatrics
Division of Adolescent Medicine
Stanford University School of Medicine
Chief, Division of Adolescent Medicine
Lucile Packard Children's Hospital at Stanford
Palo Alto, CA, USA

Estherann Grace MD
Clinical Chief, Division of Adolescent and Young
    Adult Medicine
Boston Children's Hospital;
Clinical Associate Professor of Pediatrics
Harvard Medical School
Boston, MA, USA

Jennifer A. Greene MD
Assistant Professor of Obstetrics and Gynecology
University of South Carolina School of Medicine
Columbia, SC, USA

Marjorie Greenfield MD
Professor of Obstetrics and Gynecology
Case Western Reserve University School of
    Medicine
Cleveland, OH, USA

Donald E. Greydanus MD, Dr HC (ATHENS)
Professor, Pediatrics and Human Development
Western Michigan University School of Medicine
Kalamazoo, MI, USA

Rebecca Gudeman JD, MPA
Senior Attorney
National Center for Youth Law
Oakland, CA, USA

Zeev Harel MD
Professor of Pediatrics
Division of Adolescent Medicine
Hasbro Children's Hospital;
Rhode Island Hospital;
Warren Alpert Medical School of Brown University
Providence, RI, USA

S. Paige Hertweck MD
Chief of Gynecology
Director of Pediatric and Adolescent Gynecology
Kosair Children's Hospital;
Clinical Faculty
Department of Pediatrics, and Obstetrics and
    Gynecology
University of Louisville
Louisville, KY, USA

Geri D. Hewitt MD
Associate Professor of Obstetrics, Gynecology and
    Pediatrics
Nationwide Children's Hospital; Ohio State
    University College of Medicine
Columbus, OH, USA

Paula J. Adams Hillard MD
Professor, Department of Obstetrics and Gynecology
Stanford University School of Medicine
Stanford, CA, USA

Christopher P. Houk MD
Associate Professor of Pediatrics
Medical College of Georgia
Augusta, GA, USA

Anne Hsii MD
Clinical Fellow
Department of Pediatrics
Division of Adolescent Medicine
Stanford University School of Medicine
Mountain View, CA, USA

Jill S. Huppert MD, MPH
Associate Professor of Obstetrics and Gynecology,
    Pediatrics
Cincinnati Children's Hospital Medical Center
Cincinnati, OH, USA

Michelle M. Isley MD, MPH
Assistant Professor in Obstetrics and Gynecology
The Ohio State University
Columbus, OH, USA

Mary Anne Jamieson MD
Associate Professor
Obstetrics, Gynecology and Pediatrics
Queen's University
Kingston, ON, Canada

John Jarrell MD, MSc, FRCSC
Professor of Obstetrics and Gynecology
University of Calgary
Calgary, AB, Canada

Susan Jay MD
Professor of Pediatrics
Medical College of Wisconsin
Children's Hospital of Wisconsin
Milwaukee, WI, USA

Jessica A. Kahn MD, MPH
Division of Adolescent Medicine
Cincinnati Children's Hospital Medical Center
Cincinnati, OH, USA

Kristin L. Kaltenstadler MD
Private Physician
Suburban Pediatrics Associates
Cincinnati, OH, USA

Kelly Kantartzis MD
Fellow, Female Pelvic Medicine and Reconstructive
    Surgery
University of Pittsburgh School of Medicine
Pittsburgh, PA, USA

Paul B. Kaplowitz MD, PhD
Chief of Endocrinology
Children's National Medical Center
Professor of Pediatrics
George Washington University
School of Medicine and the Health Sciences
Washington, DC, USA

Andrew M. Kaunitz MD
Professor and Associate Chairman
Department of Obstetrics and Gynecology
University of Florida College of
    Medicine-Jacksonville
Jacksonville, FL, USA

Jennifer C. Kelley MD
Pediatric Endocrine Fellow
Children's Hospital of Philadelphia
Philadelphia, PA, USA

Nancy D. Kellogg MD
Professor of Pediatrics
University of Texas Health Science Center at San
    Antonio
San Antonio, TX, USA

Sari Kives MD, FRCSC, MSc
Associate Professor
University of Toronto
Hospital for Sick Children
Toronto, ON, Canada

Linda M. Kollar RN, MSN, CPNP
Cincinnati Children's Hospital Medical Center
Cincinnati, OH, USA

Melissa Kottke MD, MPH, MBA
Assistant Professor of Gynecology and Obstetrics;
Director
Jane Fonda Center for Adolescent Reproductive
    Health
Emory University School of Medicine
Atlanta, GA, USA

Eduardo Lara-Torre MD
Vice Chair for Academic Affairs
Associate Professor
Residency Program Director
Department of Obstetrics and Gynecology
Virginia Tech-Carilion School of Medicine
Roanoke, VA, USA

Peter A. Lee MD, PhD
Professor of Pediatrics
Riley Hospital for Children
Indiana University School of Medicine
Indianapolis, IN, USA;
Department of Pediatrics
The Milton S. Hershey Medical Center
Penn State College of Medicine
Hershey, PA, USA

Corinne Lehmann MD, MED
Associate Professor of Pediatrics and Internal
    Medicine
University of Cincinnati;
Cincinnati Children's Hospital Medical Center
Cincinnati, OH, USA

Sharon Levy MD, MPH
Assistant Professor of Pediatrics
Harvard Medical School
Boston Children's Hospital
Boston, MA, USA

Kaylene J. Logan MD
Chief Resident
Department of Obstetrics and Gynecology
Virginia Tech-Carilion School of Medicine
Roanoke, VA, USA

Jennifer Louis-Jacques MD, MPH
Clinical Fellow
Division of Adolescent/Young Adult Medicine
Children's Hospital Boston;
Clinical Fellow in Pediatrics
Harvard Medical School
Boston, MA, USA

Meredith Loveless MD
Kosair Children's Hospital;
Clinical Faculty
Department of Pediatrics, and Obstetrics and
    Gynecology
University of Louisville
Louisville, KY, USA

James L. Lukefahr MD
Professor of Pediatrics
Division of Child Abuse Pediatrics
University of Texas Health Science Center at San
    Antonio
San Antonio, TX, USA

Maureen Lynch MD, MS
Assistant Clinical Professor
Chief of Pediatrics at Harvard University Health
    Services
Harvard University
Cambridge, MA, USA

Courtney A. Marsh MD, MPH
Clinical Fellow
Division of Reproductive Endocrinology and
    Infertility
University of Michigan Health System
Ann Arbor, MI, USA

Sofya Maslayanskya MD
Post-Doctoral Fellow
Division of Adolescent Medicine
Albert Einstein College of Medicine
Children's Hospital at Montefiore
Bronx, NY, USA

Colleen McNicholas DO
Clinical Fellow – Family Planning
Department of Obstetrics and Gynecology
Washington University School of Medicine in St.
    Louis
St. Louis, MO, USA

Seema Menon MD
Assistant Professor
Department of Obstetrics and Gynecology
Children's Hospital of Wisconsin;
Medical College of Wisconsin
Milwaukee, WI, USA

Diane F. Merritt MD
Department of Obstetrics and Gynecology
Division of Pediatric and Adolescent Gynecology
Washington University School of Medicine in St.
    Louis
Barnes Jewish Hospital
St. Louis Children's Hospital
Missouri Baptist Medical Center
St. Louis, MO, USA

Amy B. Middleman MD, MSEd, MPH
Associate Professor of Pediatrics
Baylor College of Medicine
Houston, TX, USA

Comfort Momoh MBE, RN, RM, BSC, MSc in
    Public Health
FGM/Public Health Specialist
King's College London
University of London
London, UK

Samantha E. Montgomery MD, MSc
Department of Pediatric and Adolescent Gynecology
Cincinnati Children's Hospital Medical Center
Cincinnati, OH, USA

Melanie Nathan MD
Instructor, Obstetrics and Gynecology
Tufts Medical Center
Boston, MA, USA

Rebecca Flynn O'Brien MD
Division of Adolescent/Young Adult Medicine
Children's Hospital Boston
Assistant Professor of Pediatrics
Harvard Medical School
Boston, MA, USA

Hatim A. Omar MD
Professor, Pediatrics & Obstetrics/Gynecology
Chief, Division of Adolescent Medicine
Department of Pediatrics
Kentucky Children's Hospital
Lexington, KY, USA

Melanie Ornstein MD, FRCSC
Assistant Professor, Department of Obstetrics and
    Gynecology
University of Toronto
Toronto East General Hospital
Toronto, ON, Canada

Sherine Patterson-Rose MD
Clinical Fellow
Division of Adolescent Medicine
Cincinnati Children's Hospital Medical Center
Cincinnati, OH, USA

Jeffrey F. Peipert MD, PhD
Robert J. Terry Professor of Obstetrics and
    Gynecology
Washington University School of Medicine in St.
    Louis
St. Louis, MO, USA

Samantha M. Pfeifer MD
Associate Professor
Obstetrics and Gynecology
Perelman School of Medicine at University of
    Pennsylvania
Philadelphia, PA, USA

Rachael Phelps MD
Medical Director
Planned Parenthood of the Rochester/Syracuse
    Region
Clinical Instructor Pediatrics
Clinical Instructor in Obstetrics and Gynecology
University of Rochester
Rochester, NY, USA

Anne-Marie Priebe DO
PAG Fellow
University of Missouri Kansas City
Children's Mercy Hospital
Kansas City, MO, USA

Elisabeth H. Quint MD
Clinical Professor in Obstetrics and Gynecology
University of Michigan Medical School
Ann Arbor, MI, USA

Anita Radix MD, MPhil, MPH
Director of Research and Education
Callen-Lorde Community Health Center
New York, NY, USA

Valerie S. Ratts MD
Professor
Department of Obstetrics and Gynecology
Division of Reproductive Endocrinology and
    Infertility
Washington University School of Medicine in St.
    Louis
St. Louis, MO, USA

Ellen S. Rome MD, MPH
Professor of Pediatrics
Cleveland Clinic Lerner College of Medicine
Head, Center for Adolescent Medicine
Cleveland Clinic Children's Hospital
Cleveland, OH, USA

Robert L. Rosenfield MD
Emeritus Professor of Pediatrics and Medicine
The University of Chicago Pritzker School of
    Medicine
Section of Pediatric Endocrinology
Chicago, IL, USA

Mandakini Sadhir MBBS
Adolescent Medicine Fellow
Department of Pediatrics
Division of Adolescent Medicine
Children's Hospital of Wisconsin
Medical College of Wisconsin
Milwaukee, WI, USA

Patricia Schram MD
Developmental and Behavioral Pediatrics
Harvard Medical School
Boston Children's Hospital
Boston, MA, USA

Taraneh Shafii MD, MPH
Assistant Professor of Pediatrics
Division of Adolescent Medicine
University of Washington School of Medicine
Seattle, WA, USA

Avni C. Shah MD
Clinical Assistant Professor
Stanford University and the Lucile Packard
  Children's Hospital at Stanford
Pediatric Endocrinology and Diabetes
Stanford, CA, USA

Sejal Shah MD
Clinical Instructor
Pediatric Endocrinology and Diabetes
Stanford University and the Lucile Packard
  Children's Hospital at Stanford
Stanford, CA, USA

Yolanda R. Smith MD, MS
Professor of Obstetrics and Gynecology
Division of Reproductive Endocrinology and
  Infertility
University of Michigan Health System
Ann Arbor, MI, USA

Noam Smorgick-Rosenbaum MD, MSc
Fellow in Pediatrics and Adolescent Gynecology
University of Michigan Health System
Ann Arbor, MI, USA

Michael G. Spigarelli MD, PhD
Professor of Pediatrics;
Chief, Division of Adolescent Medicine
University of Utah
Salt Lake City, UT, USA

Stephanie Stockburger MD
Division of Adolescent Medicine
Department of Pediatrics
University of Kentucky
Lexington, KY, USA

Julie L. Strickland MD, MPH
Professor of Obstetrics and Gynecology
University of Missouri Kansas City
Children's Mercy Hospital
Kansas City, MO, USA

Gina Sucato MD, MPH
Associate Professor of Pediatrics and Adolescent
  Medicine
University of Pittsburgh School of Medicine
Pittsburgh, PA, USA

Stephanie B. Teal MD, MPH
Associate Professor of Obstetrics and Gynecology;
Director, Fellowship in Family Planning
University of Colorado
Denver School of Medicine
Aurora, CO, USA

Claire Templeman MD
Assistant Professor
Department of Obstetrics and Gynecology
University of Southern California
Los Angeles, CA, USA

Maria Trent MD, MPH
Associate Professor of Pediatrics
Department of Pediatrics
Johns Hopkins School of Medicine
Baltimore, MD, USA

Amy M. Vallerie MD
Clinical Instructor of Obstetrics and Gynecology
Department of Pediatrics
Division of Adolescent Medicine
New York Medical College
Valhalla, NY, USA

Michelle Vichnin MD
Medical Director
Merck Vaccines
West Point, PA, USA

Terri Warren BA, BSN, MED, MSN
Nurse Practitioner
Westover Heights Clinic
Portland, OR, USA

Sara E. Watson MD
Fellow Pediatric Endocrinology and Diabetology
Riley Hospital for Children
Indiana University School of Medicine
Indianapolis, IN, USA

Bree Weaver MD
Assistant Research Professor of Medicine
Indiana University School of Medicine
Indianapolis, IN, USA

Amy K. Whitaker MD, MS
Assistant Professor
The University of Chicago
Department of Obstetrics and Gynecology
Section of Family Planning and Contraceptive
    Research
Chicago, IL, USA

Lea E. Widdice MD
Division of Adolescent Medicine
Cincinnati Children's Hospital Medical Center
Cincinnati, OH, USA

Matthew B. Wintersteen PhD
Assistant Professor
Department of Psychiatry & Human Behavior
Thomas Jefferson University
Philadelphia, PA, USA

Sophia Yen MD, MPH
Assistant Professor
Stanford University School of Medicine
Department of Pediatrics
Division of Adolescent Medicine
Stanford, CA, USA

Jennie Yoost MD
Assistant Professor of Obstetrics and Gynecology
Pediatric and Adolescent Gynecology
Marshall University School of Medicine
Huntington, WV, USA

Katherine A. Zakhour BA, MBBS
Imperial College
London, UK

Andrea L. Zuckerman MD
Associate Professor of Obstetrics and Gynecology
Division Director
General Obstetrics and Gynecology and Pediatric &
    Adolescent Gynecology
Women's Care at Tufts Medical Center
Boston, MA, USA

SECTION 1
Prepubertal girls

1

Initial assessment

Maureen Lynch

Health Services, Harvard University, Cambridge, MA, USA

Infants are ideal patients. The first gynecologic exam should occur in the nursery, when the patient is the most co-operative. Obviously, what can be described at that time is the anatomy and patency of the system.

The primary care provider, who will form a relationship with the child and family over time, is the ideal person to perform routine gynecologic assessments, including inspection of the external genitalia in the context of a routine physical exam. Making the genital exam a part of the general physical exam dispels forbidden boundaries and provides an opportunity for education about normal anatomy and hygiene, and discussions of body changes, when appropriate. It is also a time to open discussions about accurately identifying body parts in order to relieve their stigma. Although parents and children should be having age-appropriate discussions about sexuality during the prepubertal years, specialist expertise may be needed on occasion.

The most common presenting complaints of the genital area in the infant and prepubertal child concern anatomy and development, labial agglutination, dermatologic issues, itching and discharge, bleeding, and sexual abuse. In order to evaluate and diagnose the prepubertal child, you need to take a problem-focused history and perform a physical exam while allaying anxiety and fears.

History

The history is best taken while the child is comfortably dressed in her own clothes. It is always good to

> ★ **Tips and tricks**
>
> • Make no mistake, a successful visit with a young child requires the provider to dispel some assumptions – a child is not a small adult and the provider is not in total control. The patience, flexibility, and playfulness of the clinician are keys to engaging and examining the prepubertal child, a challenging undertaking that, when successful, is very rewarding.
> • Inspection of the external genitalia should be a routine part of a general physical exam.
> • The history is best taken while the child is comfortably dressed in her own clothes.
> • When it comes to the physical exam, it is imperative to explain to the child what you will be doing in a way that she can understand. It is always good first to do a general exam, including height and weight, as going straight to the genital area, which may not have been examined before, may appear threatening.

> ✋ **Caution**
>
> If the provider has a question about sexual abuse, it should be asked before proceeding to the physical exam so as not to create a situation in which the parent/caregiver assumes that the provider saw something to initiate the question.

talk to the child in an age-appropriate way and to note and comment on something personal, like her shoes, dress, barrette, or a security toy that she brings. Obtaining any history from the child and parents about masturbation or infections in the family, such as Strep or pinworms, can be helpful.

You should find out when the presenting problem started and whether it is persistent or intermittent. Has anything been tried to treat it, and did this help? If concerns about sexual abuse have been expressed, ask about any behavioral changes that have been noted, such as sleeping problems, bedwetting, abdominal pain, or inappropriate acting out. If the complaint is vaginal bleeding, it is important to find out about growth and development, trauma, odor or previous history of a foreign body. Actually asking the young girl directly if she has ever put anything in her vagina can be revealing. Finally, it is important to obtain a history for any exposure to hormonal creams or patches.

Taking a history also provides an opportunity to describe normal and anticipated changes and to answer questions. At the end of the history, it is good to ask if the parent or child has any questions.

Physical exam

When it comes to the physical exam, it is imperative to explain to the child what you will be doing in a way that she can understand. It is always good to first perform a general exam, including height and weight, as going straight to the genital area, which may not have been examined before, may appear threatening. Children are comfortable and familiar with their chests and hearts being listened to and their tummies examined. Give the child choices: not whether or not she will get undressed, but what gown to wear and whether she wants to sit on the table or stay in her parent's lap. It is also good to introduce the light and gloves as things you will be using and allow the child to touch and play with them a little. If you will be using a colposcope, allowing the child to look at something through the scope can demystify the experience. Moreover, the pace of the exam is important: if you rush the child, you can forfeit her co-operation.

Reinforce, particularly to the parents, that you will not do anything to change the anatomy and that mostly you will just be inspecting the anatomy without inserting any instruments. It is important to state clearly that the exam will be painless.

The physical exam also provides an opportunity to look for any nongenital skin problems, pigmentation, breast development, hernias, or signs of early puberty, which may explain the presenting complaint.

Then, depending on how the child is doing, you can give the child a description of the choice of positions you would like her to take: butterfly, frog, or lying on mom or dad on the table, in or out of stirrups. Children familiar with horse riding may choose the stirrups. Once the child has chosen a position, simple inspection without touching can reveal lichen sclerosis or evidence of a previous or current vulvovaginitis or excoriations, and the clinical question may be answered. Always inspect the anal area for lesions or excoriation.

You should always identify the anatomy carefully, even if the presenting complaint is an obvious skin condition, because the child may have an additional problem, such as imperforate hymen, that has not been previously noted.

In order to examine the genitalia further, it is important to desensitize the child by first touching her legs and then maybe her inner thighs with your gloved hand. Engaging the child to use her own hands to assist you can be very helpful. They sometimes like to put gloves on as well. Sometimes gentle retraction laterally and downward can reveal labial agglutination or provide a better view of the anatomy, including the clitoris, urethra, and hymen. If you cannot define the anatomy of the hymen, retracting the labia gently forward and asking the child to cough can open things up further. When the vagina is visible, sometimes the clinician can see a discharge or can smell anaerobic organisms. The vagina may be estrogenized or there may be clear hygiene issues.

You can sometimes make a game of placing the child in the knee–chest position (on her knees with her shoulders on the table and bottom up in the air). Spreading her legs and gently spreading the labia can allow you to look up into the vagina for evidence of discharge or foreign bodies such as toilet paper. Before doing this, it is important to tell the child that you are not going to put anything into her bottom and to show her the light you will use. Getting the child to "pant like a puppy" or cough also can help to relax the vagina.

You always need to be particularly sensitive if the child has been sexually abused or had other exams that that did not go well. If, for instance, someone has previously tried to do a vaginal culture with a standard swab used for throat cultures, it is almost impossible to convince a child that the tiny Calgiswab you are going to use is different. Getting her to cough (which distracts the child and can also relax the hymen and open the vagina) and not touching the hymenal ring usually provides a very good vaginal (as opposed to vulvar or vaginal vestibule) culture.

> ### ✋ Caution
>
> If, after following these suggestions, the visit is not going well and the problem is not acute, you will save your relationship with the child by suggesting simple common solutions to the problem (e.g. hygiene, topical "butt creams", changes in clothing and sleep wear, etc.) and scheduling a future visit.

It is important to praise the young child constantly for what a good job she is doing. This is an exam for which you should allow extra time if needed. If the child becomes upset, a time out for everyone to regroup can salvage the appointment that day. If things do not go well, it is still important to identify and acknowledge something that the child did well. Sometimes parents become very frustrated and angry because they have taken time off work for the visit and just want to fix what is going on. It is critical that the child not be punished if she has tried her best, even if it does not work. Sometimes it is best to schedule another visit when the child has eaten or is not tired after school.

> ### ✋ Caution
>
> Depending on the urgency of the complaint and the need to obtain an adequate exam sooner rather than later, an exam under anesthesia may be required. However, for most nonacute issues, if you cannot accomplish what is needed at the first visit, you can schedule a follow-up visit; on the second occasion the child may be more familiar with the office.

Working with children is not only a challenging but also a humbling experience, especially for those of us who usually like to be in control. A good visit can be very satisfying, but sometimes, in spite of all our best intentions, patience, and planning, we may not accomplish everything that was requested or that we set out to do during a visit. The clinician will inevitably develop their own unique approach and personal tricks for success. Do not be afraid to act a little like an adult child. Children have a radar for honesty and caring. Making the first experience a good one lays the groundwork for future success for everyone.

Further reading

Emans SJ. Office evaluation of the child and adolescent. In: Emans SJ, Laufer MR, Goldstein DP, eds. *Pediatric and Adolescent Gynecology*, 5th edn. Philadelphia: Lippincott Williams & Wilkins, 2005.

2 Ambiguous genitalia in the neonate and infant

Sejal Shah and Avni C. Shah

Stanford University and the Lucile Packard Children's Hospital at Stanford, Pediatric Endocrinology and Diabetes, Stanford, CA, USA

Disorders of sex development (DSD) are defined according to the 2006 Lawson Wilkins Pediatric Endocrine Society (LWPES) Consensus Guidelines as "congenital conditions in which development of chromosomal, gonadal, or anatomic sex is atypical." DSD can be further classified into three categories:
- **46, XX DSD:** e.g. congenital adrenal hyperplasia (CAH), *in utero* exposure to androgens or progestational agents, gonadal dysgenesis, vaginal atresia
- **46, XY DSD:** e.g. androgen insensitivity syndrome, 5-alpha reductase deficiency, disorders of testosterone biosynthesis, gonadal dysgenesis
- **Sex chromosome DSD:** e.g. Turner syndrome, Klinefelter syndrome, sex chromosome mosaicism.

It is important to keep in mind that a majority of virilized 46, XX infants have CAH (the most common is 21-hydrxoylase deficiency), while only 50% of 46, XY infants with a DSD receive a definitive diagnosis (Figure 2.1).

Ambiguous genitalia, which are usually immediately apparent at birth, are a significant type of DSD, affecting 1:4500–5000 live births.

The finding of ambiguous genitalia in the newborn is rarely anticipated by the parents and always stressful and distressing. A prepared and well-informed physician can have a positive influence on the life of the family and infant faced with ambiguous genitalia. There are many possible etiologies of ambiguous genitalia, and the diagnostic process is often prolonged and may not yield a clear diagnosis. There are many challenges with short- and long-term care of the newborn. The universal parental question of "is it a boy, or is it a girl?" requires the medical practitioner to have a basic understanding of embryologic and fetal development, and to develop a sensitive approach to diagnosis and management. Paramount to the immediate and long-term management of a neonate with ambiguous genitalia is involvement of a multidisciplinary team.

> ## ✋ Caution
>
> - Ambiguous genitalia should be addressed as a medical emergency.
> - Although infants with ambiguous genitalia appear medically stable in the first few days of life, if not addressed urgently, they can medically decompensate, causing significant morbidity and mortality.
> - Appropriate initial steps include consultation with experts in the field and an evaluation focused on identifying causes of ambiguous genitalia that are associated with glucocorticoid (cortisol) deficiency and salt-losing crisis (occurs in the first 4–15 days of life).
> - Many of these infants may require immediate high-dose hydrocortisone while the work-up is being carried out.
> See Figure 2.5 and the "Obtaining a consultation" section later.

Practical Pediatric and Adolescent Gynecology, First Edition. Edited by Paula J. Adams Hillard.
© 2013 John Wiley & Sons, Ltd. Published 2013 by John Wiley & Sons, Ltd.

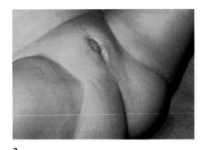

a

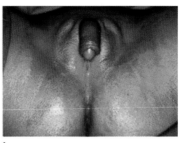

b

Figure 2.1 Masculinization in a 46, XX female with congenital adrenal hyperplasia. (a) Minor clitoral enlargement. (b) More severe virilization with a phallic urethra and a single perineal opening of a urogenital sinus.

Reproduced from Arthur R, R. In Baert, Albert L, *Encyclopedia of Diagnostic Imaging*, Springer, 2008, Chapter 59, with kind permission from Springer Science + Business Media.

⚘ Science revisited

- Male and female internal structures originate from common primordial ducts (Figure 2.2). Bipotential gonads are present at 4–6 weeks. Under the influence of the sex-determining gene on the Y chromosome (*SRY*), the gonads will develop into testes and secrete testosterone and anti-Müllerian hormone, leading to preservation of the Wolffian structures and regression of the Müllerian ducts.

- External genital structures arise from a common genital tubercle, labioscrotal folds, and ureteral folds, which are formed by 9 weeks (Figure 2.3). Under the influence of testosterone converted to dihydrotestosterone (DHT), male external structures are fully formed by 14 weeks. Female structures are fully developed by 20 weeks.

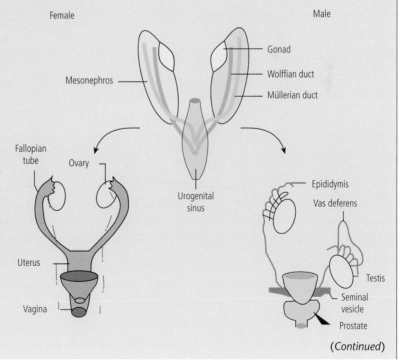

Figure 2.2 Differentiation of the internal genitalia of the human fetus.
Reproduced from *Textbook of Endocrine Physiology* edited by Griffin & Ojeda (1996) Adapted Figure: Differentiation of the internal genitalia of the human fetus. By permission of Oxford University Press; Adapted from *Goldman: Goldman's Cecil Medicine*, 24th edn. Copyright © 2011 Saunders, An imprint of Elsevier.

(*Continued*)

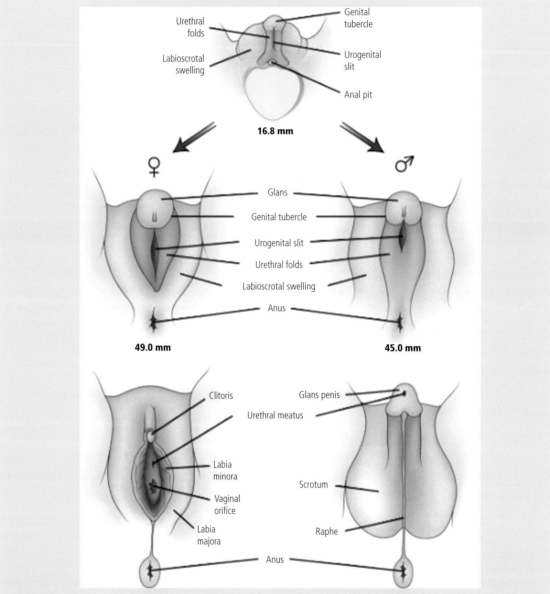

Figure 2.3 Differentiation of male and female external genitalia.
Adapted courtesy of Carnegie Institute from Spaulding MH. The development of the external genitalia in the human embryo. *Contrib Embryol Carnegie Inst* 1921;13:69–88. Kronenberg.

What is considered ambiguous? Ambiguous genitalia occur when there is a discordance between the external genitalia, gonads, and chromosomal sex. Examples include clitoromegaly, penoscrotal transposition, labial–scrotal fusion, and microphallus with cryptorchidism. Isolated microphallus is *not* ambiguous if it is a normally formed penile structure without hypospadias and with palpable testes. Isolated first- or second-degree hypospadias is *not* ambiguous if there is a normally formed penis with palpable testes. Unilateral cryptorchidism is unlikely to be a sign of ambiguous genitalia if the penile structure is normally formed and there is normal positioning of the meatus; however, if bilateral, then severely virilized CAH should be considered.

Diagnosis

To start the diagnostic process, key aspects in the maternal and perinatal history and physical exam of the neonate are needed to help guide an efficient laboratory and imaging evaluation. Unfortunately, the differential diagnosis for ambiguous genitalia is broad with no set protocol. In addition, the work-up, diagnosis, and treatment can potentially be a prolonged and controversial process. Therefore, at the center of any evaluation that is undertaken, there should be an expert multidisciplinary team available to guide you at your facility and so help you provide a uniform, yet comprehensive picture to the family.

It is important to evaluate for any maternal history of exposure to androgenic or progestational agents while the neonate was *in utero*, as well as any maternal virilizing symptoms. Evaluation of the family history should focus on any family members with CAH, history of neonatal death, aunts or other relatives with amenorrhea and/or infertility, as well as history of parental consanguinity.

Throughout the physical exam, gender neutral terms should be used (Table 2.1). While a thorough exam of the neonate is important, we will focus on key aspects that will guide the diagnostic evaluation. The general health of the neonate should be evaluated, including weight, blood pressure, hydration status, and urine output. You should look for signs of adrenocorticotropic hormone (ACTH) excess shown by hyperpigmentation of the skin (axilla, areola, skin folds/creases), and other midline defects (central incisor, heart defects) or other syndromic features.

Table 2.1 Gender neutral terms

Male	Neutral	Female
Boy/he	Your baby	Girl/she
Penis	Phallus	Clitoris
Testes	Gonads	Ovaries
Scrotum	Labioscrotal folds	Labia
Urethra	Urogenital sinus	Vagina, urethra

It is important to note that the genitourinary physical exam can be similar regardless of sex; therefore, a DSD diagnosis cannot be made solely by physical exam. Evaluation of the genitourinary region should begin with palpation of any gonadal tissue, assessing for symmetry, size, texture, and location. For improved sensitivity, the examiner should use clean, bare hands rather than gloved hands for the exam and begin the exam in the inguinal canal to evaluate for any gonads that are more proximal in the canal. The phallic structure, if present, should be measured while fully stretched, with the ruler pressed against the pubic ramus to the tip of the glands.

Another important aspect of the exam is evaluation of the degree of posterior fusion and virilization. There are many ways to describe the degree of virilization; one example is the Prader scale (Figure 2.4). An anogenital ratio [distance from the anus to the posterior fourchette (AF) divided by the distance from the anus to the base of the phallic structure (AC); AF/AC] greater than 0.5 indicates posterior fusion. The position of the urogenital opening is important – is there a common opening or separate openings?, where is the urethral opening located?, where does the urine stream originate?

A careful history, physical exam, and consultation with an expert DSD team will help guide appropriate laboratory testing. Our proposed algorithm is outlined in Figure 2.5. The initial work-up is critical as certain hormone levels such as 17-hydroxyprogesterone are needed to understand if immediate medical treatment, such as hydrocortisone, is required to prevent life-threatening salt-losing crisis. Primary testing includes a karyotype with FISH for SRY

> ✱ **Tips and tricks**
>
> **Physical exam**
> • Take care when assessing premature infants as they may have physiologic labial atrophy or clitoral edema.
> • If the meatus is not normally positioned, further evaluation may be warranted before circumcision is performed.
> • It is generally accepted that a penile length of less than 2.5 cm in a term male and a clitoral length of greater than 6 mm in a term female are abnormal. There is variation by gestational age and ethnicity.
> • In cases with microphallus, consider panhypopituitarism. Growth hormone is synergistic with testosterone during the last trimester to increase phallus length, so a deficiency can cause a microphallus and even hypoglycemia.

> ✋ **Caution**
>
> • Be aware of which lab tests should be performed after 24 hours of life. Evaluation of androgens before 24 hours of life could capture a physiologic immaturity of the adrenal gland leading to falsely elevated levels.
> • Often the result of the drawn STAT 17-hydroxyprogesterone level (17-OHP) will return before the newborn screen results. However, you should check with your institution about obtaining an expedited result for the newborn screen 17-OHP value.
> • Preterm infants can have a slightly elevated 17-OHP value on the newborn screen, so if the infant is stable with normal electrolytes and genitalia, you can repeat the 17-OHP value and discuss this with a pediatric endocrinologist.

(this should be done even when prenatal karyotype is available) and measurement of a STAT 17-hydroxyprogesterone, testosterone, luteinizing hormone, follicle stimulating hormone, and anti-Müllerian hormone; and serum electrolytes and urine analysis to evaluate for renal anomalies.

An abdominal/pelvic ultrasound is important to evaluate for uterine and gonadal structures located in the pelvis or inguinal canal. The ultrasound is also helpful in evaluating the adrenal glands and the kidneys for any structural abnormalities. The ability of an ultrasound to detect intra-abdominal gonads

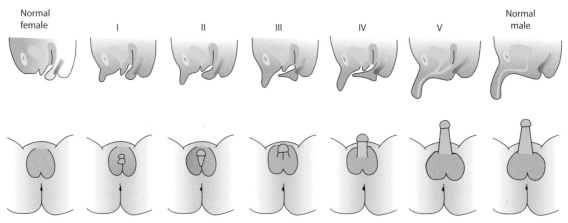

Normal female   I   II   III   IV   V   Normal male

Figure 2.4 Schematic representations of normal female and male anatomy flank a series of schematics illustrating different degrees of virilization of females, graded using the scale developed by Prader. The uterus (shaded) persists in virilized females even when the external genitalia have a completely masculine appearance (Prader grade V).

Adapted with permission from Prader A. Der Genitalbefund beim Pseudohermaphroditismus femininus der kengenitalen adrenogenitalen Syndroms. *Helv Paediatr Acta* 1954;9: 231–248. Société suisse de pédiatrie/Schwabe Verlag; Adapted from *Goldman: Goldman's Cecil Medicine*, 24th edn. Copyright © 2011 Saunders, An imprint of Elsevier.

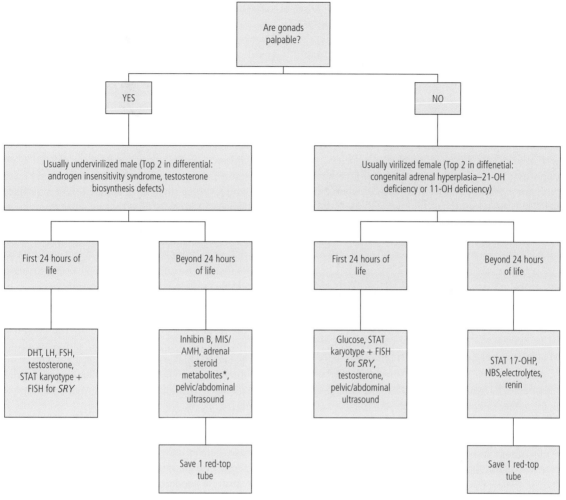

Figure 2.5 Preliminary diagnostic algorithm.
*Adrenal steroid metabolites [progesterone, 17-OH pregnenolone, 17-OH-progesterone (17-OHP), androstenedione, DHEA (dehydroepiandrosterone), 11-desoxycortisol, deoxycorticosterone]. DHT, dihydrotestosterone; LH, luteinizing hormone; FSH, follicle-stimulating hormone; FISH, fluorescence *in situ* hybridization; MIS/AMH, Müllerian-inhibiting substance/ anti-Müllerian hormone; NBS, newborn screening.

is limited and operator dependent. A more detailed evaluation of the internal anatomy may require cystoscopy/genitogram, magnetic resonance imaging and/or laparoscopy, for which you will be instructed through the input from a multidisciplinary team, which usually includes urologists and radiologists. If the infant is to be transferred to the institution where the DSD multidisciplinary team is located, then you may be asked to hold off on some of these procedures until then.

Discussion with the parents

When ambiguity of the genitalia is being considered, you, the healthcare professional, need to objectively tell the parents or caregivers, in layman terms, what is unexpected about the development of their infant. The information needs to be delivered with the utmost honesty and sensitivity. This is a traumatic event and many families will feel scared, shocked, and ashamed. Reassurance should be given that they did not cause this and they should be encouraged to share information with family members and friends for support. Most of all, the family should know that despite the sexual ambiguity, the child has the potential to be a well-adjusted, functional member of society. It is important to explain that in order to move forward with the work-up, you have contacted experts in the field and the parents will be involved and informed in the process.

✴ Tips and tricks

Talking to parents/caregivers

• You could start by saying, "There has been a problem in the complex system that directs genitalia development. So, it is difficult to tell the sex of your child by examining the external genitalia." Then, objectively show the parents the genitalia of their baby alongside pictures of nonambiguous genitalia.

• Remember to use gender neutral terms in discussions with the family (Table 2.1).

• Advise the parents to delay naming the infant, announcing the baby's birth, and registering the birth until more information becomes available. Ensure that your medical staff and hospital medical record system also know not to assign gender (you may need to relay to them what gender neutral terms to use).

• There are web-based sources of information, such as http://www.aboutkidshealth.ca/EN/HOWTHEBODYWORKS/SEXDEVELOPMENTANOVERVIEW (basic understanding of sexual development), http://www.accordalliance.org (also has a Handbook for Parents), and http://www.caresfoundation.org (CARES Foundation – Congenital Adrenal Hyperplasia Education & Support).

Obtaining consultation

Not only does concern over ambiguity of the genitalia need to be conveyed to the family promptly, it also must be discussed with a center that has a DSD multidisciplinary team. You should assure the parents that you and your team are going to take care of their needs and those of their child by consulting with DSD experts, and they will remain involved and informed in the process.

Children with DSD require patient-centered care, preferably from an experienced multidisciplinary team and with resources that are generally found in tertiary care centers. A typical DSD team includes the following services: pediatric endocrinology, urology and/or surgery, psychology/psychiatry, pediatric gynecology, genetics, neonatology, radiology, social work, nursing, and medical ethics. The core team will vary according to DSD type, local resources, and location.

Upon the initial phone contact (usually with the pediatric endocrinologist), the team will educate you on appropriate initial management for the newborn and the family. We have given you our suggestions of a general initial work-up (Figure 2.5). The team will direct you on further steps, which may require transfer to or follow up as an outpatient at their institution.

After the diagnostic work-up has been completed and the DSD team with family input has discussed the case, gender assignment and treatment (medical and surgical) plan options will be evaluated. The goal is to ensure a gender-appropriate appearance, sexual function, fertility, healthy gender identity, and long-term psychological and social well-being. The timing of treatment depends on the specific DSD type and situation. Many controversies and uncertainties surround medical and surgical management; therefore, full disclosure along with psychological and genetic counseling, and support groups will help enhance psychosocial adaptation long term. Long-term happiness in quality of life for the family and child is of priority, with its foundation laid as soon as ambiguous genitalia are considered.

Further reading

Ahmed SF, Achermann JC, Arlt W, *et al.* UK guidance on the initial evaluation of an infant or an adolescent with a suspected disorder of sex development. *Clin Endocrinol* 2011;75:12–26

Lee PA, Houk CP, Ahmed SF, Hughes IA. International Consensus Conference on Intersex. Consensus Statement on Management of Intersex Disorders. *Pediatrics* 2006; 118(2):e488–e500.

Murphy C, Allen L, Jamieson MA. Ambiguous genitalia in the newborn: An overview and teaching tool. *J Pediatr Adolesc Gynecol* 2011;24:236–250.

3 Vaginal discharge and odor

Corinne Bazella and Marjorie Greenfield

Case Western Reserve University School of Medicine, Cleveland, OH, USA

Vaginal discharge and odor are the most common symptoms that bring prepubertal girls to the gynecologist. The symptoms may be vague, but usually include one of the following: discharge, erythema, soreness, pruritus, dysuria, odor, or staining of the underwear. Prepubertal girls with vaginal complaints should always be evaluated for sexual abuse.

The etiology of discharge and odor differs in prepubertal girls from adults and adolescents due to the difference in secondary sexual development, estrogenization of the vagina, and lifestyle factors.

Prepubertal girls have limited labial development with no labial fat pads or pubic hair to protect the vagina. The lack of estrogen also results in a thin vaginal epithelium and alkaline pH. Prepubertal girls have unique hygiene issues, such as diapers or poor toilet habits, which may expose the vagina to colonic flora. Personal products like bubble baths and harsh soaps have the potential to irritate perineal skin. Nonabsorbent tight clothing like bathing suits, nylon leotards, and blue jeans can potentiate the problem. The current obesity epidemic in children is also making vulvovaginal complaints more common. Although the etiology of some cases can be discovered from the history or physical exam, in many patients a specific cause cannot be found.

✋ Caution

- An evaluation for sexual abuse should be performed in any child who presents with vulvovaginal complaints. Sexually-transmitted infections (STIs) and human papillomavirus (HPV) in children older than age 3 years give reasonable cause to suspect child abuse and should be immediately reported.
- All US states require by law that care providers report suspected child abuse by contacting a state or local child protection service agency.
- Forensic exams should be performed by an experienced clinician.
- Diagnostic laboratory tests sent from the exam must have high specificity to be admissible in court.
- Culture for *Neisseria gonorrhoeae* is done on modified Thayer-Martin medium. Chlamydia and herpes culture should be sent in viral culture media.
- Culture should be used over nucleic acid amplifications tests (NAATs) due to the possibility of false-positive results with NAATs. If cultures are unavailable, a second NAAT probing a different nucleic acid sequence can be done for confirmation.

Practical Pediatric and Adolescent Gynecology, First Edition. Edited by Paula J. Adams Hillard.
© 2013 John Wiley & Sons, Ltd. Published 2013 by John Wiley & Sons, Ltd.

Science revisited

- The vagina of prepubertal girls is atrophic, and is colonized by different bacteria from the well-estrogenized, glycogen-rich mucosa of an adolescent or adult woman.
- The normal pH is alkaline at approximately 6.5–7.5.
- Few data are available on what comprises normal vaginal flora in this age group, but it may contain *Staphylococcus epidermidis*, *Streptococcus viridans*, diptheroids, mixed anaerobes, enterococci, lactobacillus, and *Escherichia coli*.

Differential diagnosis

Nonspecific vulvovaginitis

Nonspecific vulvovaginitis occurs in 25–75% of girls presenting with symptoms of discharge and odor. Symptoms usually resolve within 2–3 weeks with changes in hygiene and lifestyle (Table 3.1). Persistent symptoms require further evaluation.

Foreign body

A foreign body (FB) in the vagina presents with foul smelling discharge and/or bleeding. Common items that are retained in the vagina are toilet paper,

Table 3.1 Nonspecific vulvovaginitis hygiene care

- Wear only cotton underwear
- Sleep without underwear or pajama bottoms
- Launder underwear with hypoallergenic detergent, double rinse, and avoid fabric softeners and dryer sheets
- Wear loose fitting clothing
- Change bathing suits quickly after swimming
- Take daily tepid water soaks/baths
- Eliminate chemical irritants, including bubble baths, bath salts, and scented soaps
- Supervision of toileting and front to back wiping (from behind)
- Use petroleum jelly or zinc oxide for skin protection
- Use cool compresses or cool water soaks for acute exacerbations

toys, hair accessories, and paper clips. Diagnosis and treatment can be accomplished by irrigating the vagina with warm water or saline after the hymen is treated with lidocaine jelly. Calgiswabs can be used to remove small objects. With the patient under sedation, fiberoptic vaginoscopy with a hysteroscope or cystoscope can be performed for larger foreign bodies or if a more thorough examination is necessary. Most children do not recall or do not admit to inserting anything into the vagina. One study has suggested a strong association between a vaginal FB and sexual victimization. This may be due to the perpetrator inserting objects or, more likely, due to unusual insertional behaviors following sexual abuse. Evaluation for the possibility of sexual victimization should be performed during the work-up for vaginal FB.

Respiratory and enteric pathogens

Children can self-inoculate the vagina with respiratory and enteric flora, which can cause a purulent or mucoid discharge. The most common respiratory pathogen is *Streptococcus pyogenes* or Group A strep. Other less common bacteria are *Haemophilus influenzae*, *Staphylococcus aureus*, *Streptococcus pneumoniae*, *Branhamella catarrhalis*, and *Neisseria meningitides*. Enteric pathogens like shigella and yersinia can also cause vaginal discharge that may or may not be associated with diarrhea. Vaginal cultures should be collected to streamline treatment. Discussion with your microbiology lab is necessary, as routine adult vaginal cultures do not plate respiratory or enteric flora. Group A streptococcus is treated with penicillin. *H. influenzae* and *S. aureus* may resolve with hygiene changes, but if symptoms do not resolve, antimicrobial treatment is advised. *S. pneumoniae* can be treated with penicillin, but resistance is quite common and sensitivities should be obtained. Shigella and yersinia should be treated with trimethoprim–sulfamethoxazole or ampicillin for 5 days, but may need prolonged courses.

Yeast

Candida vaginitis is relatively rare in prepubertal girls. Risk factors for yeast include recent antibiotic courses, immunosuppression, diabetes mellitus, and diapers. Yeast is over-diagnosed in this age group, and in most cases should be low on the differential.

Sexually-transmitted infections

STIs in children include *N. gonorrhoeae, Chlamydia trachomatis, Trichomonas vaginalis*, herpes simplex, and human papillomavirus (HPV). The presence of an STI in children most commonly results from abuse, but only 3.7% of abuse victims acquire an STI.

Gonorrhea infections usually present with green purulent discharge and are rarely asymptomatic. Children with vaginitis who fail to respond to typical therapy should be cultured. Routine culturing of asymptomatic victims of sexual abuse is of low yield.

C. trachomatis can be transmitted through sexual contact or perinatally. Persistence of a perinatal infection past the age of 2 or 3 years is rare due to treatment with antibiotics for other medical problems. Chlamydia infections are frequently asymptomatic and most cases are associated with abuse.

Trichomonas can be transmitted perinatally; however, the infection usually spontaneously resolves. If an infection is confirmed by wet mount or culture, sexual contact is likely.

Treatment of *N. gonorrhoeae, C. trachomatis*, and trichomonas is described in Table 3.2.

Herpes simplex virus (HSV) type 1 is typically oral in location, but can be transmitted to the vulva through self-inoculation during a primary infection. HSV type 2 is typically from a genital source. Both HSV types 1 and 2 can be sexually transmitted. If lesions are noted on a prepubertal child, the potential for sexual abuse must be evaluated.

HPV subtypes 6 or 11 can cause warts in the genital or perianal area, and can be transmitted at birth from the mother. Infections of children older than 2–3 years should prompt an evaluation for sexual abuse as HPV is rarely a persistent perinatal infection. Resolution of perinatal HPV usually occurs within 5 years with expectant management. Treatment with imiquimod cream is easier for the patient than other topical treatments, but skin reactions are common. Trichloroacetic acetic (TCA) and laser treatment are also options; however, sedation is required for the laser, and TCA is painful.

Table 3.2 Treatment for sexually-transmitted infections in prepubertal girls

Neisseria gonorrhoeae	<45 kg Ceftriaxone 125 mg IM single dose >45 kg Ceftriaxone 250 mg IM single dose plus Azithromycin 1 g single dose
Chlamydia trachomatis	<45 kg Erythromycin 50 mg/kg/day PO divided QID for 14 days >45 kg Azithromycin 1 g PO single dose or Doxycycline 100 mg PO BID for 7 days if older than 8 years
Trichomonas	Metronidazole 15 mg/kg/day PO divided TID for 7 days

Ectopic ureter

An ectopic ureter from a duplex collecting system or a dysplastic kidney can cause wetness, purulent discharge, and irritation that can be thought to be coming from the vagina. Ectopic ureters are typically located near the normal urethra, but can insert into the vagina, the urethra, or even the upper reproductive tract. On exam, urine can be seen at the opening of the ectopic ureter after the child drinks a large amount of fluid. Diagnostic testing includes ultrasound and intravenous pyelogram with special attention to the contour of the kidney. Treatment is surgical.

Evaluation (see also Appendices 1.1.1 and 1.1.2)

It is important to elicit a detailed history about the quality, duration, discharge color and odor, cleansing products, hygiene habits, and behavioral changes like enuresis. Past medical history of dermatologic diseases, allergies, recent pharyngitis, upper respiratory tract infection, or diarrhea helps to narrow the differential diagnosis as well. Behavioral changes like nightmares, withdrawal, sexualized behaviors, or complaints of chronic pain may suggest abuse or physiologic stressors.

On first presentation for vaginal discharge, an external examination and instructions on hygiene changes should be reviewed (Table 3.1). If the discharge is persistent, further work-up with external examination, examination of the vagina in the knee–chest position, collection of wet prep and cultures, and if necessary, a rectal examination. A rectal examination is usually necessary only if there is bleeding, persistent abdominal pain, or discharge. Masses in the vagina, including tumors and larger foreign bodies, may be palpated on rectal exam. If the vagina and cervix are not adequately visualized, an exam under sedation with fiberoptic vaginoscopy and saline irrigation is the final step in evaluation. Persistent bleeding should prompt vaginoscopy to rule out rare tumors and masses.

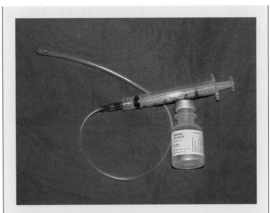

Figure 3.1 Catheter and syringe for collection of a vaginal wash/irrigation sample.

Further reading

Emans SJ, Laufer MR, Goldstein DP. *Pediatric and Adolescent Gynecology*, 5th edn. Philadelphia: Lippincott, Williams & Wilkins, 2005.

Girardet RG, Lahoti S, Howard LA, *et al.* Epidemiology of sexually transmitted infections in suspected child victims of sexual assault. *Pediatrics* 2009;124:79.

Stricker T, Navratil F, Sennhauser FH. Vulvovaginitis in prepubertal girls. *Arch Dis Child* 2003;88:324.

★ Tips and tricks

In the evaluation of vaginal discharge in a prepubertal girl, a sample of the discharge is needed for a wet mount with saline and potassium hydroxide and for cultures. There are several techniques that make collecting the samples more tolerable for the child.

• Pretreatment of the hymen with lidocaine jelly followed by insertion of a Calgiswab can easily be done if only wet mount is necessary.

• A vaginal wash/irrigation sample can also be collected using a trimmed 4-cm red rubber catheter over a butterfly catheter attached to a syringe (Figure 3.1). Non-bacteriostatic saline is instilled into the vagina and the fluid can then be aspirated and sent for study. This device can then be used to irrigate the vagina and flush out a foreign body.

4 Vaginal bleeding

Valerie S. Ratts

Department of Obstetrics and Gynecology, Washington University School of Medicine in St. Louis, St. Louis, MO, USA

Vaginal bleeding in infants and prepubertal children is rare and should always be evaluated.

A thorough history should be obtained, including onset, duration, and description of the bleeding. A check should be made for any history of trauma and if there were eye witnesses, as well as evaluation for associated symptoms of headache, vision changes, abdominal pain or dysuria.

Next, a comprehensive exam should be performed in the office or emergency room setting, looking for signs of sexual precocity, marks of trauma, and abnormalities of the genital examination including dermatologic conditions, structural abnormalities, vaginal discharge, foreign body, and/or lesions. Sedation or general anesthesia may be required. The goal of the exam is to establish and document the site of bleeding, although commonly there is only an undocumented history with no obvious source.

Differential diagnosis (Table 4.2)

Vulvovaginitis (see Chapters 3 and 7)

Vulvovaginitis may be caused by respiratory, oral, and fecal pathogens, as well as sexually-transmitted infections and parasites. Pediatric patients are at increased risk for vulvovaginitis due to their hypoestrogenic status producing a thin vaginal mucosa without benefits of protective lactobacilli colonization, limited protection of the less developed labia, and

---

✋ Caution

- The use of noninvasive imaging may be helpful in identifying radiopaque foreign objects.
- However, imaging:
  - Does not rule out a foreign object
  - Does not address possible abuse
  - Is not helpful for identifying malignancy.
- Persistent vaginal bleeding or discharge despite a normal simple office exam requires an examination under anesthesia (EUA; Table 4.1) with vaginoscopy and cystoscopy in prepubertal girls.

Table 4.1 Indications for examination under anesthesia (EUA)

- Removal of foreign body that cannot be removed in the office
- Evaluation of the extent of vulvovaginal trauma that cannot be adequately assessed in the office or emergency department
- Repair of vulvovaginal trauma
- Unexplained vaginal bleeding
- An expanding vulvar or vaginal hematoma
- Concomitant injuries that require EUA
- Patient is young, too frightened, or uncooperative

Practical Pediatric and Adolescent Gynecology, First Edition. Edited by Paula J. Adams Hillard.
© 2013 John Wiley & Sons, Ltd. Published 2013 by John Wiley & Sons, Ltd.

Table 4.2 Differential diagnosis of prepubertal vaginal bleeding

---

- Vulvovaginitis
- Foreign objects
- Dermatologic conditions, including lichen sclerosus, eczema, psoriasis, excoriations
- Trauma
- Urinary tract source, including urethral prolapse, urinary tract infection, urethral prolapse
- Vulvar/vaginal neoplasms
- Factitious bleeding
- Exogenous estrogen exposure
- Endometrial sloughing in the neonate
- Endocrine causes, including precocious puberty, hypothyroidism
- Autonomously functioning ovarian dominant follicle
- Ovarian neoplasm
- Premature menarche (see Chapter 15)

---

often poor or improper hygiene. The purulent or sero-sanguineous drainage leads to vulvar irritation with excoriations. Treatment involves standard perineal hygiene measures, avoiding topical irritants, and application of bland emollients such as zinc oxide or petroleum jelly. Culture for organisms is helpful to guide antibiotic treatment.

Vaginal foreign objects

Foreign objects are a common cause of vaginal bleeding often associated with foul odor, vaginal discharge, pruritus or burning. Shreds of toilet paper are a commonly-found foreign body. Vaginal foreign bodies seen in the office can sometimes be removed with flushing technique using warm saline or water with a syringe and feeding tube or IV catheter within a urethral catheter (see Figure 3.1), Alternatively, EUA and vaginoscopy allows direct inspection and removal.

> ### ★ Tips and tricks
>
> - A fingertip placed in the rectum can sometimes detect a foreign body in the vagina.
> - A foreign object in the vagina can sometimes be removed by "milking" the object towards the introitus.
> - 2% lidocaine jelly placed at the introitus can facilitate removal.

Dermatologic conditions

Dermatologic conditions are often associated with bleeding, including lichen sclerosus, lichen simplex chronicus, lichen planus, atopic dermatitis, hemangiomas, genital condylomata [human papillomavirus (HPV)], and acute genital ulcers. Lichen sclerosus (see Chapter 11) is characterized by chronic inflammation and intense pruritus. Characteristic exam findings include thinning or whitening of the vulvar and perianal skin in a keyhole or butterfly pattern. Petechia and blood blisters are also common and may be mistaken for a sign of sexual abuse. Management involves use of potent topical steroids. Findings of HPV (see Chapter 44.2) and/or genital ulcers (see Chapter 10.2) require appropriate evaluation.

Accidental trauma

Accidental trauma or unintentional genital trauma in young girls can produce injuries with vaginal bleeding (see Chapter 12). If the extent of the injury cannot be assessed or there is concern for penetrating trauma or transection of the hymen, then most patients will require at least conscious sedation or an EUA for evaluation and possible repair.

Disorders of the urinary tract

Disorders of the urinary tract can present with vaginal bleeding. Gross hematuria can be seen with a urinary tract infection or trauma. Urethral polyps can also be a source of "vaginal bleeding." However, the most common urinary-related etiology of prepubertal vaginal bleeding is urethral prolapse (Figure 4.1). This occurs when the intraurethral mucosa protrudes beyond the urethral meatus. Risk factors for urethral prolapse include estrogen deficiency, increased intra-abdominal pressure, trauma, urinary tract infection, and redundant mucosa or other anatomic defects. The urethral prolapse can be mild (minimal or segmental prolapse without inflammation), moderate (circumferential prolapse with edema), or severe (severe hemorrhagic inflammation with necrosis or ulceration of the prolapse).

Urethral prolapse is usually treated nonsurgically with sitz baths to reduce the inflammation and swelling, and the use of topical estrogen cream. Surgical therapy is reserved for symptomatic prepubertal patients when conservative therapy does not work.

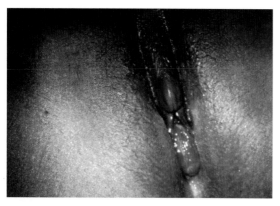

Figure 4.1 Urethral prolapse.

★ **Tips and tricks**

Distinguishing between urethral prolapse and a vaginal mass
- Place traction on the vulva and attempt to see into the vagina.
- Alternatively, identify the meatus at the center of the edematous tissue by asking the patient to void on a bedpan and observing urine exiting from the center of the mass.
- If these maneuvers are unsuccessful, place a small catheter to obtain urine.

Tumors

Tumors as a cause of bleeding are extremely rare. Pediatric perineal hemangiomas can be part of a larger (pelvis) syndrome, including external genitalia malformations, lipomyelomeningocele, vesicorenal abnormalities, imperforate anus, and skin tags. MR imaging should be performed in infants with segmental perineal hemangiomas to evaluate for spinal abnormalities. Rare tumors that cause vaginal bleeding include yolk sac (endodermal sinus) tumors, which arise from the vagina, and embryonal rhabdomyosarcomas (botryoid tumors), which can arise in the uterus, cervix or vagina. These types of lesions are typically diagnosed by EUA. Lesions should be biopsied to make an appropriate diagnosis and guide therapy.

Endocrine disorders

Endocrine disorders or estrogen-related exposure may also produce prepubertal vaginal bleeding. Normal neonatal endometrial sloughing is seen in infants, usually within the first 7–10 days of life. Exposure to *in utero* placental estrogens can result in breast budding and vaginal discharge from cervical mucus in the neonate. The dropping estrogen levels at birth cause physiologic endometrial shedding. Vaginal bleeding after this time requires further work-up.

Exogenous estrogen exposure

Exogenous estrogen exposure can also produce prepubertal vaginal bleeding. This can be seen if there has been accidental ingestion of estrogens, such as oral contraceptive pills, exposure to a menopausal relative's topical estrogen gel or products containing hormones, such as performance-enhancing shower gels or shampoos, or prolonged exposure to estrogen cream, such as in the treatment of labial adhesions.

Precocious puberty

Prepubertal vaginal bleeding can also be seen in association with precocious puberty (see Chapter 15). Precocious puberty can have a peripheral or central etiology. Peripheral precocious puberty is a condition where estrogen is produced without the central control of gonadotropin hormones and thus, is considered gonadotropin independent. Idiopathic autonomously functioning ovarian cysts can briefly produce bursts of estradiol that are enough to stimulate the endometrium and cause endometrial shedding. Sometimes, the follicular structures can be seen on ultrasound, but often by the time vaginal bleeding occurs the follicle has collapsed and resolved. Primary hypothyroidism, resulting in cross-reactivity of thyroid-stimulating hormone (TSH) with ovarian follicle-stimulating hormone (FSH) receptors can cause peripheral precocious puberty. A clue to this etiology is the absence of a growth spurt and delayed skeletal maturation with breast development. Treatment for hypothyroidism will result in resolution of the pubertal symptoms. McCune–Albright syndrome with the triad of fibrous dysplasia, café-au-lait spots, and precocious puberty is due to somatic mutations in G protein. In this syndrome, ovarian tissue is autonomously activated and produces estradiol which can act to produce central precocious puberty. Finally, ovarian tumors can produce hormones that result in precocity. Granulosa cell tumors of the ovary are most common, but other tumors of the ovary that can induce vaginal bleeding include human chorionic gonadotropin (hCG)-producing tumors, cystadenomas, gonadoblastomas, Sertoli–Leydig cell tumors, lipoid cell tumors, and thecomas. Feminizing adrenal tumors can also produce estrogen and symptoms. When an ovarian tumor is suspected, a pelvic ultrasound is indicated followed by lab evaluation including LH, FSH, TSH, free thyroxine, hCG, and estradiol. If signs of hirsutism are present, lab evaluation of testosterone, dehydroepiandrosterone sulfate (DHEAS), and 17-hydroxyprogesterone (17-OHP) may also be indicated. High estradiol levels with low LH or FSH levels suggest an ovarian cyst or tumor.

Central precocious puberty (see Chapter 15) may be due to central nervous system (CNS) dysfunction from a CNS tumor, post infection or head injury. However, most cases are idiopathic due to premature enhancement of hypothalamic gonadotropin-releasing hormone (GnRH) pulsatile release.

Summary

Vaginal bleeding in prepubertal children requires assessment. The most common etiologies of bleeding are vulvovaginitis, trauma, urethral prolapse, benign autonomously functioning follicular ovarian cyst, ovarian tumors, and precocious puberty; rarely the etiology is a vaginal tumor. The key part of evaluation is an adequate examination, which often requires sedation to determine the source of bleeding. If no source is found on exam, endocrine etiologies need to be considered. Assessment then includes pelvic ultrasound and laboratory tests for LH, FSH, estradiol, TSH, and hCG. Central and peripheral precocious puberty should be ruled out.

Further reading

Huh WW, Skapek SX. Childhood rhabdomyosarcoma: new insight on biology and treatment. *Curr Oncol Rep* 2010; 12(6):402–410.

Merritt DF. Genital trauma in children and adolescents. *Clin Obstet Gynecol* 2008;51(2):238.

Metry D. Epidemiology; pathogenesis; clinical features; and complications of infantile hemangiomas. *UpToDate* 18.3. www.uptodate.com

5 Ovarian masses

Julie L. Strickland and Anne-Marie Priebe

University of Missouri Kansas City, Children's Mercy Hospital, Kansas City, MO, USA

When a parent hears their child has an ovarian mass, for many, the first concern is cancer. Historically, any palpable mass in a prepubertal girl was concerning for malignancy and necessitated surgical exploration. Today, with ever improving ultrasound technology and the availability of tumor markers, there is often a role for watchful waiting as an alternative to immediate radical surgery. Ovarian preservation, when possible, enables future fertility.

From fetal development to puberty, the most common abnormal finding is an ovarian cyst. Development of ovarian cysts is influenced by several different factors that change as a child grows. Fetal life is influenced by maternal factors along with the rapid growth and eventual decline in the number of oocytes by birth, the neonatal period is influenced by remaining maternal hormones, and childhood is marked by a quiescent time with increasing activity when approaching puberty.

Masses detected antenatally

Routine fetal ultrasounds suggest that the incidence of fetal ovarian cysts is 30–70%. Fetal ovarian cysts seem to be more common in offspring of mothers with diabetes, polyhydramnios, pre-eclampsia, and isoimmunization. A unilateral follicular cyst develops when maternal estrogen crosses the placenta and stimulates the fetal ovary; fetal gonadotropin production further influences cyst development. Other

🔅 Science revisited

Ovarian development

• Functional development of the ovary begins along the urogenital ridge at approximately 6–8 weeks' gestation. The ovary functions to produce hormones and germ cells. Mitosis of these germ cells leads to the development of oogonia. Primitive oogonia peak at 6–7 million by 20 weeks' gestation, followed by formation of oocytes through meiosis. Follicular development then begins between 16 and 20 weeks' gestation with peak oocyte counts occurring around 22–24 weeks' gestation. Atresia of the follicles at all stages of development occurs at a rapid rate, leaving only one to two million germ cells at birth. After birth and well into adulthood, follicular development and atresia continue in the ovary.

• The origin of the ovary begins at the level of the tenth vertebra and migrates into the true pelvis by puberty. This explains the ovarian blood supply from the aorta just below the renal artery. The venous drainage of the ovary on the right returns to the inferior vena cava and the left vein drains into the left renal vein.

• From fetal life into childhood, ovarian masses are found in the abdomen due to the lack of development of a true pelvis.

Practical Pediatric and Adolescent Gynecology, First Edition. Edited by Paula J. Adams Hillard.
© 2013 John Wiley & Sons, Ltd. Published 2013 by John Wiley & Sons, Ltd.

Table 5.1 Other causes of intra-abdominal cystic masses in fetuses and neonates

Gastrointestinal origins
Meconium cyst
Mesenteric cyst
Duodenal atresia
Enteric duplication cyst
Volvulus

Genitourinary origins
Renal cyst
Megaloureter
Megalocystitis
Urinary tract obstruction
Urachal cyst
Cloacal anomaly
Hydrometrocolpos
Ovarian cyst

Miscellaneous origins
Lymphangioma
Neuroblastoma
Anterior meningocele
Presacral cystic teratoma
Adrenal cyst
Splenic cyst
Pancreatic cyst
Choledochal cyst

Reproduced with permission from Emans SJ, Laufer MR, Goldstein DP. Benign and malignant ovarian masses. In: *Pediatric and Adolescent Gynecology*, 2005, pp. 685–728.

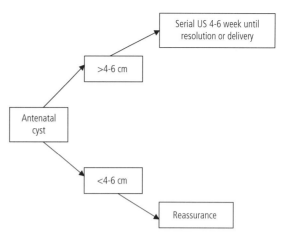

Figure 5.1 Management of an antenatal cyst. Based on Strickland JL. Ovarian cysts in neonates, children and adolescents. *Curr Opin Obstet Gynecol* 2002;14:459–465, with permission.

pathologic conditions can be mistaken for an ovarian cyst (Table 5.1).

At the time of diagnosis, it is important to further qualify fetal ovarian cysts as simple or complex, along with the diameter in order to determine both an antenatal and postpartum management plan. The majority of fetal cysts are functional cysts and will resolve without intervention, but large cysts (>4–6 cm) should be followed with serial ultrasounds until resolution or delivery (Figure 5.1). In addition to delivery dystocia, a large cyst may occupy enough space to cause lung hypoplasia and respiratory distress after birth. Obstruction to the gastrointestinal tract or the urinary system may occur with large cysts. If the cyst ruptures, hemorrhage leading to anemia can occur. Enlarged ovaries are also at risk of torsion. If this

happens during the fetal period, the ovary can become necrotic, be absorbed, or calcify.

Although there is a theoretical risk of delivery dystocia if the cyst is larger than 6 cm, there is no literature to support the superiority of cesarean section for mode of delivery. Percutaneous drainage of a fetal ovarian cyst is another proposed treatment option, but it remains controversial. This is often a technically difficult procedure to perform and exposes both the mother and baby to potential risk of infection, premature rupture of membranes, and maternal–fetal morbidity. If a clear diagnosis cannot be made, percutaneous drainage should be avoided during the fetal period.

Masses detected neonatally

During the neonatal period, most ovarian cysts are found incidentally by ultrasound. Rarely, they will present with enlarging abdominal circumference or failure to thrive. Secondary to the shallow pelvis, neonatal ovarian masses are most often found in the mid or upper abdomen. As a result of the ovarian mobility and tethering of the vascular supply, torsion may occur. The most common ovarian mass is a unilateral functional ovarian cyst due to the persistent effect of maternal hormones. The majority of the functional cysts are simple and will resolve with no intervention. Less commonly, functional cysts are complex, but resolution may be expected in a small portion of these cases.

The differential diagnosis for neonates is similar to fetal ovarian cysts (Table 5.1). As in fetal life, it is essential to clarify the origin of the cyst prior to intervention. Typically, ultrasound is adequate to both qualify and assess the size of the mass. Occasionally, MRI may be helpful to clarify the etiology of the cyst. Complex cysts can be a result of torsion or hemorrhage *in utero*, but they are seldom germ cell tumors. Rarely a cyst can autonomously secrete sex steroids and presents with premature thelarche and/or vaginal bleeding. Management of an ovarian mass in neonates is outlined in Figure 5.2.

Masses detected in childhood

The ovary is less active during childhood due to the hypogonadotropic state; the finding of a large ovarian cyst is less common than in other stages of life. There is an incidence of 2.6 cases per 100 000 girls, representing 1% of all childhood cancers. Ovarian cysts (Figure 5.3) are more likely to present with abdominal complaints or other nonspecific signs, including nausea, vomiting, abdominal fullness, and urinary frequency or retention. A patient may present with acute pain, a surgical abdomen, or intermittent episodic pain that could suggest complete or intermittent ovarian torsion. Occasionally, an ovarian cyst will be palpated by the clinician on routine office visits. Rarely, increasing abdominal girth is noted.

Although the ovary is less active during childhood than in the fetal, neonatal, or adolescent age groups, the most common cause of an ovarian mass is a follicular cyst. Occasionally these cysts can be hormonally active and cause precocious puberty. McCune–Albright syndrome or polyostotic fibrous dysplasia includes café-au-lait skin spots, multiple disseminated cystic bone lesions that easily fracture, and gonadotropin-independent ovarian cysts. If a child has an ovarian cyst without signs of precocious puberty, hypothyroidism must also be considered.

Management

Management of ovarian masses depends on the suspected etiology and presence of symptoms. If there is

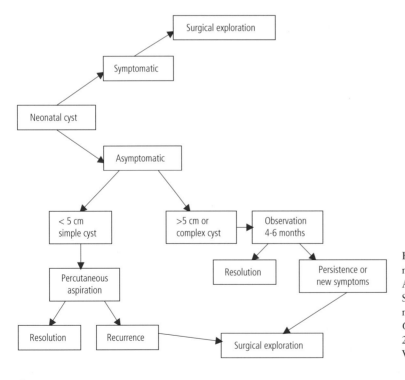

Figure 5.2 Management of a neonatal cyst.
Adapted with permission from Strickland JL. Ovarian cysts in neonates, children and adolescents. *Curr Opin Obstet Gynecol* 2002;14:459–465. Lippincott Williams & Wilkins.

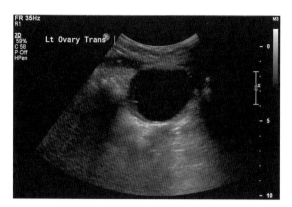

Figure 5.3 Ultrasound finding of childhood ovarian cyst. Courtesy of JL Strickland.

clinical and sonographic suspicion for torsion, surgical exploration by diagnostic operative laparoscopy or laparotomy is necessary, with ovarian conservation if possible. Suspected functional cysts should be observed with ultrasound. Rarely, simple cysts may

---

☆ Tips and tricks

Torsion

- Ovarian torsion is a complication of an ovarian mass and occurs in 3% of ovarian masses in prepubertal girls. This is considered a gynecologic emergency, requiring decisive action to restore ovarian blood supply and anatomic position to preserve ovarian tissue.
- Fetal and neonatal torsions are most commonly caused by a functional cyst. Childhood torsions are rare because of the limited function of the ovary during this time period. The incidence increases as girls near menarche due to functional cyst formation and elongation of the utero-ovarian ligament during development.
- Half of ovarian torsions in prepubertal girls are found in normal ovaries.
- Ovaries greater than 5 cm are thought to be at high risk of torsion; parents should be given precautions including symptoms of torsion.
- Strenuous exercise and increased abdominal pressure have been linked to torsion.

- Torsion in the right ovary is more common than the left, likely because of the presence of the sigmoid colon on the left which may limit ovarian mobility.
- Ultrasound can be helpful in the evaluation of suspected ovarian torsion:
  - Note ovarian size, characteristics of the cyst, and vascular flow
  - Torsion can be present even if flow is demonstrated
  - The most common ultrasonic finding is unilateral enlarged ovary
  - The classic finding is peripheral follicles with stromal edema.
- Management of suspected ovarian torsion includes a diagnostic laparoscopy (Figure 5.4); if torsion is present, untwisting or detorsing the ovary is indicated. Speedy diagnosis and management are needed to attempt to save the ovary. Delaying diagnosis can lead to ovarian necrosis, peritonitis, infertility or death. Detorsion is a safe option and, rather than oophorectomy, should be attempted to preserve ovarian function.

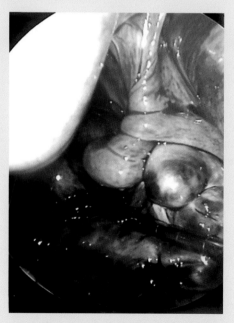

Figure 5.4 Laparoscopy of ovarian torsion. Courtesy of JL Strickland.

✋ Caution

- Malignant masses of the ovary account for 1% of all childhood cancers (Table 5.2).
- Ovarian tumors in children are most commonly germ cell in origin (see Chapter 48.2).

- These are typically benign cystic teratomas (dermoid cysts).

Table 5.2 Malignant ovarian masses

Germ cell tumors	Sex cord-stromal tumors	Epithelial tumors
Teratomas	Sertoli–Leydig cell tumor	Serous
Gonadoblastoma	Granulosa cell tumor	Mucinous
Choriocarcinoma	Gynandroblastoma	Small cell
Dysgerminoma	Lipid cell tumors	Clear cell
Embryonal carcinoma		Endometrioid
Polyembryoma		Transitional
Endodermal sinus tumor		Brenner
Mixed forms		Mixed malignant
		Mesodermal
		Undifferentiated
		Metastases to ovary

Based on the World Health Organization's International Histologic Classification of Ovarian Tumors. Reproduced from Emans SJ, Laufer MR, Goldstein DP. Benign and malignant ovarian masses. In: *Pediatric and Adolescent Gynecology*, 2005, pp. 685–728.

⚙ Science revisited

Dermoid tumor

- Dermoid tumors, also known as mature cystic teratomas, are the most common ovarian tumor in childhood.
- 20–25% of ovarian neoplasms have a germ cell origin, of which 95% are dermoid cysts. These account for 50% of pediatric tumors.
- They are comprised of several cell types and may include hair, sebaceous fluid, or calcifications such as teeth (Figure 5.5). Due to the multiple tissue types present, dermoid tumors are often characterized by ultrasound (Figure 5.6) as complex ovarian masses.
- Most dermoids are benign, but their malignant potential is due to the histologic differentiation of the neural tissue present. If malignancy is present, it is termed an immature teratoma, which represent less than 1% of all teratomas.

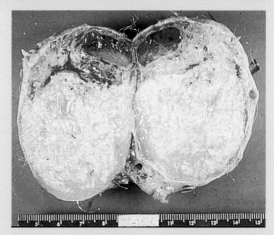

Figure 5.5 Courtesy of Pr E. Friedlander MD, Kansas City University of Medicine and Biosciences. From http://www.pathguy.com/~dlaporte/dermoid.htm

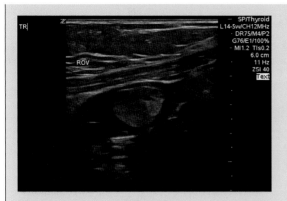

Figure 5.6 Ultrasound of dermoid.
Courtesy of Pr E. Friedlander MD, Kansas City
University of Medicine and Biosciences. From
http://www.pathguy.com/~dlaporte/dermoid.htm

- Another rare complication is a hormonally-active teratoma containing thyroid tissue. These are called struma ovarii. Hormone production can lead to thyrotoxicosis.
- 10–20% of dermoid cysts are bilateral.
- Treatment is surgical. There is continued debate over mini-laparotomy versus a laparoscopic approach. The goals of surgery are to preserve as much ovarian tissue for future fertility while removing the dermoid cyst intact to prevent a chemical peritonitis from spillage. If dermoid rupture occurs during cystectomy, copious irrigation of the abdomen and pelvis will decrease risk of adhesions from a chemical or granulomatous peritonitis.

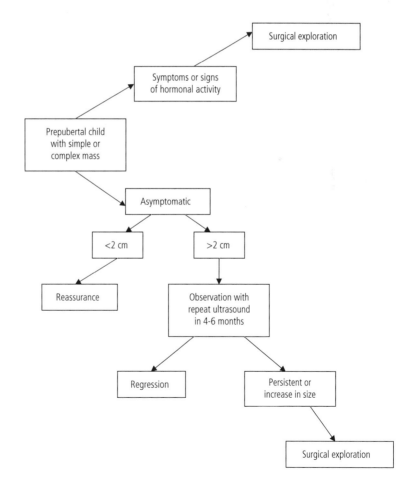

Figure 5.7 Management of
prepubertal cyst.
Adapted with permission from
Strickland, JL. Ovarian cysts in
neonates, children and adolescents.
Curr Opin Obstet Gynecol
2002;14:459–465. Lippincott
Williams & Wilkins.

rupture, causing sudden increase in pain that is usually self-limited and resolves within 1–2 days. Purely cystic lesions with few internal echoes or debris suggest hemorrhage and may be followed with ultrasound. Laparoscopy or laparotomy may be warranted if symptoms persist, if the cyst is greater than 5 cm, or if the cyst is complex on imaging. During surgery, simple cysts may be fenestrated or can be removed via cystectomy, allowing for ovarian preservation, which is standard of care. For complex cysts, a cystectomy or oophorectomy should be considered in order to remove the ovarian mass intact. Cyst aspiration may be considered for ovarian cysts secondary to precocious puberty that persist after treatment is initiated. An algorithm for the management of prepubertal cysts is shown in Figure 5.7.

Summary

The ovary is a dynamic organ that develops and changes throughout a child's life, leading to the possibility of the development of a functional ovarian mass. Although malignancy is rare, it is important to develop proper management plans to ensure resolution of ovarian masses with preservation of ovarian tissue when possible. If persistent, ovarian masses need surgical exploration and pathologic diagnosis to provide optimal care.

♀ Pearls

- Ovarian cysts occur during all stages of ovarian development.
- Simple cysts less than 5 cm in diameter can be managed with close follow-up with serial ultrasounds.
- Cysts greater than 5 cm in diameter are at higher risk for torsion.
- The majority of ovarian cysts are functional in nature but a malignant process has to be kept in the differential diagnosis.

Further reading

Emans SJ, Laufer MR, Goldstein DP. Benign and ovarian masses. In: *Pediatric and Adolescent Gynecology*, 5th edn. Philadelphia: Lippincott, Williams & Wilkins, 2005, pp. 685–728.

Guthrie BD, Adler MD, Powell EC. Incidence and trends of pediatric ovarian torsion hospitalizations in the United States, 2000–2006. *Pediatrics* 2010;125:532–538.

Strickland JL. Ovarian cysts in neonates, children and adolescents. *Curr Opin Obstet Gynecol* 2002;14:459–465.

6

Labial adhesions

Jane E. D. Broecker

Ohio University Heritage College of Osteopathic Medicine, Athens, OH, USA

Adhesions of the labia minora are a common pediatric condition and are usually identified during routine examination or when girls present with urinary or vulvar complaints. As many as 1–3% of prepubertal girls may have this condition, with many of them asymptomatic. Labial adhesions are never present at birth, most common in young girls, and rarely occur after puberty. Chronic inflammation of the labia in the setting of prepubertal estrogen levels is believed to create an environment that can result in adhesion between the delicate epithelial surfaces of the labia minora.

Labial adhesions are often asymptomatic, particularly when they are minimally obstructive. Urinary or vulvar symptoms due to the inflammatory response and irritation of the vulvovaginal area can include discharge, odor, pruritus, pain, dysuria, or post-void dribbling. Examination will often uncover a diagnosis of labial adhesions with vulvovaginitis, although determination of which condition was the initial one is often impossible. Not only can adhesions cause vulvovaginitis due to irritation by trapped urine and vaginal secretions but also, chronic vulvovaginitis can lead to labial adhesions. Diaper rash, poor hygiene, tight clothing, or other causes of irritation may lead to labial adhesions.

> ## ⚙ Science revisited
>
> - Inflammation, combined with the normally low estrogen levels in prepubertal girls, is the likely mechanism of adhesion formation. The inflammatory response results in sloughing of the epithelial cells of the labia minora and overactivation of macrophages. The result is the formation of an avascular bridge of tissue between the labia minora.
> - The initial thin membrane-like connection between the labia may become thicker over time, and involve more of the length of the labia. This process may occur anywhere along the labia, and the length of the adhesions can vary from just a few millimeters to complete agglutination of the entire length of the labia minora, from the level of the clitoris to the posterior forchette.
> - Treatment includes topical estrogens and corticosteroid ointments, which are believed to work by maturing the vulvar epithelium and decreasing inflammation, respectively.
> - Labial adhesions are never present at birth due to exposure to maternal estrogen levels *in utero*.

✋ Caution

- Do not assume that a complaint of dysuria is due to a simple urinary tract infection (UTI). An exam will reveal the underlying etiology of labial adhesions or other genital pathology.
- Labial adhesions can cause urinary obstruction severe enough to result in complete inability to void. This is a surgical emergency and the labia must be manually or surgically separated to restore normal urinary function. Anesthesia or sedation should be used in this situation to avoid unnecessary pain.
- Concurrent vulvovaginitis should be treated using antibiotics and/or aggressive hygiene measures (see Table 3.1).

Evaluation

Labial adhesions may be noticed at the time of diaper changes. For a child who is potty trained, new-onset incontinence, complaints of pain with urination, or an odor may be the primary complaints. Inadequate hygiene in older girls who are showering may lead to labial adhesions, while younger girls may be using soaps and bubble baths which initiate an inflammatory response. Because labial adhesions may sometimes be the result of the chronic inflammatory response of vulvovaginitis, you should ask questions regarding hygiene practices, such as bathing, wiping, and time in occlusive or damp clothing (tights/swimsuits). History obtained from both the child and parent (or other responsible adult) will be very helpful. Always remember to screen for abuse.

A gentle approach to the pediatric vulvar exam is essential for successful diagnosis and follow-up (see Chapter 1). For infants in diapers, a "changing table" position and exam is simple. For toddlers, "frog-leg" positioning on a parent's lap may be the most reassuring. For older girls, positioning on the examination table with knees and feet apart can give you the opportunity to educate the parent on the findings you identify and to point out what to expect with successful treatment. Some girls will welcome the opportunity to look using a hand mirror. You should use gentle lateral and downward traction on the labia majora to separate the labia minora. Be sure to differentiate labial adhesions from imperforate hymen, congenital absence of the vagina, severe lichen sclerosus or other abnormalities. If at any point the patient is significantly unco-operative or uncomfortable, do not hold her down or forcefully examine her; instead, schedule an exam under anesthesia.

★ Tips and tricks

- Use an anatomically correct doll to explain the exam.
- Find out what words the family uses for the girl's anatomy and use those terms to describe how you will be doing the exam.
- Use the child's colloquial phrases to ensure understanding, but also introduce and define anatomically correct language as appropriate.

✋ Patient/parent advice

- Address the parent's potential concerns regarding the use of estrogen cream and corticosteroid ointment, and discuss side effects.
- Estrogen cream often causes transient side effects, such as erythema of the vulva, estrogenization of the hymen, and (very rarely) breast budding or vaginal bleeding.
- Steroid ointment may cause local irritation.
- Labial adhesions may recur until a girl has entered puberty.
- After separation of adhesions, use of topical emollient, such as petroleum jelly or an ointment containing vitamins A and D, may prevent recurrences and may be necessary until puberty.
- Continued attention to proper hygiene may prevent recurrences, and baths in plain water can help maintain genital health.

There are three main descriptors for adhesions:
- **Length of involvement** using a percent method: 100% adhesed describes complete occlusion; 75% fairly extensive adhesions involving three-quarters of the total length of the labia, and so on.
- **Thickness of adhesions,** such as very thick, thick (dense in appearance), thin (almost translucent) or very thin.

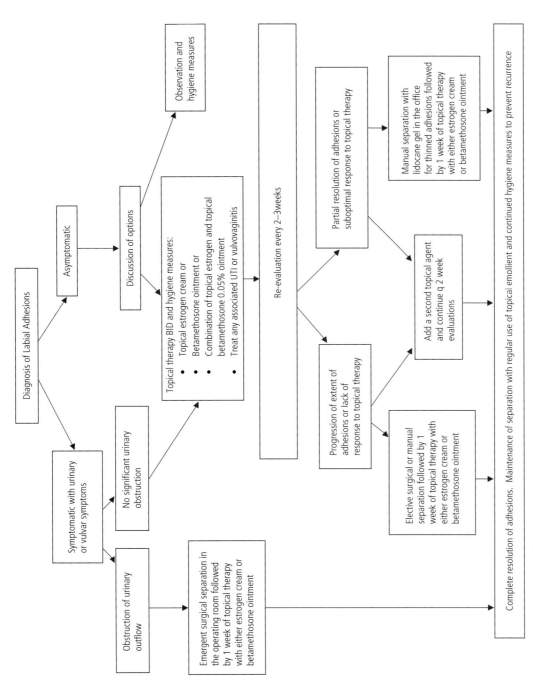

Figure 6.1 Management of labial adhesions.

• **Anatomic location** in relation to the associated anatomy, using the clitoris, urethra, introitus, and posterior forchette as anatomic landmarks.

Sometimes adhesions are multifocal and can have a fenestrated appearance. A simple anatomic drawing documenting location and length of adhesions is an effective way of documenting findings. While photographs can be very useful for accurate documentation, you must be sensitive to privacy concerns and discuss with parent and child.

Management

Asymptomatic and minimal adhesions may resolve with time and hygiene measures, so observation is an option for minor asymptomatic labial adhesions. Symptomatic patients or those with extensive but asymptomatic adhesions should be treated medically. Topical application of conjugated estrogens and/or corticosteroid ointment may be used to treat most labial adhesions, even those that are thick and extensive. Surgical separation is infrequently required, and is reserved for those with urinary obstruction or refractory adhesions after adequate treatment. The initial response to twice-daily application of topical treatments can be re-assessed every 2–3 weeks. Rarely should adhesions be manually separated in the office due to patient discomfort. Very thin translucent adhesions may be separated manually after application of 2% lidocaine jelly if necessary. Any associated vulvovaginitis should be treated with hygiene measures and antibiotics, such as amoxicillin. Figure 6.1 outlines the management options.

Further reading

Eroğlu E, Yip M, Oktar T, Kayiran SM, Mocan H. How should we treat prepubertal labial adhesions? Retrospective

Evidence at a glance

• Topical estrogen cream BID has been the traditional treatment modality, with separation occurring in over 75%. The duration of treatment required may vary from days to weeks, with most labial adhesions resolving within 12 weeks.
• Recent studies have evaluated the efficacy of betamethasone ointment 0.05% and report similar or improved success, with about 75% of adhesions resolving with BID or TID applications. Duration of treatment may be similar or shorter than that for estrogen cream.
• A combination of estrogen cream and betamethasone 0.05% may eventually prove to be the most effective topical regimen, with a recent study showing similar separation rates, similar time to resolution, and possibly lower recurrence rates.
• Recurrence after surgical separation can occur in over 10%.

comparison of topical treatments: estrogen only, betamethasone only, and combination estrogen and betamethasone. *J Pediatr Adolesc Gynecol* 2011;24(6):389–91.

Leung AK, Robson WL, Kao CP, Liu EK, Fong JH. Treatment of labial fusion with topical estrogen therapy. *Clin Pediatr (Phila)* 2005;44(3):245–247.

Mayoglou L, Dulabon L, Martin-Alguacil N, Pfaff D, Schober J. Success of treatment modalities for labial fusion: a retrospective evaluation of topical and surgical treatments. *J Pediatr Adolesc Gynecol* 2009;22(4): 247–250.

7

Pediatric vulvovaginitis

Sari Kives

University of Toronto, Hospital for Sick Children, Toronto, ON, Canada

Vulvovaginitis is one of the most common gyneco-logic complaints in prepubertal girls. It is also often quite easy to treat with the elimination of risk factors and simple hygiene measures. Infrequently, the symp-toms are particularly troublesome or recurrent and referral to a specialist is required.

The symptoms primarily include vulvar irritation or burning with or without discharge, and occasion-ally bleeding. Girls may complain of burning with urination, sometimes making distinction from a urinary tract infection (UTI) challenging.

Behavioral factors may also play a role as children have a tendency for poor hygiene and a natural curi-osity of exploring their own bodies. Chronic consti-pation may also be a contributing factor.

Most often the etiology is nonspecific irritation, but occasionally a bacterial infection, sexually transmit-ted infection due to abuse or foreign body may be the offender (Table 7.1).

The history that should be elicited is described in Table 7.2.

Diagnosis

The physical exam can usually be limited to an exter-nal genital exam with adequate exposure of the hymen in the frog-legged position or knee–chest posi-tion. Tanner staging and the absence or presence of estrogen in the vagina should be documented. If dis-charge is present, a vaginal culture should be obtained. If there is any suggestion of sexual abuse, cultures from the vagina for *Chlamydia trachomatis*, *Neisseria gonorrhoeae* or *Trichomonas vaginalis* should be obtained as well.

In addition, examination should look for the pres-ence of vulvar swelling, vesicular lesions or ulcera-tions, secondary excoriations, evidence of trauma, whitish discoloration, and labial adhesions. Any abnormalities of the hymen should be documented.

The entire body should be inspected for any other dermatologic conditions that may involve irritation in the vulvar area, particularly eczema, allergic reac-tions, and dermatitis (Table 7.3).

The differential diagnosis is listed in Table 7.4.

Practical Pediatric and Adolescent Gynecology, First Edition. Edited by Paula J. Adams Hillard.
© 2013 John Wiley & Sons, Ltd. Published 2013 by John Wiley & Sons, Ltd.

Table 7.1 Characteristics and treatment of vulvovaginitis

Type	Frequency	Etiology	Symptoms	Treatment
Nonspecific vulvovaginitis	75%	Irritation from bubble baths, perfumed detergents, and poor hygiene	Protracted history of scant to copious foul smelling discharge, red irritated vulva; vagina is often spared	Improved hygiene
Streptococcal vaginitis	5%	Respiratory infection	Short history (<1 week) of purulent discharge and erythematous vulva, vagina, and perianal area	Amoxicillin
Sexually-transmitted vaginitis	Rare	History of sexual abuse	Copious yellow to green discharge	Treat the specific organism and report suspicion of abuse to child protective services as required per state law
Foreign body	5%	Prior history	Bloody malodorous and persistent discharge	Remove foreign body

Table 7.2 History of vulvovaginal symptoms in prepubertal girls

- Duration of symptoms
- Time of day when symptoms are worse
- Presence of discharge:
  - Color
  - Presence of foul odor
- Vaginal bleeding
- Itching
- Dysuria
- Burning and/or vulvar pain
- Irritant exposure including:
  - Bubble baths
  - Harsh detergent
  - Poor wiping techniques
- Prior home or prescribed regimens:
  - Recent antibiotics
  - Recent steroid use (inhaled or topical)
- Voiding habits
- Bowel habits

> ★ **Tips and tricks**
>
> - The main objective of the examination is to distinguish between the common nonspecific vulvovaginitis, which accounts for the majority of cases, and a specific vulvovaginitis. The history is typically of symptoms that have waxed and waned over several months or more.
> - Vulvovaginitis due to a specific pathogen is usually associated with significant erythema of the vagina and perianal area, as well as a vaginal discharge (often bloody, yellow, or greenish). The history often includes a recent (<1 week) and more abrupt onset than is seen with a nonspecific vulvovaginitis.

To obtain a culture, a small sterile, saline moistened Calgiswab (cervical or urethral) should be carefully introduced into the vagina. Careful attention should be given to avoiding touching the hymen as this can cause significant discomfort. In younger children, a feeding tube or urethral catheter can be used to introduce a small amount of saline (1 mL) into the vagina and this is then aspirated using an attached syringe (see Figure 3.1). The specimen should be sent for culture and sensitivity as well as a wet mount to identify a specific bacterial pathogen.

If bleeding or a recurrent malodorous discharge is present, a foreign body should be suspected. Vaginal irrigation with saline can be performed in the office, using a catheter within a catheter technique (urethral catheter through which a small angiocath tubing has been threaded), attached to a 60-mL Luer lock syringe (Figure 7.1); this will often dislodge one of the most

Table 7.3 Review of systems for prepubertal girls with vulvovaginal symptoms

- History of trauma
- Topical allergies
- Atopy
- Skin conditions:
  ○ Eczema
  ○ Psoriasis
- Potential risk of sexual abuse
- Signs of early puberty
- History of previous or current urinary tract infections,
- Recent gastroenteritis
- Enuresis
- Encopresis
- Recent respiratory infection

Table 7.4 Differential diagnosis

- Nonspecific vulvovaginitis
- Specific vulvovaginitis
- Dermatologic skin disorders, e.g. lichen sclerosus
- Vaginal foreign bodies
- Sexually-transmitted infections
- Urinary tract infection
- Ectopic ureter
- Sexual abuse
- Pinworms
- Systemic disorders, e.g. Kawasaki disease
- Vulvodynia – rare
- Congenital enteric fistula

✋ Caution

- Normal children harbor a mixture of vaginal bacteria including bowel flora (e.g. *Escherichia coli, Staphylococcus aureus, Streptococcus viridans, Pseudomonas aeruginosa*) in the absence of lactobacillus (Table 7.5).
- It is therefore paramount that a culture only be performed in a symptomatic child with vulvovaginitis and discharge.

Table 7.5 Normal flora in prepubertal vagina

Anaerobes	Aerobes
Gram positive	**Gram positive**
Actinomyces	*Staphylococcus aureus*
Bifidobacteria	*Streptococcus viridans*
Peptococcus	*Enterococcus foecalis*
Peptostreptococcus	Corynebacteria or
Propionibacterium	diphtheroids
Gram negative	
Veillonella	
Bacteroides	
Fusobacteria	
Gram-negative cocci	

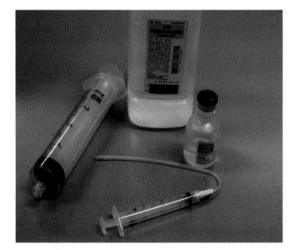

Figure 7.1 Equipment for vaginal irrigation.

common vaginal foreign bodies, a small piece of toilet paper. Vaginoscopy under sedation or general anesthetic may be required if this office procedure is not effective.

Management

The mainstay of therapy is improved perineal hygiene with particular focus on front-to-back wiping.

An emollient such as petroleum jelly or vitamin A and D ointment may offer symptomatic as well as psychological relief. With severe inflammation, topical estrogen and/or a topical low-dose hydrocortisone ointment may facilitate healing and help break the itch–scratch cycle. Antibiotics are rarely indicated unless a specific pathogen is discovered.

☝ Patient/parent advice

- Avoid contact irritants: perfumed bath products and/or detergents.
- Dry the vulva meticulously after bathing with a blow dryer on a gentle setting.
- Baths are more soothing and provide better cleansing than showers:
  - At least 10–15 min daily or twice daily
  - Do not scour the vulva
  - Warm water is all that is necessary for good hygiene
  - Never allow the child to sit in soapy water; hair washing should be reserved for the end of the bath and the child should stand to have her hair rinsed
  - Mild soaps such as Aveeno or Dove may be used if necessary.
- Use plain white toilet paper and white cotton underwear, and do not use fabric softeners or antistatic sheets.
- Have the child void with their legs wide open.
- No underwear at bedtime.
- Avoid tight-fitting clothing (e.g. ballet leotards), nylon clothing, and prolonged exposure to wet bathing suits.

⬡ Science revisited

- The most common specific causes of vulvovaginitis are *Streptococcus pyogenes* and *Haemophilus influenzae*:
  - A positive culture may occur in up to 25% of children with vulvovaginitis.
- *S. pyogenes* (Group A beta-hemolytic strep) is a Gram-positive bacterium found in the upper airways of 5–92% of asymptomatic girls:
  - It is not uncommon for the child to have a history of an upper respiratory infection preceding the vulvovaginitis which typically includes a purulent or bloody discharge
  - Treatment is with amoxicillin.
- *H. influenzae* is a Gram-negative coccobacillus that can be associated with a concomitant otitis media or conjunctivitis:
  - The history usually includes a greenish purulent discharge
  - Treatment is with amoxicillin.

✋ Caution

- Candida is rarely the culprit in pediatric vulvovaginitis because of the lack of both lactobacilli and an acidic environment.
- Candida should be considered only in the following scenarios: diaper use, a recent course of antibiotics (rare even with this history) and/or corticosteroids, diabetics or other immunocompromised states.

Specific causes

If nighttime itching is the predominant complaint, pinworms (*Enterobius vermicularis*) should be suspected. A tape test to the anal area can be performed overnight to allow for microscopic examination of the ova. Empiric treatment with 100 mg of mebendazole orally and repeated 2 weeks later can be used. Underwear and bedding should also be carefully laundered.

Other less common specific causes of vulvovaginitis include: *Yersinia enterocolitica* and *Shigella flexneri*. Treatment is with trimethoprim and sulfamethoxazole if susceptible.

Other opportunistic pathogens may cause symptoms. Amoxicillin/clavulanic acid is the antibiotic most commonly used for *S. aureus*. Other treatments should include oral probiotics, sitz baths, and topical antiseptics. Antibiotic treatment should be limited to the most severe cases, given the potential for organisms to develop resistance.

In rare cases, a sexually-transmitted pathogen may be the cause of the vulvovaginitis. Although perinatal transmission is possible up to 3 years of age, sexual abuse must always be considered with vulvovaginal symptoms. Treatment is with antibiotics specific to the pathogen.

Recurrent vulvovaginitis

If symptoms of vaginal discharge do not resolve or recur after a short period of time, reconsideration of the initial diagnosis is warranted. Ensuring that the family implemented the current treatment as well as ruling out other potential sources, i.e. a foreign body and dermatologic conditions, is necessary.

Recurrence of symptoms after treatment for *H. influenza* or *S. pyogenes* may necessitate alternative treatment or protracted treatment, i.e. bedtime dosing for 1 month. This recurrence is often secondary to asymptomatic carriage in the child or a family member.

Follow-up

As the majority of cases of vulvovaginitis are nonspecific, the prognosis is usually excellent with the establishment of good hygiene measures. A preprinted hand out in your office can be helpful. If the diagnosis is unclear, the parents require additional reassurance, or, if the condition does not respond to either nonspecific treatment or specific treatment options, referral to a specialist may be warranted.

Further reading

Dei M, Di Maggio F, Di Paola G, Bruni V. Vulvovaginitis in childhood. *Best Pract Res Clin Obstet Gynaecol* 2010 Apr;24(2):129–137.

Merkley K. Vulvovaginitis and vaginal discharge in the pediatric patient. *J Emerg Nurs* 2006;32(6):535–540.

Van Eyk N, Allen L, Giesbrecht E, *et al.* Pediatric vulvovaginal disorders: A diagnostic approach and review of the literature. *J Obstet Gynaecol Can* 2009;31(9):850–862.

8 Sexual abuse

Nancy D. Kellogg and James L. Lukefahr
University of Texas Health Science Center at San Antonio, San Antonio, TX, USA

Each year approximately 88 000 US children are confirmed victims of sexual abuse. It is common for abuse to occur for several weeks or months and to progress to penetration before detection. Sexual abuse in childhood has been associated with long-term deleterious outcomes, including depression, suicide, eating disorders, relationship violence, obesity, illicit drug use, and poor parenting skills.

Child sexual abuse is not commonly detected during clinician evaluation. Most cases of child sexual abuse first present to a clinical setting after a child discloses their abuse to another person. Currently, most regions in the US have specialized programs and protocols to evaluate children who have made a disclosure of sexual abuse. These programs can usually be identified by contacting a Children's Advocacy Center, or a regional hospital. Sometimes, however, children will present to clinicians with physical symptoms or behaviors that are concerning for sexual abuse.

Physical symptoms that may indicate sexual assault or ongoing sexual abuse include vaginal or penile discharge, anogenital bruising, abrasions or lacerations, and anogenital lesions such as verrucous growths, vesicles, or ulcers (Table 8.1). Parents sometimes present with their children for other physical symptoms such as "redness" or "her opening looks too big," but only about 15% of children referred for sexual abuse examination with physical symptoms but no disclosure of abuse have findings concerning for sexual abuse or sexually-transmitted infection (STI).

Young children often present to clinicians with sexual behaviors that raise concern for sexual abuse. Sexual behaviors are two to three times more common in children who have been sexually abused when compared to children who have not been abused. However, sexual behaviors are also associated with physical abuse, neglect, domestic violence, conduct disorders, and exposure to sexually explicit material or nudity. Sexual behavior can also be normal, especially among preschool-age children. When sexual behaviors are coercive, occur between children 4 or more years apart, or could potentially result in physical or emotional harm, a report should be made to child protection agencies so the safety of all children involved can be evaluated; it is also appropriate to refer these children to a mental health specialist for further assessment and treatment.

Diagnosis

There are four components in the medical assessment of suspected child sexual abuse: history, physical examination and inspection for injuries, testing for STIs, and forensic evidence collection.

The history from the child is usually the most important factor in the diagnosis and treatment of sexual abuse. A history can be gathered from children

Practical Pediatric and Adolescent Gynecology, First Edition. Edited by Paula J. Adams Hillard.
© 2013 John Wiley & Sons, Ltd. Published 2013 by John Wiley & Sons, Ltd.

Table 8.1 Causes of anogenital signs and symptoms in children

Sign or symptom	Trauma	Infection	Inflammation	Other
Genital or anal bleeding	Abusive trauma Accidental trauma, e.g. straddle injury	Shigella Group A beta-hemolytic strep Candidiasis	Intravaginal foreign body Excoriation due to irritants, hygiene, diaper dermatitis	Anal fissures Dehisced labial adhesions Urethral prolapse
Genital or anal bruising	Abusive blunt trauma Accidental blunt trauma, e.g. straddle injury		Lichen sclerosus et atrophicus	Hemangiomas Urethral prolapse Bruise mimics (nevi, Mongolian spots)
Genital or anal erythema	Abusive abrasive trauma	N. gonorrhoeae C. trachomatis Candidiasis Streptococcus or staphylococcus infections	Irritants, including soaps, fecal material, diaper dermatitis Folliculitis Psoriasis Lichen sclerosus et atrophicus	Normal prepubertal mucosa
Scarring of the hymen, vestibule or anus	Healed abusive blunt force or penetrative trauma			Labial adhesion Linea vestibularis Anatomic variants (usually midline), e.g. linea vestibularis, diastasis ani, failure of midline fusion
Dilatation of hymenal or anal openings	Uncommon, nonspecific finding for abuse			Obesity in females Decreased sphincter tone due to neurologic condition or sedation Presence of stool in rectal vault Encopresis Prolonged exam or change in exam position
Genital discharge	Healing genital trauma	N. gonorrhoeae C. trachomatis T. vaginalis Streptococcal infection Bacterial vaginosis Candidiasis	Intravaginal foreign body Overgrowth of normal vaginal flora	Semen Physiologic leukorrhea Smegma
Vesicles		Herpes simplex virus 1 or 2 Varicella zoster virus Epstein-Barr virus Impetigo	Behçet disease Pyoderma gangrenosum	
Papules and nodules		Condylomata acuminata Molluscum contagiosum Condylomata lata	Crohn disease Perianal pseudo-verrucous papules and nodules	Anal skin tags Urethral/peri-urethral cysts

as young as 4 years, and should be taken out of the presence of the parent. Children may look to their parent for cues, or may be protective and reluctant to verbalize information that could upset their mother or father. Clinicians should be careful not to ask suggestive or leading questions, especially in this younger age group, who may be eager to answer questions that are not clearly understood.

★ Tips and tricks

- Urine samples rather than vaginal swabs can be submitted when testing for gonorrhea and chlamydia with nucleic acid amplification tests (NAATs); this reduces the trauma of the exam for many children.
- It is important to talk with the child out of the presence of the parent; children may be reluctant to disclose hurtful details of the abuse for fear of upsetting their mother.
- Having the child talk to you while you are doing the genital examination tends to be more effective than talking to the child at another time.
- The prone knee–chest position allows the clinician to visualize the vaginal vault and cervix without using a speculum; this is effective in looking for foreign bodies.

For purposes of medical diagnosis and treatment, it is important to establish:
- Who abused the child (family or non-family member).
- What types of sexual contact occurred (which part or parts of the abuser's body touched which part or parts of the child's body).
- Last sexual contact (if within 72 hours, forensic evidence collection may be indicated).
- Any imminent threats to safety (Does the abuser still have access to the child? Does the nonabusing parent support/believe the child? Has the abuser been violent to family members?).

While young children may only be able to describe who abused them and what happened, children who are aged 8 years and older can elaborate on physical and emotional symptoms, their feelings about the abuse, and their parents' response to learning about the abuse. The parents and the child should independently be asked about: pain or bleeding during or following the abuse, including dysuria, and pain on defecation, discharge from the genitals, and painful or painless bumps, blisters, or lesions of anogenital structures. Behavioral symptoms may also be reported by the child or parent: nightmares, particularly about the abuser, abuse or family members being hurt; school difficulties, such as trouble focusing because of intrusive thoughts about the abuse; and feeling sad or thinking about dying. Family members may describe the child as more withdrawn, showing regressive behaviors, or being more "clingy"; other child victims may become aggressive verbally, physically or sexually with others. Not all abused children, however, have behavioral changes. It is important to inform parents that just because their child is acting "normally," this does not mean that they were not abused or did not suffer emotional trauma.

✋ Patient/parent advice

- Sexual behaviors that do not mimic intercourse, such as touching own genitals, touching adult breasts, and trying to view parent nudity are common sexual behaviors in children 5 years and younger, and do not necessarily indicate abuse.
- Sexual behavior that is not appropriate for the child's age, or that causes emotional distress or physical pain, is not normal; parents should seek the advice of a clinician.
- If a child discloses sexual abuse to a parent or other trusted adult, it is vitally important for that adult to show complete support to the child. Only enough information to make a report of the abuse should be gathered, and verification of the child's statement should be left to the investigators.

The physical examination should include a careful "head-to-toe" inspection, and any signs of bodily injury should be noted. Positions and techniques for the anogenital examination include:
- Supine frog-leg or lithotomy positions: use labial separation and gentle traction to reveal the hymen,

urethra, and vestibule. Inspection of male genitalia can be done with the patient lying supine with legs straight and slightly parted so testicles can be inspected and palpated.

• Lateral decubitus position: if anal samples are needed, the child should be placed in a lateral decubitus position with the knees drawn up.

• Prone knee–chest position: children with a history of anal penetration or who appear to have healed hymenal transections in supine position should be examined in the prone knee–chest position. The child should first get on her hands and knees, and while keeping the hips directly above the knees, arch the lower back and place the side of the head and shoulders on the table. The hymen is visualized by placing both thumbs at the level of the posterior commissure and lifting the labia and perineum to reveal the hymen. The prone knee–chest position also permits visualization of the vaginal canal and cervix without instrumentation.

Most (>90%) of examinations of sexually-abused prepubertal children will be normal or show only nonspecific signs, such as erythema. Sexual abuse may not result in visible tissue trauma, or superficial trauma may heal quickly and completely. Findings considered indicative of sexual abuse include: hymenal bruising, lacerations, or healed transections; posterior vestibule or perineal lacerations or scars; bitemarks to the penis; and anal lacerations and scars (other than superficial anal fissures).

Forensic evidence collection kits are usually provided by state agencies and contain specific and detailed instructions for collecting evidence, including clothing, linens, secretions, debris, fingernail scrapings, hair, blood, and patient norm samples. Most forensic evidence collected from prepubertal children is recovered within 24 hours of sexual contact, although in rare instances material has been recovered as late as 96 hours.

If the child gives a history of genital–genital, genital–anal, or genital–oral contact, has symptoms of an STI, or appears reluctant or too scared to provide complete details of the abusive contact, then strong consideration should be given to testing for *Neisseria gonorrhoeae* and *Chlamydia trachomatis*. Although culture techniques have been considered the "gold standard" and do provide antibiotic susceptibility data, many laboratories are utilizing nucleic acid amplification tests (NAATs) instead, due to

better sensitivity. One swab sample can be submitted for both chlamydia and gonorrhea testing; urine can also be submitted for testing and may be optimal for prepubertal children. While *Trichomonas vaginalis* is uncommon in prepubertal children, a culture or polymerase chain reaction (PCR) can be submitted if a discharge is visualized on examination. Cultures or PCR for herpes simplex virus type 1 or 2 can be submitted if there are vesicles or ulcers. Testing for human immunodeficiency virus (HIV), syphilis, and hepatitis is recommended for children who are diagnosed with one STI, who have symptoms, or if patient or parent anxiety can be assuaged with testing. Since several STIs, notably *Condylomata acuminata*, may take weeks or months to present clinically; follow-up examinations should be carefully planned.

✋ Caution

• Most sexually-abused prepubertal children do not have STIs; presumptive antibiotic therapy prior to receiving the results of STI testing is not recommended.
• However, STI testing is strongly recommended, since most children who do have chlamydia or gonorrhea infections will not have obvious symptoms.
• Most children presenting with genital bleeding or bruising and no history of sexual abuse will have causes other than sexual abuse trauma.

⚗ Science revisited

• Most examinations of sexually-abused children are normal or nonspecific.
• Most injuries associated with sexual abuse/assault heal quickly and completely.
• "Normal" does not mean "nothing happened."
• The history from the child is the most important evidence.
• NAATs detect more chlamydia and gonorrhea infections than culture techniques, but antibiotic sensitivity cannot be determined with NAATs.

Management

The first step in management is to report suspected abuse to child protection agencies. In some states, if the abuser is not a family member, law enforcement should be notified.

The physician can provide important education, support, and reassurance to the child and family. A normal examination does not mean "nothing happened," and reassuring the child of physical integrity can be a relief. The family should also be provided with counseling resources.

Presumptive antibiotic prophylaxis is not recommended in prepubertal children because few children contract STIs and very few present for evaluation within hours of sexual contact.

Prompt referral to a mental health professional qualified to assess and provide psychotherapy in child trauma victims is essential.

Further reading

Adams JA, Kaplan RA, Starling SP, *et al.* Guidelines for medical care of children who may have been sexually abused. *J Pediatr Adolesc Gynecol* 2007;20:163–172.

Hammerschlag MR. Sexual Aasault and abuse of children. *Clin Infect Dis* 2011;53(S3):S103–109.

Kellogg ND, The Committee on Child Abuse and Neglect. Clinical Report: The Evaluation of Sexual Behaviors in Children. *Pediatrics* 2009;124:992–998.

Concerns in prepubertal girls and in adolescents

Normal hymen and hymenal variations

Amy D. DiVasta[1,2] and Estherann Grace[1]

[1]Division of Adolescent and Young Adult Medicine, Boston Children's Hospital, Boston, MA, USA
[2]Division of Pediatric and Adolescent Gynecology, Boston Children's Hospital, Boston, MA, USA

The development of the female genital tract is a complex process, resulting in the potential for clinical variations. All newborn female infants are born with hymens. The hymen should be carefully inspected during an external vaginal exam, as it can demonstrate a multitude of normal variants (Figure 9.1). First, the hymen should be assessed for estrogen effect. Well-estrogenized hymens appear light pink and thickened. Hymens appear well-estrogenized in the newborn period (reflecting stimulation by maternal hormones) and with puberty. During late infancy and through the prepubertal period, the hymen is thin and translucent, with smooth edges.

The shape of the hymen varies. The most common hymen configuration is annular, completely surrounding the introitus (hymenal tissue extending from 12 o'clock to 12 o'clock). A crescentic hymen, with a shape like a half moon (hymenal tissue not appearing between 11 o'clock to 1 o'clock), is also a normal variant. Other fimbriated hymens have a "ruffled" appearance due to redundant tissue that folds into itself.

Congenital hymen anomalies

Congenital hymen anomalies include imperforate, microperforate, septate, and cribriform hymens (Figure 9.2).

> ### ★ Tips and tricks
>
> • To best examine the vaginal introitus and hymen configuration, the patient should be placed in either the frog-leg position or lithotomy position.
> • The labia majora can be gently retracted down and laterally for optimal visualization.
> • Often, a moistened soft Q-tip or Calgiswab can be used to gently run around the edges of the hymen, to evaluate for hymenal tags, irregularities, and openings.
> • An especially redundant hymen may initially appear to have no opening; however, when the skin is retracted and stretched, the opening will usually become apparent.

Imperforate hymen

This malformation is one of the most common obstructive lesions of the female genital tract. When detected at birth, the bulging imperforate hymen is due to a mucocolpos formed in response to maternal estradiol stimulating vaginal secretions in the infant. Should the imperforate hymen diagnosis be missed, the secretions are reabsorbed. If there is no further inspection of the genitalia, the diagnosis may then be

---

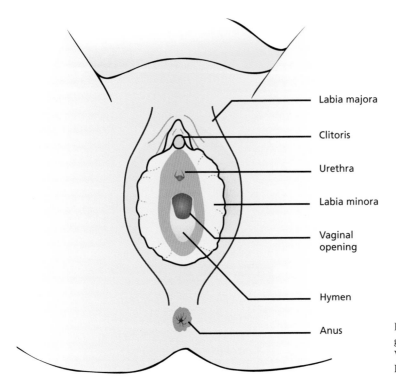

Labia majora

Clitoris

Urethra

Labia minora

Vaginal
opening

Hymen

Anus

Figure 9.1 Based on Normal female genital anatomy. Center for Young Women's Health, Boston Children's Hospital.

Science revisited

- Initially, the hymen is the membrane that separates the vaginal lumen from the urogenital sinus.
- The hymen usually ruptures before birth as a consequence of the degeneration of the central epithelial cells, leaving a fold of membrane around the vaginal introitus, which is attached to the vaginal wall.
- When the epithelial cells fail to degenerate, hymenal anomalies result.

delayed until puberty. Typically, if not diagnosed earlier, an adolescent girl will present with primary amenorrhea and cyclic abdominal or pelvic pain. The pain may be referred to the back and may worsen with urination and/or defecation. Inspection of the vulva reveals a bulging, bluish hymenal membrane due to hematocolpos.

Treatment response is facilitated by estrogen exposure to the tissues. The best timing for surgical repair is in the newborn period or just prior to menarche. Under anesthesia, an elliptical incision allows for evacuation of the collected materials. The excess hymenal tissue is excised, and the vaginal mucosa is sutured to the hymenal ring to prevent recurrence of the obstruction.

Incomplete fenestration

Incomplete fenestration of the hymen includes microperforate, septate, and cribriform hymens. These lesions may all remain undiagnosed until the patient attempts tampon insertion or coitus.

The microperforate hymen, while allowing some menstrual flow, may cause post-menstrual spotting and discharge due to poor drainage related to partial obstruction to flow. When there is retained menstrual blood in the vagina, infection can develop and result in a tubo-ovarian abscess. Treatment of the microperforate hymen requires a surgical procedure to resect the excess hymenal ring.

The septate hymen occurs when bands of tissue bisect the hymenal orifice, creating two or more

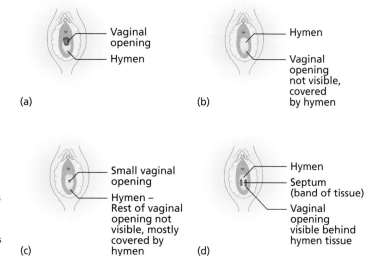

Figure 9.2 Based on Congenital variations of the hymen (a) normal; (b) imperforate; (c) microperforate; (d) septate. Center for Young Women's Health, Boston Children's Hospital.

smaller openings. A septate hymen is frequently responsible for the difficult removal of a saturated tampon. Classically, but depending on the width of the septum, the adolescent is able to insert the dry, slender tampon by displacing the septum to one side. However, after absorption of moisture occurs, the tampon expands. Then, attempts to remove the tampon are met with pain and resistance. as the septum may block the opening. With time, the septum may adequately stretch secondary to tampon use and/ or coitus. However, for full correction, surgery is recommended. Depending on the thickness of the hymenal septum/band and the tolerance of the patient, this can frequently be incised with local anesthesia as an office procedure.

The cribriform hymen has multiple small holes. This configuration allows for more efficient menstrual flow than the single opening of the microperforate hymen. However, surgical correction is required to provide a fully functional introitus.

Acquired anomalies

Hymenal skin tags are common findings. These usually regress, and treatment is not needed for asymptomatic lesions.

Acquired abnormalities of the hymen may occur from sexual contact; accidental trauma very rarely involves the hymen. Importantly, most girls with a history of substantiated sexual abuse have a normal genital exam. In the adolescent female, hymenal clefts may result from consensual or nonconsensual intercourse, or from painful insertion of a tampon. Clefts of the lower hymen below the 2 o'clock and 10 o'clock line are seen in the majority of sexually-active adolescents, but have also been noted in nonsexually active pad and tampon users. Notches occurring below the 4 o'clock to 8 o'clock line are more common in girls with a history of sexual activity, or those reporting a history of difficult tampon insertion. Hymenal measurements lack both specificity and sensitivity for establishing the likelihood of sexual contact.

> ### ✋ Caution
>
> A normal external genital exam does not mean that sexual abuse has not occurred. The majority of girls with a history of substantiated sexual abuse have a normal genital exam.

When to refer?

- Microperforate, septate, cribriform, or imperforate hymen identified
- Patient's inability to use a tampon or have coitus
- Primary amenorrhea

🖐 Patient/parent advice

For teens and parents, information and illustrations of the various hymen configurations can be found at: www.youngwomenshealth.org/hymen.html

♀ Pearls

- Various configurations of the normal hymen occur: annular, crescentic, fimbriated.
- Congenital abnormalities of the hymen commonly occur. All females need an external genital exam.
- The hymen and vaginal tissues are extremely resilient. There are no physical findings that can definitively exclude sexual contact, consensual or nonconsensual.

Further reading

Berenson AB, Grady JJ. A longitudinal study of hymenal development from 3 to 9 years of age. *J Pediatr* 2002; 140(5):600–607.

Center for Young Women's Health, Children's Hospital Boston. www.youngwomenshealth.org

Emans SJ, Woods ER, Allred EN, Grace E. Hymenal findings in adolescent women: impact of tampon use and consensual sexual activity. *J Pediatr* 1994;125:153.

Pillai M. Genital findings in prepubertal girls: what can be concluded from an examination? *J Pediatr Adolesc Gynecol* 2008;21:177–185.

Acknowledgements

Funding sources include NICHD K23 HD060066 and Project 5-T71-MC-00009-14 from the Maternal and Child Health Bureau.

10.1 Overview of vulvar signs and symptoms

Paula J. Adams Hillard

Department of Obstetrics and Gynecology, Stanford University School of Medicine, Stanford, CA, USA

Vulvar signs and symptoms are among the most common complaints of girls of all ages – from the diaper rash of infants through other conditions of childhood, puberty, and adolescence. The clinician needs to know that while some conditions occur in both prepubertal and adolescent girls (Table 10.1.1), pubertal growth leads to changes in the anatomy, microbiology, and microbial flora of the vulvovaginal area, and the risks of exposures to sexually-transmitted infections. In a prepubertal child with vulvovaginal symptoms, the possibility of sexual abuse must at least be considered, and correlated with the history and findings on exam. Additionally, the child may not be able to adequately describe her symptoms, which may range from pruritus, to tenderness/pain, to dysuria; parents' descriptions of the appearance of the area and the child's behavior are important. Urinary tract infection (UTI) must be in the differential. Specific details of perineal hygiene should be assessed (bathing versus showers; use of soaps, creams, vigorous scrubbing, etc.). The possibility of a vaginal foreign body must be considered, and the child's history of having placed a foreign body in another orifice should be elicited.

No matter the cause of vulvar symptoms, good hygiene can facilitate healing and minimize the risks of subsequent discomfort.

This chapter is not intended to be comprehensive, but rather to help the clinician to think about common causes of vulvar signs (findings and physical exam) and symptoms (presenting complaints), starting with what they see in the office: a child of a given age and pubertal status, with specific history of symptoms that will need to be correlated with the findings on a careful physical exam (see also Appendices 1.1.1–1.1.3, and 1.4). More common conditions will be covered in specific chapters that will be referred to for details.

> **✋ Patient/parent advice**
>
> • A daily bath helps to clean the genital area better than a shower.
> • Use plain water of a comfortable temperature.
> • Avoid bubble baths, harsh soaps, and vigorous scrubbing of the genitals, as these can be irritating, particularly to the vaginal area of young girls.
> • If the area is particularly red or painful, sitting in a bathtub of warm water can be soothing.
> • Gently wash between the labial folds using a washcloth to remove any secretions.
> • Dry carefully between the labial folds.
> • If the area is sore or irritated, use a hair dryer at a comfortable temperature to dry the labia.

Table 10.1.1 Vulvar conditions that may present in girls of any age

- Lichen sclerosus
- Condyloma
- Contact irritant
- Epidermoid cysts (also termed sebaceous cysts)
- Molluscum contagiosum
- Pigmented nevus
- Psoriasis
- Vulvar abscess
- Vulvar vestibulitis
- Vulvar ulcers

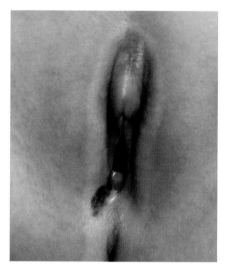

Figure 10.1.1 Lichen sclerosus in a prepubertal girl. Courtesy of Paula JA Hillard, MD.

Prepubertal girls

Vulvar itching

Vulvar itching in prepubertal girls is a nonspecific symptom that can be associated with any number of conditions, including a mixed bacterial vulvovaginitis (see Chapter 7) that is associated with poor hygiene and frequently occurs with odor and discharge. Other causes of vulvar itching include specific skin conditions (such as psoriasis) than can occur elsewhere on the skin as well. Anal or vaginal pinworms can cause intense itching. A sticky-tape test will reveal the eggs; instruct the parent to press the sticky side of a piece of tape over the anal area for a few seconds. The tape is then placed on a glass slide, sticky side down, which when examined under a microscope will reveal the eggs that have been deposited overnight.

An examination may reveal classic signs of lichen sclerosus (Figure 10.1.1). Vulvar lichen sclerosus typically responds well to high-potency topical corticosteroid ointment.

While vulvar itching is frequently attributed to a "yeast infection" similar to what is common in adolescents and adults, once a girl is out of diapers, a true yeast vulvitis is quite uncommon or even rare prior to puberty.

Vulvar itching must be distinguished from normal or potentially excessive self-exploration or stimulation. Parents can shape behaviors if they suspect that the child is exploring pleasurable feelings by suggesting that touching is OK in "private," but not in public; true vulvar itching will occur involuntarily, and may quickly become painful rather than itchy.

✶ Tips and tricks

- A prepubertal girl with complaints of vulvar itching without vaginal discharge or odor strongly suggests the diagnosis of lichen sclerosus (see Chapter 11). Findings associated with lichen sclerosus include:
  - "Cigarette paper" skin changes (crinkling of vulvar skin) with architectural distortion (obliteration of interlabial folds)
  - Splitting of the skin
  - "Figure of eight" distribution in vulvar and perianal skin
  - Subepithelial hemorrhage ("blood blisters") due to skin fragility.
- Prepubertal girls rarely get true fungal/candida yeast infections.

Vaginal discharge

Prepubertal girls typically develop a vulvitis and may secondarily develop a vaginitis, while adolescents typically develop a vaginitis that secondarily becomes a vulvitis. Any condition causing a vaginal discharge (see Chapter 7) can present with vulvar itching and inflammation as well. A vaginal foreign body should be considered if there is a foul smelling or bloody discharge, or when the discharge persists in spite of

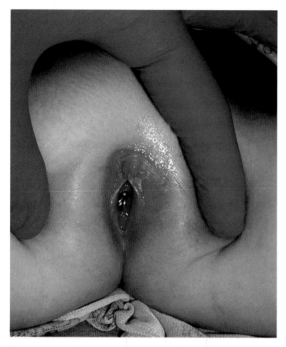

Figure 10.1.2 Removal of a vaginal foreign body. Courtesy of Paula JA Hillard, MD.

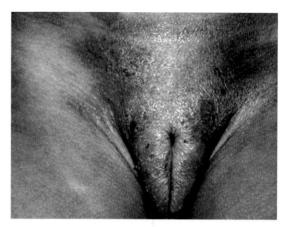

Figure 10.1.3 Psoriasis of the vulva in a prepubertal girl. Courtesy of Jill S Huppert, MD, MPH.

treatment. Removal of a vaginal foreign body may require sedation or general anesthesia (Figure 10.1.2). The most common foreign body is a piece of toilet paper that has found its way into the vagina, rather than having been intentionally placed within the vagina. Toilet paper can often be flushed from the vagina using a red rubber catheter (see chapter 3).

> ### ★ Tips and tricks
>
> • A *recurrent* discharge with on/off symptoms is most likely a mixed bacterial, hygiene-related vulvovaginitis.
> • A *persistent* discharge that does not improve with treatment should prompt consideration of a vaginal foreign body, particularly if the discharge is foul-smelling or bloody.

Vulvar rash

Vulvar candidiasis can occur in girls who are still in diapers, and is typically characterized by marked ery-

> ### Evidence at a glance
>
> • Multiple studies reviewing the microbiologic causes of vulvovaginal symptoms indicate that once a child is out of diapers, yeast infections *rarely* occur in otherwise healthy children.
> • In prepubertal girls, most vulvar irritation is related to poor hygiene and the multiple bacteria (including fecal bacteria) that are a resident part of the vulvovaginal ecosystem.

thema with peripheral satellite lesions. Other pediatric causes of a vulvar rash include atopic, irritant or allergic contact dermatitis (bubble baths or vaginal hygiene products designed for adults); lichen sclerosus; psoriasis; perianal and vulvovaginal (perineal) streptococcal infections.

Vulvar psoriasis involves a well-demarcated, symmetrical plaque (Figure 10.1.3); other sites of lesions (scalp, extensor surfaces of limbs, and pitting of the nails) may suggest the diagnosis. Nonvulvar psoriasis often has scaly plaques. Psoriasis occurs in up to 3% of adults, and often has its onset in childhood. There is a genetic predisposition to psoriasis, and a family history should be sought. Topical steroids are typically used as initial treatment.

Perineal streptococcal infections, caused by Group A beta-hemolytic streptococci, is characterized by marked erythema with mostly well-defined margins and signs of inflammation (edema, induration, and tenderness), pain, bleeding, and fissures that can be present for extended periods of time. Treatment includes oral penicillin and topical mupirocin for 14–21 days. Less common lesions include staphylococcal folliculitis, vulvar bullous pemphigoid, and scabies. Vulvar manifestations of systemic diseases may include varicella, inflammatory bowel disease, staphylococcal scalded skin syndrome, and Henoch-Schönlein purpura. Pigmented nevi and hemangiomas (which may be ulcerated) also occur in the vulvar area.

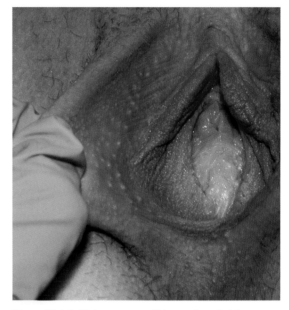

Figure 10.1.4 "Sebaceous cysts" in a pubertal girl. Courtesy of Paula JA Hillard, MD.

⚛ Science revisited

Psoriasis
- Psoriasis is an immunologically mediated disease with hyperproliferation and abnormal differentiation of the epidermis, plus inflammatory cell infiltrates.
- T lymphocytes and dendritic cells are key components of the process.
- Newer therapies for psoriasis include monoclonal anti-TNF antibodies (infliximab and adalimumab) and a TNF receptor.

Lumps, bumps, and lesions

Specific dermatologic descriptions of vulvar lumps (papules or plaques, depending on size) or tumors can occur. A very common lesion in both prepubertal and pubertal girls and women is often termed a "sebaceous cyst". These small, firm, round, mobile, flesh-colored to yellow or white subcutaneous bumps beneath the surface of the skin are due to a proliferation of epidermal cells within the dermis (Figure 10.1.4). They are usually without symptoms, but can become infected and enlarge, with erythema and pain; they may then rupture with a cheese-like material extruding, or they may resolve spontaneously. Reassurance is typically all that is required.

The lesions of molluscum contagiosum are due to a viral innoculation, and can be recognized by their characteristic pearly appearance with a pink or flesh-colored umbilicated dome-shaped papule (Figure 10.1.5), although they may be confused with genital warts (Figure 10.1.6). Genital warts, caused by

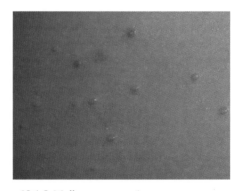

Figure 10.1.5 Molluscum contagiosum. Courtesy of L Sperling, CDC, Walter Reed Army Medical Center at http://www.cdc.gov

human papillomavirus (HPV), can be perinatally acquired and can present up to 2–3 years of age. Sexual abuse should be considered beyond this, and any parental suspicions should be explored with referral to appropriate sexual abuse evaluation teams (see Chapter 8). Other lesions, such as urethral prolapse, can initially appear to be a vaginal mass (Figure 10.1.7). While not a true mass, vulvar asymmetry with painless enlargement of one labium has been

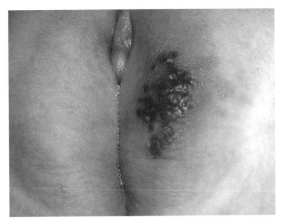

Figure 10.1.8 Vulvar ulcers due to herpes simplex virus. Courtesy of Jill S Huppert, MD, MPH.

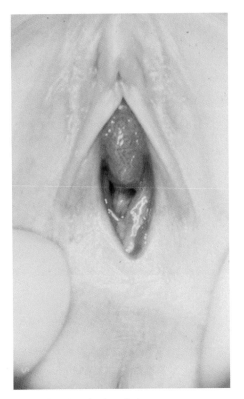

Figure 10.1.6 Periurethral genital warts. Courtesy of Paula JA Hillard, MD.

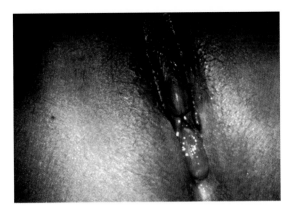

Figure 10.1.7 Urethral prolapse. Courtesy of Jill S Huppert, MD, MPH.

described as CALME syndrome (childhood asymmetric labium majus enlargement).

Vulvar pain

Vulvar pain in prepubertal girls can be caused by any inflammatory lesion. It is not uncommon for dysuria to be a primary complaint; distinction between an "internal" dysuria due to UTI and an "external" dysuria due to a vulvitis is difficult for adult women to make, and almost impossible for young girls to describe. UTI should be ruled out with a urinalysis and/or culture if necessary. Vulvar abscesses, while uncommon in prepubertal girls, can occur and be a cause of pain (see Chapter 10.4). Vulvar ulcers due to herpes simplex virus (HSV) can occur in prepubertal girls, and may be due to autoinnoculation from oval lesions or to abuse (Figure 10.1.8); culture should be performed to confirm the diagnosis. Vulvar aphthosis is another uncommon cause of pain with ulceration (see Chapter 10.2).

Pubertal and adolescent girls

Vulvar itching

The most common cause of vulvar itching in pubertal and adolescent girls is a yeast vulvovaginitis, typically caused by *Candida albicans* vaginal infection, which then secondarily becomes a vulvitis (see Chapter 43.1). Other causes of vaginal discharge (bacterial

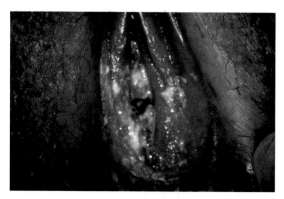

Figure 10.1.9 Yeast.
Courtesy of Paula JA Hillard, MD.

vaginosis, sexually-transmitted infections) can cause vulvar irritation and itching. Lichen sclerosus can present initially during adolescence.

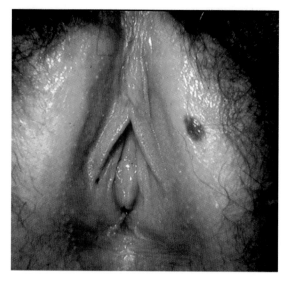

Figure 10.1.10 Vulvar nevus.
Courtesy of Jill S Huppert, MD, MPH.

Vulvar rash

The most common cause of a vulvar rash in adolescents is a yeast vulvitis (see Chapter 43.1), presenting with vulvar erythema (with satellite lesions; Figure 10.1.9), edema, and itching. A folliculitis due to shaving is not rare. Psoriasis and lichen sclerosus (see Chapter 11) cause characteristic vulvar lesions. Pigmented nevi of the vulva are common (Figure 10.1.10) and, while they are invariably asymptomatic, the site is difficult to monitor, and an excisional biopsy has been recommended. Other pigmented lesions include: lentigines, malignant melanoma, hemangioma, hematoma, or endometriosis. Contact dermatitis may be due to soaps, body wash, "vaginal hygiene" products, or other topical or intravaginal agents such as over-the-counter medications (Figure 10.1.11).

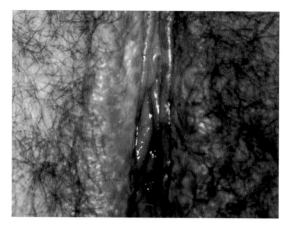

Figure 10.1.11 Contact dermatitis.
Courtesy of Jill S Huppert, MD, MPH.

Lumps, bumps, and lesions

The most common vulvar lesion in an adolescent who has been sexually active are vulvar condylomas (Figure 10.1.12) (see Chapter 44.2). Vaginal intercourse is not required for the acquisition of these lesions, as skin-to-skin contact can result in viral transmission. HPV vaccination with the quadrivalent vaccine at the recommended age of 11–12 years can markedly reduce the risks of acquisition of this virus

that causes discomfort, itching, bleeding, and embarrassment. Vulvar tumors, cysts, and abscesses are less common (see Chapter 10.3). Vulvar skin tags can grow to a large size (Figure 10.1.13). Ectopic breast tissue can be present in the vulvar area. Rare benign lesions include granular cell tumors, neurofibromas, vascular hemangiomas, lymphangiomas, lipomas, rhabdomyomas, fibromas, and vulvar intraepithelial neoplasia. Syringomas, which are benign tumors of

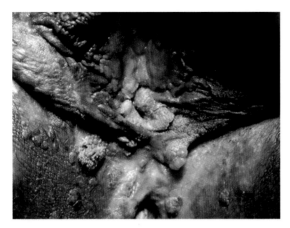

Figure 10.1.12 Vulvar condylomas.
Courtesy of Paula JA Hillard, MD.

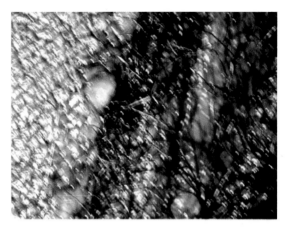

Figure 10.1.14 Syringoma.
Courtesy of Paula JA Hillard, MD.

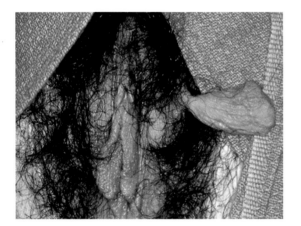

Figure 10.1.13 Vulvar skin tag.
Courtesy of Paula JA Hillard, MD.

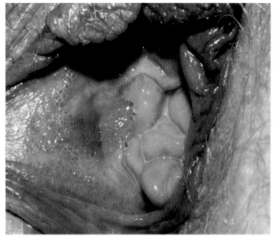

Figure 10.1.15 Vulvar vestibulitis.
Courtesy of Paula JA Hillard, MD.

the eccrine sweat glands, are also rare (Figure 10.1.14). Malignant vulvar lesions are even rarer still in this age group.

Vulvar pain

Vulvar pain in adolescents can be caused by any inflammatory lesion, and the difficult distinction from UTI can still be challenging in an adolescent. Vulvar pain may be due to inflammation and local irritation from soaps, detergents, douching, benzocaine (in Vagisil®, an over-the-counter anti-itching topical), neomycin (in triple antibiotic ointment), or latex condoms. Vulvar abscesses, including a Bartholin's or Skene's gland abscess or a clitoral abscess are painful, and like any other abscess, may require drainage (see Chapter 10.3).

Vulvar ulcers can be exquisitely painful (syphilitic ulcers are painless). Ulcers can be caused by STIs (herpes; see Chapter 44.1) or vulvar aphthosis (see Chapter 10.2). One additional cause of vulvar pain is an uncommon condition officially termed localized provoked vulvodynia, but also referred to as vulvar vestibulitis. This condition does not have a

55

clear etiology (and thus no clearly and universally effective therapy), but is associated with characteristic findings of pinpoint erythema in the hymenal sulcus which is tender to touch with a Q-tip (Figure 10.1.15). This condition can be a cause of pain with intercourse or attempted insertion of a tampon (which is most commonly due to inexperience and is associated with vaginismus, or to the presence of a hymenal band, but which can be due to vulvar vestibulitis as well).

Summary

Clinicians should be aware that vulvar symptoms can be nonspecific, and that a symptom such as itching may have many causes. The causes of symptoms often differ by age and pubertal status. A careful history, thorough examination of all skin in addition to the genital area, and visual recognition of common lesions may lead to a diagnosis that will then direct therapy (see Appendices 1.1.1–1.1.3, and 1.4). Unusual lesions and those that do not respond to therapy should prompt referral.

Further reading

Fiorillo L. Therapy of pediatric genital diseases. *Dermatol Ther* 2004;17(1):117–128.

Jamieson MA. A photo album of pediatric and adolescent gynecology. *Obstet Gynecol Clin North Am* 2009; 36(1):1–24.

Van Eyk N, Allen L, Giesbrecht E, *et al.* Pediatric vulvovaginal disorders: a diagnostic approach and review of the literature. *J Obstet Gynaecol Can* 2009;31(9):850–862.

10.2 Vulvar ulcers and aphthosis

Helen R. Deitch

WellSpan Medical Group, York Hospital, WellSpan Women's Specialty Services, York, PA, USA

Acute vulvar ulcerations (AVUs) in young female patients occur infrequently, but their presence can cause excruciating pain and severe emotional distress. The most common diagnosis in a sexually-active female is herpes simplex virus (HSV); however, in a never sexually active or abused adolescent or pre-teen patient, the presence of AVUs inevitably raises the suspicion for HSV, and with that diagnosis, an inquiry into sexual abuse. Once HSV has been excluded, the most likely of the remaining differential diagnosis, for AVU (Table 10.2.1) is vulvar aphthosis.

Vulvar aphthosis has not been well studied and its incidence is unknown. Nonsexually transmitted AVUs were first described in 1913 by Lipschutz as a series of gangrenous, self-limited, nonrelapsing ulcers in virginal women that were associated with systemic symptoms. Since then, there have been many case series and case reports associating AVU with infectious causes such as Epstein–Barr virus (EBV), cytomegalovirus, influenza A, *Salmonella paratyphi*, mumps and Group A strep, but often a concurrent systemic illness cannot be identified. An acute illness, either viral or bacterial, triggers the immune response that is responsible for the aphthosis, which explains the similar presentation for a variety of etiologies.

A patient with vulvar aphthosis will commonly report prodromal symptoms such as fever, malaise, headache, cough, and gastrointestinal complaints. Vulvar discomfort and contact dysuria precede the severe pain that develops as the aphthotic lesions

> ### 🔅 Science revisited
>
> • The pathogenesis of vulvar aphthosis is unknown.
> • It is suspected that an underlying systemic infection, either viral or bacterial, triggers an immune response in the vulva that leads to microthrombi formation in the epidermis, causing ischemia, necrosis, and skin ulcerations.

develop and ulcerate. If the patient or her parent has inspected the vulva, they may describe purple or blackish blood blisters that scab and then open up into ulcerations (Figures 10.2.1 and 10.2.2). Severe vulvar pain and dysuria are the most common complaints and the most challenging symptoms to manage.

Diagnosis

The patient history should concentrate on the exclusion of voluntary sexual activity or abuse, and identification of other infectious processes. Patients should be questioned privately about sexual experiences, including oral–genital and genital–genital contact. Signs and symptoms associated with Behçet disease, such as a history of oral ulcerations, previous vulvar ulcerations, skin rashes, or visual disturbances, should

Practical Pediatric and Adolescent Gynecology, First Edition. Edited by Paula J. Adams Hillard.

Table 10.2.1 Differential diagnoses for AVU

Ulcerating sexually-transmitted infections
- Herpes simplex virus (HSV)
- Syphilis
- Lymphogranuloma venereum
- Human immunodeficiency virus (HIV)
- Chancroid
- Granuloma inguinale

Ulcerating nonsexually-transmitted disorders
- Vulvar aphthosis
- Behçet disease
- PFAPA (periodic fever, aphthous stomatitis, pharyngitis, adenitis)
- Crohn disease
- Cyclic neutropenia
- Autoimmune progesterone dermatitis
- Pemphigoid
- Pemphigus
- Lichen sclerosus
- Drug reactions

Associated infections
- Epstein–Barr virus (EBV)
- Cytomegalovirus (CMV)
- Influenza A
- Group A strep
- Paratyphoid
- Mumps

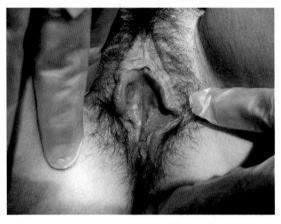

Figure 10.2.2 The same patient on day 14 after the onset of vulvar symptoms.

also be elicited. The family history should include the presence of autoimmune disorders such as Crohn or Behçet disease.

A comprehensive physical exam including evaluation of the oral mucosa, oropharynx, skin for rashes, and vulva is recommended. The vulva should be inspected gently; a speculum exam should *not* be performed. HSV cultures should be obtained directly from the ulcerations, and bacterial cultures considered if localized erythema and edema suggest secondary bacterial infection. Ulcerations are found most commonly on the minora and bilateral "kissing" lesions are not unusual.

The lab evaluation of a patient presenting with acute vulvar ulcerations should concentrate on excluding sexually-transmitted infections, and identifying the underlying disease process. Viral cultures for HSV should be obtained in all patients, even those without a history of sexual contact. Testing for EBV, human immunodeficiency virus (HIV), syphilis, and cytomegalovirus should be ordered, as should HSV type I- and II-specific IgG and IgM. A complete blood count is useful for screening for neutropenia. Any additional evaluations should be symptom based (stool cultures if significant diarrhea is present, Group A strep culture for pharyngitis, influenza A testing).

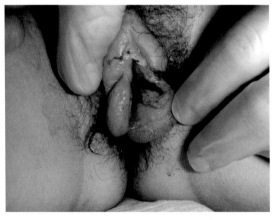

Figure 10.2.1 Vulvar aphthosis 2 days after the onset of vulvar symptoms.

Management

Treatment should focus on pain management and management of the underlying illness. Outpatient pain

> **⚠ Caution**
>
> • Vulvar biopsy is not recommended as part of a routine evaluation.
> • Nonspecific, nondiagnostic biopsy results have been reported in the literature.

management with nonsteroidal anti-inflammatory drugs (NSAIDs), topical lidocaine jelly 2%, and topical sulcrafate (1 g/10 mL solution) applied directly to the lesions can ameliorate some of the discomfort, but oral narcotics may also be necessary. Dysuria may be severe enough to cause urinary retention, so urination in warm bath water may help to ease the passage of urine. Twice-daily sitz baths are helpful to decrease the accumulation of fibrinous exudate on the lesions.

Bacterial superinfection of the lesions is common, and treatment with a broad-spectrum antibiotic is often necessary. Modification of the inflammatory response with topical steroid ointment such as beta-methasone or triamcinalone, or oral steroids in the form of a Medrol dose pack has been described.

Most patients can be managed in the outpatient setting; however, severe pain and urinary retention may require intravenous pain medication and bladder catheterization. In some cases the precipitating illness may be severe enough to necessitate inpatient management. Surgical debridement of the ulcers has been reported, but its value in expediting healing is uncertain and not routinely recommended.

The lesions should resolve spontaneously without scarring over several weeks. A recurrence rate of up to 60% has been described; fortunately the recurrences tend to be less severe. A patient with recurrent vulvar aphthosis or any other manifesta-tions of Behçet disease should be evaluated by a rheumatologist.

> **★ Tips and tricks**
>
> • Avoid a speculum exam, especially in virginal patients. Vaginal ulcerations may be present but identification will not change the management.
> • The recurrence rate is as high as 60%.
> • A recurrence of the vulvar ulcerations should prompt a rheumatologic evaluation for Behçet disease.

> **⚠ Patient/parent advice**
>
> • Patients and parents should be reassured that the ulcerations are not sexually transmitted, and that the patient did nothing to cause the ulcerations.
> • Complete healing may take 3–6 weeks.

Further reading

Huppert JS. Lipschutz ulcers: evaluation and management of acute genital ulcers in women. *Dermatol Ther* 2010; 23:533–540.

Huppert JS, Gerber MA, Deitch HR, *et al*. Vulvar ulcers in young females: A manifestation of aphthosis. *J Pediatr Adolesc Gynecol* 2006;19:195–204.

Lehman JS, Bruce AJ, Wetter DA, Ferguson SB, Rogers RS 3rd. Reactive nonsexually related acute genital ulcers: Review of cases evaluated at Mayo Clinic. *J Am Acad Dermatol* 2010;63(1):44–51.

10.3 Vulvar tumors, cysts, and masses

Meredith Loveless

Kosair Children's Hospital and Department of Pediatrics, and Obstetrics and Gynecology, University of Louisville, Louisville, KY, USA

Diagnosis

The typical presentation is an enlarging mass. The mass may be solid, polypoid or cystic. It may be asymptomatic or cause discomfort or pain. Rarely, it may present with a chronic scar or ulceration. It may have an acute onset or have been present for a long period of time.

Vulvar masses may be associated with underlying medical conditions such as neurofibromatosis or inflammatory bowel disease. A complete past medical history can guide the diagnosis.

The physical exam should begin with a complete skin exam and inspection of the mucosal surfaces, including the buccal mucosa. Other skin findings should be looked for, such as café-au-lait macules as seen in neurofibromatosis. A complete vulvar exam should be performed, paying attention to skin and hair patterns. The mass should be palpated to determine if it is fluid-filled, cystic or solid, and its location, size, and extent. The mass should be measured and tenderness, fluctuance, and color documented.

A perineal/pelvic ultrasound can be useful to determine the nature of the mass (whether fluid filled, solid, or cystic); document the internal anatomy; and exclude an inguinal hernia if suspected. If the genitalia appear ambiguous, a karyotype and testosterone level should be obtained to exclude testicular origin of the mass. Vascular magnetic resonance imaging

Evidence at a glance

- Vulvar cysts are closed epithelium-lined cavities which may contain liquid or semisolid material.
- Cysts may be congenital or appear after the hormonal stimulation of puberty. Vulvar cysts are common.
- Tumors of the vulva, characterized by the growth of tissue in which cell multiplication is uncontrolled and progressive, are uncommon, and most are benign.
- Malignant vulvar tumors in children occur in approximately 0.5 cases per million children.

(MRI) may be used to evaluate vascular lesions such as hemangiomas.

The differential diagnosis is listed in Table 10.3.1.

Management

Epidermoid inclusion cyst

This is a benign inclusion cyst that presents as a firm, nodular mass and is usually asymptomatic. It is rare in children, but may be seen in adolescents, or in

Practical Pediatric and Adolescent Gynecology, First Edition. Edited by Paula J. Adams Hillard.
© 2013 John Wiley & Sons, Ltd. Published 2013 by John Wiley & Sons, Ltd.

Table 10.3.1 Vulva: masses and cysts

Masses
- Congenital or acquired hernia
- Crohn disease (rare)
- Fibroepithelial polyp (acrochordon)
- Hamartoma (rare)
- Malignant tumors:
  - Embryonal rhabdomyosarcoma (sarcoma botryoides)
  - Endodermal sinus tumor
  - Primitive neuroectodermal tumor (PNET)
  - Squamous cell carcinoma
  - Malignant melanoma
  - Adenocarcinoma
  - Embryonal carcinoma
- Mesenchymal tumors:
  - Smooth muscle: leiomyoma (rare)
  - Striated muscle: rhabdomyoma/rhabdomyosarcoma
  - Fat: lipoma
  - Fibrous tissue: fibroma
  - Lymphatics: lymphangioma
  - Neural :
    - Granular cell myoblastoma
    - Neurofibromatosis
  - Vascular: hemangioma
- Supernumerary nipple (rare)
- Teratoma (rare)
- Vulvar varicosities

Cysts
- Embryonic or gonadal remnants:
  - Periurethral cyst
  - Hymenal cyst
  - Mesonephric (Gartner duct) cyst
  - Canal of Nuck cyst
  - Bartholin's duct cyst
- Epithelial inclusion cyst
- Folliculitis
- Vestibular mucous cyst

should be excised after the acute infection has resolved.

Fibroepithelial polyp (acrochordon or skin tag; see Fig. 10.1.13)

This is a benign polypoid mass with a fibrovascular core covered by skin. It is soft and feels like an empty sac. It is usually asymptomatic and no treatment is required. Symptoms such as discomfort along clothing lines may prompt removal; excision under local anesthesia or ligation at the base can be performed.

Folliculitis

This is a papulomacular eruption from inflammation of the superficial hair follicle. Pruritus and tenderness

> **Science revisited**
>
> **Infectious folliculitis:**
> - Infectious folliculitis is usually caused by *Staphylococcus aureus* (impetigo) or *Streptococcus pyogenes*.
> - Multiple pustules and/or superficial red papules, often with a white central crust, are seen (Figure 10.3.1).
> - Bacterial culture and a potassium hydroxide preparation may be necessary to evaluate for fungal etiology.
> - Oral antibiotics or antifungals that cover the infecting agent usually eradicate the infection, but reoccurrences are common.
>
>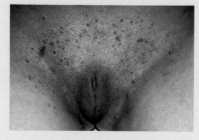
>
> **Figure 10.3.1** Infectious folliculitis. This rash consists of follicular papules and crust. Reproduced with permission from Trager Jonathan D.K. Pubic hair removal – pearls and pitfalls. *J Pediatr Adolesc Gynecol* 2006;19:117–123. Elsevier.

individuals who have undergone female genital mutilation. The risk of malignancy is extremely low. If asymptomatic, no therapy is required. If the patient desires removal, excision can be performed as drainage is not adequate therapy. Rarely, they become infected, which will result in pain, erythema, and induration of the surrounding skin. Infection is treated with oral antibiotics and warm soaks. Drainage is necessary if an abscess forms, and the cyst may occur. Mechanical folliculitis usually is a result of shaving and is not infectious. Treatment consists of low-potency topical steroid and improved shaving techniques or avoidance of shaving.

Granular cell tumor

Granular cell myoblastoma is thought to arise from the peripheral nerve sheath. It can occur in children or adults and may first appear as a small, firm globular mass. It may be single or multiple. It can mimic squamous cell carcinoma and the surface can become ulcerated. This tumor does have malignant potential and wide local excision is necessary. The patient must then be monitored as reoccurrences may occur.

Hernia

An inguinal hernia may present with a cystic mass in the groin or labium majorum. Surgical repair is indicated.

Hemangiomas

These are not true neoplasia but rather anomalous development of blood vessels. Capillary and cavernous hemangiomas occur in childhood. Hemangiomas of the vulva rarely bleed without trauma. Vascular MRI can help confirm diagnosis and define depth of a hemangioma; it can extend into the deep pelvic structures. Most hemangiomas will regress between 2 and 5 years of age and require no treatment. If medical or surgical intervention is considered, co-management with a vascular surgeon is recommended.

✋ **Caution**

- Solid vulvar lesions should be biopsied to exclude malignancy.
- Soft lesions could be vascular and imaging may be necessary to exclude a vascular etiology, such as a hemangioma.
- A vascular lesion should *not* be biopsied as bleeding may occur.

Lipoma

This fatty tumor presents as a sharply circumscribed, soft mass. If asymptomatic it can be observed; if symptomatic, it can be excised.

Lymphangioma

This is caused by localized dilation and ectasia of lymphatic vessels, and may appear as a papule or nodule. Milky discharge consistent with lymphatic fluid may be present. Diagnosis is made by biopsy. No treatment is required; recurrence is common after surgical excision.

Leiomyoma

This smooth muscle tumor is rare on the vulva. It usually presents as small, mobile masses. Diagnosis and treatment can be accomplished by excision.

Malignant neoplasia

The most common vulvar malignancies in children include embryonal rhabdomyosarcoma, usually originating from the anterior vaginal wall, and endodermal sinus tumor, usually arising from the gonad but it can occur in the vulva. An incisional biopsy is necessary, and surgical management is based on tumor type. Chronic ulcerations should be biopsied to exclude malignancy.

Neurofibromas

Neurofibromas are rare in children, but may be the presenting sign of neurofibromatosis. Suspicion is increased if café-au-lait spots are present. Lesions are usually multiple and benign. They also may occur in the bladder or vagina; cystoscopy and vaginoscopy should be performed. Expectant management is appropriate unless anatomy is distorted.

Vestibular mucous cyst

Mucous-filled cystic dilations of the minor vestibular glands located in the introitus and inferior to the hymen can occur in newborns as a painless vulvar mass, which can be confused with a Bartholin's or Skene's duct cyst. It is superficial with a smooth surface and translucent appearance. It can be single or multiple and is usually less than 2 cm. If symptomatic it can be excised. In the newborn, the cyst can be aspirated rather than excised, but only if symptomatic (such as interference with urine stream), as it will usually resolve spontaneously.

The remaining diagnoses in the differential diagnosis represent very rare processes (typically found in case reports), but should be considered when a vulva mass is encountered. Treatment guidelines are limited by lack of data, and a thorough review of the reported cases can guide management plans.

Follow-up

If a condition is benign and asymptomatic, periodic reassessment is indicated (3 months to 1 year) depending on the condition.

When to refer and to whom

Surgeries should be performed by a surgeon with experience in the management of these conditions in children. Malignancies should be managed with oncology/surgery as appropriate for tumor type. Vascular lesions should be co-managed with a vascular surgeon.

Further reading

Perlman, SE, Nakajima, ST, Hertweck PS. Labial/vulvar mass. *Clin Protocols Pediatr Adolesc Gynecol*. Oxford: The Parthenon Publishing Group, 2004.

Wilkinson E, Stone K. *Atlas of Vulvar Dermatology*, 2nd edn. Philadelphia: Lippincott Williams & Wilkins, 2008.

Williams TS, Callen JP, Owen LG. Vulvar disorder in the prepubertal female. *Pediatr Ann* 1986;15(8):588–605.

10.4 Vulvar abscesses

Jennie Yoost[1] and S. Paige Hertweck[2]

[1]Marshall University School of Medicine, Huntington, WV, USA
[2]University of Louisville, Louisville, KY, USA

An abscess of the vulva can present with mild to significant discomfort or a feeling of pelvic pressure and fullness. Hair follicles and sebaceous glands of the skin along with vulvar glands, such as Bartholin's and Skene's, can be sites for abscess formation.

Vulvar skin abscess

Hair follicles and sebaceous cysts are subject to infection. This risk increases with obesity, poor hygiene, shaving or waxing of pubic hair, and conditions of immunocompromise, including diabetes.

> ### ⚗ Science revisited
>
> - The skin of the vulva is normally colonized by *Staphylococcus aureus*, streptococcal species, *Escherichia coli*, and other Gram-negative organisms.
> - The microbiology of a vulvar skin abscess is usually polymicrobial. Anaerobic organisms can also be found.
> - Methicillin-resistant *S. aureus* (MRSA) is the most common pathogen in vulvar skin abscesses that require incision and drainage.

Patients present with symptoms of a small painful vulvar mass that typically progresses in size. They can report pain with movement, sitting, or intercourse. A vulvar abscess rarely presents with fever unless the abscess is quite large with surrounding cellulitis.

On physical exam a vulvar skin abscess usually is unilateral involving the labia majora or mons pubis (Figure 10.4.1). A tender mass ranging from 1 to 5 or more cm is palpable in the superficial skin. There is often erythema of the overlying skin, and a pustular area where the abscess has "come to a head." Laboratory studies and imaging do not contribute to making the diagnosis of a vulvar abscess.

A small (<2 cm) abscess can be treated with sitz baths or warm compresses, and antibiotics. The exception to this is in immunocompromised patients, where drainage is typically required.

Incision and drainage with local or general anesthesia involves an incision of sufficient size, drainage, irrigation, breaking up areas of loculation, and packing with gauze. As the prevalence of resistant organisms such as MRSA is increasing, it is important to collect aerobic and anaerobic cultures at the time of the procedure.

As an alternative to incision and drainage, two to four small (4–5 mm) incisions are made within the border of the abscess (Figure 10.4.2). Pus is evacuated, the abscess cavity is irrigated, and loculations

Practical Pediatric and Adolescent Gynecology, First Edition. Edited by Paula J. Adams Hillard.
© 2013 John Wiley & Sons, Ltd. Published 2013 by John Wiley & Sons, Ltd.

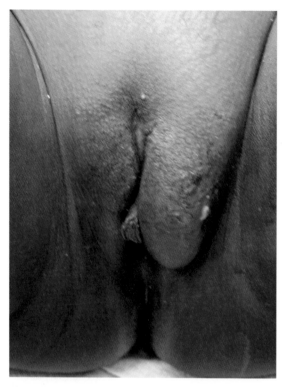

Figure 10.4.1 Vulvar skin abscess of a young adolescent patient.

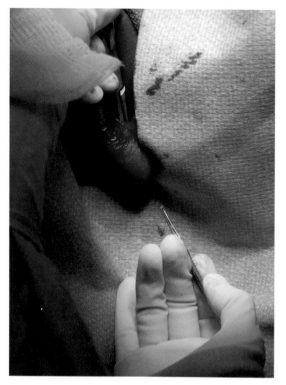

Figure 10.4.2 Incisions made at the inferior and superior margins of a large abscess.

are broken down. A sterile vessel loop or Penrose drain is then passed from one incision to the other and the ends tied together without tension (Figures 10.4.3 and 10.4.4). The drain keeps the incisions open, allowing continued drainage. It is left in place until drainage stops and cellulitis improves (approximately 7–10 days).

Antibiotics should be used for vulvar skin abscesses when there is suspicion for MRSA involvement, surrounding cellulitis, the abscess is recurrent, the abscess is large (>5 cm), or the patient is immunocompromised.

Patients should be seen a few days after initial presentation or incision and drainage procedure to determine resolution or the need for further treatment. Consultation with an experienced pelvic surgeon is appropriate if extensive debridement is required or if there is extension to another anatomic compartment (the thigh or anterior abdominal wall).

Evidence at a glance

- Trimethoprim–sulfamethoxazole (TMP–SMX) is the first-line agent as approximately 96% of MRSA isolates from vulvar abscesses are sensitive to this drug. TMP–SMX also covers the majority of Gram-negative isolates.
- Antibiotics should be continued for 7–10 days.

Bartholin's abscess

Bartholin's glands lie bilaterally at the base of the labia minora and drain through ducts that empty into the vestibule. Abscess microbiology is usually polymicrobial. *Neisseria gonorrhoeae* is the predominant aerobic pathogen, but most commonly the pathogens are anaerobes.

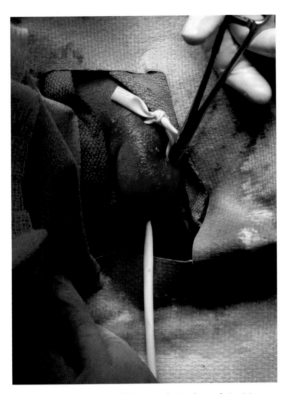

Figure 10.4.3 Passage of Penrose drain through incisions.

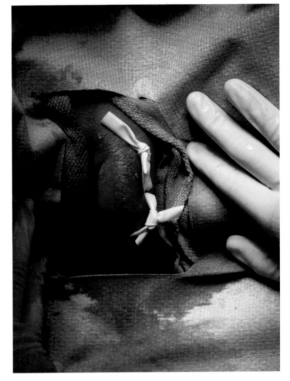

Figure 10.4.4 Penrose drain edges affixed together without tension.

✋ Caution

- Necrotizing fasciitis is rare, but should be considered in patients with significant soft tissue involvement and pain out of proportion to skin findings.
- This is a quickly progressive and severe disease that can result from vulvar skin infections and result in hemodynamic instability and fatality.
- Infection involves the skin, subcutaneous tissues, and fascial planes.
- Vulvar necrotizing fasciitis may present with woody induration, edema, and erythema surrounding a vulvar infection.
- Treatment involves intravenous broad-spectrum antibiotics and wide debridement of the necrotic tissue.

Diagnosis is based on the location of a unilateral tender cystic mass, which can expand anteriorly and be as large as 8 cm. Induration may be present as well as surrounding cellulitis. Pain is exacerbated by walking, sitting or intercourse. Imaging and laboratory tests are not needed for diagnosis.

Management may involve placement of a Word catheter (Figure 10.4.5). A 5-mm incision is made within the introitus just external to the hymenal ring in the area of the duct orifice. The abscess is drained,

★ Tips and tricks

- When placing a Word catheter, make a small stab incision with an #11 blade on the medial aspect of the abscess.
- After placing the catheter, orient it such that the free end can be tucked into the vagina for comfort.

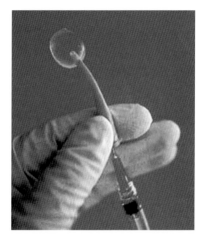

Figure 10.4.5 A Word catheter with balloon fitted.

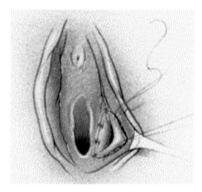

Figure 10.4.6 Marsupialization of a Bartholin's abscess. Interrupted sutures are placed to leave the abscess open for adequate drainage and healing.

the catheter is inserted, and the balloon is inflated with 2–3 mL of saline and left in place for 4–6 weeks.

The Word catheter can fall out before sufficient epithelialization, leading to recurrence; pain can also limit treatment. Sitz baths can aid comfort and healing.

Alternative management involves marsupialization, usually under anesthesia in adolescents. A 1.5–3-cm vertical incision is made in the medial aspect of the abscess in the skin of the vestibule. The cyst wall is incised and the abscess is drained (Figure 10.4.6). The cyst capsule is then sutured to the edges of the skin incision with interrupted absorbable suture. The tract will shrink and re-epithelialize over time. Sitz baths can begin on the first postoperative day. Patients

should be seen 1 week after either marsupialization or Word catheter placement.

Skene's abscess

The Skene's glands are bilateral paraurethral glands located posterior–lateral to the distal urethra. Skene's cysts or abscesses are uncommon in children and adolescents. Pathogens include *N. gonorrhoea* in sexually-active patients, but can also include Gram-positive cocci such as *S. aureus*.

A Skene's gland abscess is found as an enlargement of the anterior wall of the vagina and can cause periurethral swelling. Rarely, there are symptoms of urethral obstruction and urinary retention. A Skene's duct abscess must be distinguished from a urethral diverticulum. Compression of a Skene's duct cyst will not result in fluid extravasation.

Abscess of the Skene's ducts should be treated with simple incision and drainage under local anesthetic or general anesthesia. The site should be well irrigated and left open without packing. Cultures should be obtained at the time of incision and drainage.

Pilonidal sinus abscess

A pilonidal sinus occurs in hair-bearing areas but only rarely on the vulva. Anatomic clefts promote accumulation of hair fragments that develop into a sinus. If left untreated, hair continues to grow into the enlarging sinus, and inflammation and an abscess can develop. Presentation is similar to that of an abscess of the skin, with an erythematous mass on the labia majora or mons.

If hair is found within the mass, an oblique incision is used to excise the sinus tract. This eliminates the anatomic factor that caused hair accumulation. Antibiotics can be used if there is surrounding cellulitis.

Hidradenitis suppurativa

Hidradenitis suppurativa (HS) is a chronic, recurrent inflammatory disease that initially presents with recurrent painful, deep-seated subcutaneous nodules that then coalesce to form deep dermal painful

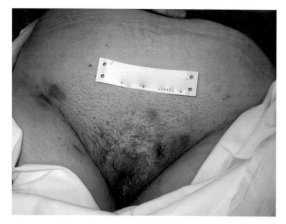

Figure 10.4.7 Early stage hidradenitis.

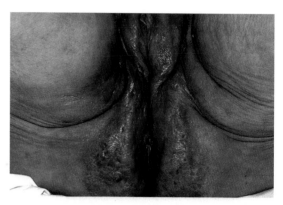

Figure 10.4.8 Advanced hidradenitis.

abscesses. The disease is thought to begin with occlusion of hair follicles. Sinus tracts develop that can be infected. Significant scarring can result (Figures 10.4.7 and 10.4.8). HS can be seen in the vulvar, inguinal, perianal, and perineal regions, as well as axillary and mammary areas. HS occurs after puberty, typically in the second or third decades, but can be seen in adolescents. Smoking and obesity may exacerbate the disease.

Diagnosis is made clinically and biopsies are unnecessary. Milder cases present with an inflammatory follicular and pustular disease and severe cases involve hypertrophic scarring, sinus and fistula formation. Diagnosis is based on location and a pattern of relapse and chronicity of typical lesions with deep-seated nodules (blind boils) and/or fibrosis. HS lesions are tender to palpation and a malodorous discharge is usually present.

✋ Patient/parent advice

- Improving the vulvar environment will assist in treatment.
- Reduce vulvar friction, heat, and sweating by wearing loose clothing; use antiseptic washes; stop smoking; and lose weight.

Antibiotics are the mainstay of medical treatment. Topical antibiotic in the form of clindamycin 1%

lotion twice daily is the first line. Oral antibiotics include tetracycline, clindamycin, doxycycline or amoxicillin/clavulanic acid used for 7–10 days. Patients with extensive inflammation can be placed on a 3-month course of clindamycin and then adjusted to a maintenance dose of daily tetracycline.

Oral contraceptive pills can be used to reduce androgens. Triamcinolone acetonide can be injected into lesions of painful early papules. Oral steroids, methotrexate, and tumor necrosis factor-α inhibitors have been used in advanced disease.

Incision and drainage should be avoided. The involvement of a dermatologist is recommended in cases of HS. Surgical excision of HS should involve a knowledgeable vulvar surgeon to excise all sinuses and fistulae with healing by secondary intention or with skin grafting.

Further reading

Alikhan A, Lynch PJ, Eisen DB. Hidradenitis suppurativa: a comprehensive review. *J Am Acad Dermatol* 2009;60(4): 539–561; quiz 562–563.

Bora SA, Condous G. Bartholin's, vulval and perineal abscesses. *Best Pract Res Clin Obstet Gynaecol* 2009; 23(5):661–666.

Tsoraides SS, Pearl RH, Stanfill AB, Wallace LJ, Vegunta RK. Incision and loop drainage: a minimally invasive technique for subcutaneous abscess management in children. *J Pediatr Surg* 2010;45(3):606–9.

11 Vulvar lichen sclerosus

Paula J. Adams Hillard

Department of Obstetrics and Gynecology, Stanford University School of Medicine, Stanford, CA, USA

Lichen sclerosus (LS) is a chronic skin condition that can affect the vulvar skin in girls and women. It is most common in postmenopausal women, but can also occur in prepubertal girls and adolescents, although it is not common in the pediatric age group. The etiology is unclear. In adults, an office vulvar biopsy is typically performed to confirm the diagnosis, but in girls and teens, diagnosis is most commonly made on the basis of symptoms and visual signs, as the likelihood of an underlying malignancy or other premalignant condition is extraordinarily uncommon. Skin lesions of LS can occur on other areas of skin, but are not commonly seen. There is likely a genetic component to this condition, as it has been described in multiple family members. In addition, an association with autoimmune conditions has been described.

Vulvar symptoms in girls and teens typically include significant vulvar itching, burning, burning with urination [an external dysuria that must be distinguished from symptoms of a urinary tract infection (UTI)], "irritation" or even bleeding. Vaginal discharge and odor are *not* seen with LS. The signs of LS classically include pale, fragile appearing skin in a "keyhole" or figure-of-eight configuration around the vagina and anus with a crinkly "cigarette paper" appearance to the skin (Figure 11.1). Subepithelial hemorrhage can occur, causing the appearance of "blood blisters." Such an appearance can be confused with intentional trauma/abuse, although with LS, minor trauma (tight jeans or bicycle riding) can cause such lesions, which may even bleed. The fragile skin is also prone to splitting, with active or healing fissures often noted directly anterior to the clitoris, in the perineal or perianal skin. Constipation can be an associated symptom.

Diagnosis

A careful history should be obtained, including the onset, duration, exacerbating or alleviating factors, as well as information about previous therapies and their success. Hygiene measures should be noted (with baths being preferable to showers). The presence of vaginal discharge or odor should be noted, and argue against LS. UTIs should be ruled out.

Physical exam should include careful inspection of all skin areas, looking for hypopigmented macules. Genital findings typically include the appearance described above. In addition, scarring and obliteration of architectural landmarks is common in advanced disease. The interlabial sulcus may be obliterated, with a linear appearance, and obliteration or scarring of the clitoral hood may also be seen, particularly with long-standing symptoms. Adult women with long-standing undiagnosed and untreated disease

---

Practical Pediatric and Adolescent Gynecology, First Edition. Edited by Paula J. Adams Hillard.
© 2013 John Wiley & Sons, Ltd. Published 2013 by John Wiley & Sons, Ltd.

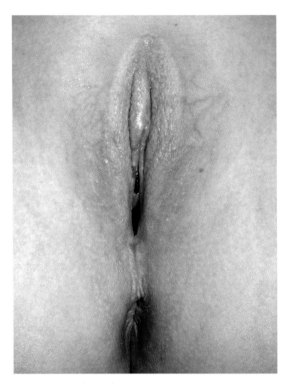

Figure 11.1 Lichen sclerosus.

can develop introital stenosis precluding intercourse or interfering with a vaginal delivery.

The differential diagnoses are listed in Table 11.1.

Management

The diagnosis and active management of LS (Figure 11.2) can greatly alleviate symptoms in the vast majority of cases. A topical ultra-high potency steroid ointment can be enormously effective in relieving symptoms and normalizing the appearance of the vulvar skin, both in gross appearance and on skin biopsy. Typically a regimen of clobetasol ointment (for better adherence in the vulvar area) is applied to the area twice daily for 4–6 weeks. While there is some controversy about the need for maintenance therapy, once scarring and vulvar architectural obliteration occur, it is irreversible, arguing for tapering the steroid potency and frequency, but maintaining a low-dose maintenance application. Ongoing use of clobetasol can cause skin atrophy or even adrenal

Table 11.1 Differential diagnosis of vulvar lichen sclerosus

- Vulvitis or vulvovaginitis in prepubertal girls: typically a mixed bacterial vulvitis due to poor hygiene, with erythema of the vaginal vestibule, and frequently associated with odor and discharge
- Vaginitis or if severe, vulvovaginitis in adolescents: yeast, bacterial vaginosis, STIs (cervicitis with gonorrhea, chlamydia, trichomoniasis) cause a primary vaginitis with a secondary vulvitis and findings of inflammation and irritation due to the presence of discharge
- Vulvar skin conditions such as psoriasis
- Pinworms: vaginal or anal can cause intense itching
- Urinary tract infections with dysuria, but also typically with urinary frequency and urgency, sometimes with incontinence

Clinical diagnosis on the basis of symptoms and signs

↓

Clobetasol ointment topically BID x 4–6 weeks

↓

Examine to assess efficacy

↓

Taper dose and frequency:

- 0.1% Triamcinolone ointment BID x 3 months
- 0.1% Triamcinolone ointment once a day x 6 months
- 0.1% Triamcinolone ointment twice weekly
-

Increase dose or frequency in stepwise fashion if symptoms recur x 2–4 week course

↓

Examination every 6 months to assess symptoms, signs, and medication adherence

Figure 11.2 Management algorithm for lichen sclerosus in childhood.

suppression, and thus caution should be exercised. A medium potency steroid ointment such as triamcinolone 0.1% can be used after clobetasol, followed by a further taper if symptoms allow.

Genital hygiene with regular baths, gentle cleansing of the interlabial folds, and avoidance of soaps, shampoos, or bubble baths that may be a chemical irritant can be helpful. Regular examinations (approximately every 6 months for maintenance) should be performed to assess the vulvar skin and reinforce ongoing use of topical therapy to prevent scarring. While some suggest that LS may resolve with pubertal growth, this does not seem to be common. It is not uncommon for preteens to discontinue their medication because of embarrassment with their pubertal growth, and then their symptoms recur. The goal of maintenance therapy is to control symptoms and prevent scarring. The prognosis for LS diagnosed in childhood is not well established. LS in adults is associated with a risk of an underlying vulvar malignancy.

✋ Caution

Lichen sclerosus, if untreated or inadequately treated, can cause scarring and obliteration of vulvar architecture that can impact sexual function.

Referral to a pediatric gynecologist or pediatric dermatologist may be indicated for recalcitrant symptoms. Other medications that may be helpful include topical tacrolimus.

✋ Patient/parent advice

Useful advice and information can be found at Fast Facts NIH: http://www.niams.nih.gov/Health_Info/Lichen_Sclerosus/lichen_sclerosus_ff.pdf

---

Further reading

Isaac R, Lyn M, Triggs N. Lichen sclerosus in the differential diagnosis of suspected child abuse cases. *Pediatr Emerg Care* 2007;23(7):482–485.

Powell J, Wojnarowska F. Childhood vulvar lichen sclerosus: An increasingly common problem. *J Am Acad Dermatol* 2001;44(5):803–806.

Smith YR, Quint EH. Clobetasol propionate in the treatment of premenarchal vulvar lichen sclerosus. *Obstet Gynecol* 2001;98:588–591.

12 Accidental trauma

Mariel A. Focseneanu[1] *and Diane F. Merritt*[1,2]

[1]Department of Obstetrics and Gynecology, Division of Pediatric and Adolescent Gynecology, Washington University School of Medicine in St. Louis; Barnes Jewish Hospital, St. Louis, MO, USA
[2]St. Louis Children's Hospital; Missouri Baptist Medical Center, St. Louis, MO, USA

The most common pediatric accidental genital trauma in females is a straddle injury. These injuries may involve the vulva, labia, clitoris, vagina, and adjacent urogenital and anogenital structures. Straddle injuries occur when the soft tissues of the vulva are compressed between an object and the underlying bones of the pelvis. A thoughtful, organized approach is essential for appropriate diagnosis, triage, and management of these injuries.

Straddle injuries in young girls are commonly seen during the warmer months, when children are wearing thin or light garments and involved in outdoor play.

> ### ✋ Caution
>
> - The clinician has an obligation to assess whether the history provided is compatible with the injuries found on the physical exam.
> - Inconsistencies between the history and physical exam should raise suspicion of sexual assault or abuse (see Appendix 1.3 and Chapter 8).

Accidents often occur due to sliding on the edge of a pool or diving board (Figure 12.1). The child may fall onto the frame of a bicycle or piece of furniture, or during climbing activities (i.e. jungle gym, sculpture, tree). Penetrating injuries occur if the child falls upon a sharp or pointed object (e.g. fence post, tent stake, furniture), resulting in impalement. It is helpful if the history can be corroborated by an eye witness. However, accidents are sometimes not witnessed, and the only history given is finding a traumatized child crying and bleeding from the vaginal area. Genital injuries often result in minor lacerations and bruising that heal rapidly. However, profuse bleeding may also occur due to the rich vascular supply in the genital area.

Diagnosis

Obtaining a detailed history of the events preceding the accident may be difficult, as the child is often traumatized or too young to provide an accurate description of how the injury occurred. Important details to obtain include the time the accident occurred, whether it was witnessed, the nature of the object/surface that was involved, and how much bleeding has occurred since the accident and whether it is increasing or decreasing. Garments worn by the child at the time of injury should also be examined for evidence. It is crucial to ask if the child has been able to void since the accident, particularly if she is being evaluated many hours after the injury occurred.

The severity of the injury and the amount of bleeding determine where and how the physical exam

Practical Pediatric and Adolescent Gynecology, First Edition. Edited by Paula J. Adams Hillard.
© 2013 John Wiley & Sons, Ltd. Published 2013 by John Wiley & Sons, Ltd.

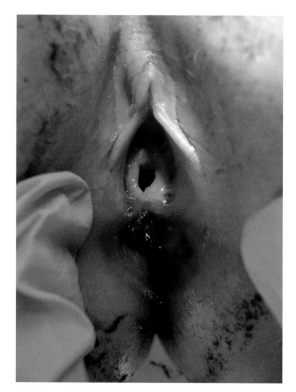

Figure 12.1 Straddle injury sustained when this child fell onto the edge of an indoor swimming pool.

The trauma of a straddle injury may result in ecchymoses (bruises), abrasions, and lacerations. Nonpenetrating injuries usually involve the mons, clitoris, and labia, and result in linear lacerations, sparing the hymen and vagina. Deep lacerations in the periurethral tissue may be seen. Penetrating injuries can cause trauma to the vagina, urethra and bladder, anus, rectum, and peritoneal cavity. Extravasation of blood into the loose areolar tissue in the labia, along the vagina, mons, or clitoral area may cause a hematoma to form. Vulvar hematomas can be very painful and may prevent a child or adolescent from urinating because of pain and swelling.

Sexual abuse (see Chapter 8) must always be considered and ruled out when evaluating a child with allegedly accidental genital injuries. The differential diagnosis of accidental genital trauma also includes dermatologic conditions of the vulva and perineum, such as lichen sclerosus and vulvovaginitis (see Chapters 10.1 and 11). In addition, normal variations in genital anatomy, such as intravaginal ridges and hymenal clefts (see Chapter 9), are often misinterpreted as evidence of old trauma or past injuries.

Management

If there is minor bleeding from an abrasion, it can often be treated with compression and ice packs. If the bleeding continues, then Gelfoam or Surgicel can be applied. Superficial lacerations that are not actively bleeding should heal without repair. Deep or bleeding lacerations may require repair under anesthesia: 1 or

should be conducted. If the injury is not severe and the child or adolescent is co-operative, she may be examined in a physician's office or emergency department. Force or restraint should never be used to achieve a pediatric genital exam. If the child is unable or unwilling to allow an adequate exam to be accomplished, conscious sedation may be necessary; this can often be done in the emergency department. General anesthesia may allow for a better exam, assessment, and repair (see Table 4.1).

Vaginoscopy is an important tool used by the pediatric gynecologist, and depending on the age and level of co-operation of the child, this procedure may be done with or without anesthesia. Placement of a pediatric cystoscope into the vagina with gentle opposition of the labia allows fluid distension to enable visualization of the vaginal vault and assessment of injuries. If there is suspected urethral involvement, the gynecologist or urologist should also perform a cysto-urethroscopy at this time (prior to the vaginoscopy).

2% lidocaine or 0.25–0.5% bupivacaine (dosed by body weight) can be injected locally with a 25-gauge needle and the repair done with #4 Vicryl interrupted sutures. Deeper lacerations are closed in layers (similar to episiotomy repair) with the goal being hemostasis and reconfiguration of anatomy. Injuries to the anal sphincter capsule, sphincter muscle, or rectal mucosa must be identified and properly repaired. When vaginal lacerations result in persistent bleeding, it is preferable to repair the injury. When this is not possible, we recommend placement of pre-moistened vaginal packing. Moistening the packing with saline or topical estrogen cream will ease removal.

⚓ Caution

It is important to determine the full extent of injuries prior to initiating repairs. If there is a penetrating rectal injury, consider a sigmoidoscopy. If the peritoneal cavity is entered, consider a diagnostic laparotomy or laparoscopy.

Vulvar hematomas can be managed conservatively with pressure over the bruise against the bony pelvis, application of ice packs (beginning immediately), and limitations on physical activities if the following conditions are met: the hematoma is not large or expanding; the perineal anatomy is not distorted; and the patient has no difficulty emptying her bladder. If the patient is unable to void after a straddle injury, a Foley catheter should be placed to avoid urinary retention. Bladder drainage should be continued until the swelling resolves. Outpatient management may be possible with ice, narcotics, a leg bag for the Foley catheter, and bed rest.

Pressure from a very large or expanding hematoma may cause necrosis of the overlying skin and result in eschar formation, tissue sloughing, and secondary infection. Evacuating the hematoma may prevent these adverse outcomes, as well as reduce pain and hasten recovery. When incising large vulvar hematomas, the incision should be along the medial mucosal surface near the vaginal orifice. Once the bed of the hematoma has been debrided of clot and devascularized tissue, and hemostasis attained, a closed system

drain (e.g. Jackson-Pratt) should be placed to prevent reaccumulation of blood, reduce pain, and reduce the risk of bacterial growth. The drain should be allowed to exit the skin in a dependent position, and the skin closed primarily. In most cases, the drain can be removed in 24 hours.

Follow-up

Vulvar swelling and ecchymotic discoloration due to straddle injuries may take several weeks to resolve (Table 12.1).

Table 12.1 Time for nonhymenal genital injuries to heal or resolve

Type of injury	Time for resolution
Abrasions	2–3 days
Edema	5 days
Ecchymoses (bruising)	2–18 days
Vulvar hematoma	2–4 weeks; may require surgical drainage
Petechia	24 hours
Blood blisters	30 days in prepubertal girl; 24 days in pubertal girl
Superficial lacerations	2 days with new vessel formation in prepubertal girls; scar tissue formation in pubertal girls
Deeper lacerations	10–14 days; may require surgical repair

Based on data from McCann J, Miyamoto S, Boyle C, *et al*. Healing of non-hymenal genital injuries in prepubertal and adolescent girls: a descriptive study. *Pediatrics* 2007;120(5):1000–1011. American academy of Pediatrics.

⚓ Patient/parent advice

Parents and patients should be reassured that healing is usually complete without residual defect or long-term adverse effects on reproductive function.

When to refer and to whom

Primary clinicians should consider referral to a pediatric gynecologist if the injuries are extensive. A general gynecologist can often manage a straightforward injury, using the guidelines noted in this chapter. Enlistment of or consultation with a qualified pediatric urologist or pediatric surgeon is indicated if the genital injury involves the anal canal above the sphincter, or if there is suspicion of a ruptured bladder or disruption of the urethra.

Further reading

Bechtel K, Santucci K, Walsh S. Hematoma of the labia majora in an adolescent girl. *Pediatr Emerg Care* 2007; 23(6):407–408.

Iqbal CW, Jrebi NY, Zielinski MD, *et al*. Patterns of accidental genital trauma in young girls and indications for operative management. *J Pediatr Surg* 2010;45(5): 930–933.

Merritt DF. Genital trauma in children and adolescents. *Clin Obstet Gynecol* 2008;51(2):237–248.

13 Female genital mutilation

Katherine A. Zakhour[1] and Comfort Momoh[2]

[1]Imperial College, London, UK
[2]King's College London (University of London), London, UK

Female genital mutilation (FGM), also termed female cutting or female circumcision, is defined by the World Health Organization (WHO) as ". . . all procedures involving partial or total removal of the external female genitalia or other injury to the female genital organs for non-medical reasons." While FGM may seem abhorrent to us in the West, in the countries where it is practiced, it is seen as an act of love – a rite of passage into womanhood that has happened for centuries. While not all family members will want it for their relative, it holds such an important place in family and societal tradition that frequently parents' or relatives' wishes not to continue the practice are ignored.

There are four different types of FGM (Figure 13.1). Type IV unclassified (not shown in Figure 13.1), includes pricking, piercing or incising of the clitoris and/or labia; stretching of the clitoris and/or labia; and cauterization by burning the clitoris and surrounding tissue.

WHO estimates that between 100 and 140 million girls and women worldwide have been subjected to FGM types I–III. There are an estimated 3 million girls in Africa at risk of undergoing FGM every year. However, not every girl from countries where FGM is practiced will have had it done, and there is evidence in some countries that the practice is in decline.

Due to rising migration, this problem is not isolated to countries where FGM is practiced. In the UK, a study by FORWARD in 2007, funded by the Department of Health, estimated there are 16 000 girls under the age of 15 at high risk of type III FGM and over 5000 at high risk of types I or II.

The main risk factor for FGM is coming from a country where the practice is prevalent (Table 13.1) and being the daughter of a woman who has undergone FGM. Even if the girl is born in the West, if her family comes from an FGM practicing community, there is still a risk that she may be subjected to FGM, e.g. while on holiday in the country of origin.

★ Tips and tricks

- Know the countries where FGM has a high prevalence to help identify girls who may have had it done.
- It may be easier to talk to the girl or her family about female circumcision, rather than FGM. FGM is a phrase that was adopted by the WHO to convey the violence and nonconsensual nature of the act, but it may alienate families.

Girls' experiences of FGM and the type of FGM they have undergone will vary greatly and depend on their country, or even area, of origin. Some girls may

---

Practical Pediatric and Adolescent Gynecology, First Edition. Edited by Paula J. Adams Hillard.
© 2013 John Wiley & Sons, Ltd. Published 2013 by John Wiley & Sons, Ltd.

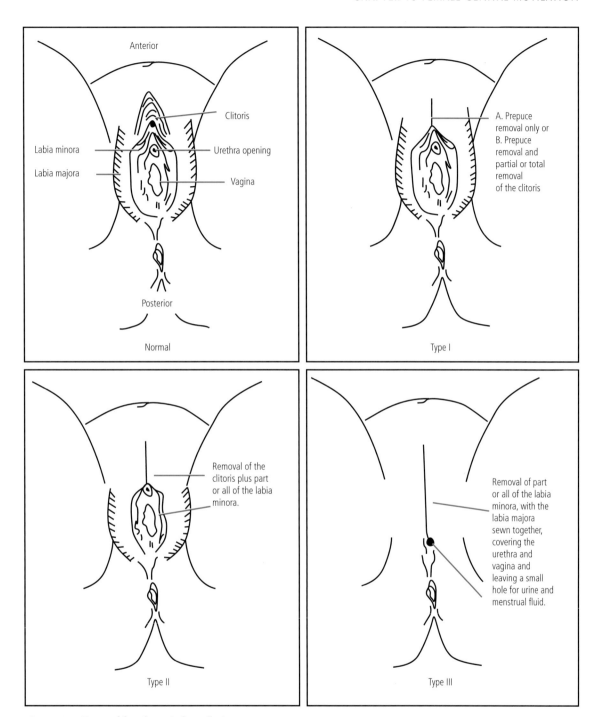

Figure 13.1 Types of female genital mutilation.

Table 13.1 Prevalence of female genital mutilation

Country	Prevalence (%)
Somalia	97
Djibouti	97
Sudan	90
Ethiopia	90
Burkina Faso	70
Egypt	50
Nigeria	50

Data from The US Department of State: Female Genital
Mutilation Individual Country Reports.

> **✋ Caution**
>
> • In the UK, FGM is illegal, as is taking girls
> abroad to perform FGM; both carry a prison
> sentence of up to 14 years.
> • In the US, federal law makes the practice
> of female genital cutting on anyone younger
> than 18 years of age illegal. It is a felony
> punishable by fines or up to a 5-year prison
> term.

have no physical symptoms, whereas others may
have pain, bleeding, urinary problems, painful
periods, difficulties with intercourse, problems conceiving, and psychological ramifications. Where FGM
is widely practiced (Table 13.1), 10% of girls and
women die from the short-term complications of
FGM, such as hemorrhage, shock, and infection, and
25% die in the long-term as a result of recurrent
urinary and vaginal infections and complications
during childbirth.

It may not be easy for the healthcare provider to
identify women and girls who have had FGM. The
symptoms that may be described are not specific to
FGM, and the diagnosis of FGM is more likely to
come from a careful and sensitive history than a
physical exam. Unless a girl, or her family, tells you
she has had FGM, recurrent urinary tract infections
(UTIs) in the prepubescent girl may be the only sign
to alert a healthcare provider to the possibility of
FGM. Awareness of the areas in which FGM is practiced is likely to help identify those girls at risk of
having had FGM (Table 13.1).

In addition to recurrent UTIs, girls may present
with difficulties in passing urine or fractures due to
excessive pressure during the procedure. Adolescents
may present with dysmenorrhea, menorrhagia, and
abdominal pain. They may also present with dyspareunia. The adult woman may present with dyspareunia or difficulty conceiving, or may only be
identified once pregnant, or even in labor.

Post-traumatic stress disorder, flash-backs, low self-
esteem, genital phobia, anxiety or depression may be
associated with FGM.

Diagnosis

It is important to have a high index of suspicion if
the girl comes from one of the prevalent countries
(Table 13.1).

If a girl has had FGM, the following information
will need to be elicited:
• How old was she when FGM was carried out? The
age can vary from months to early teens.
• How was it done? There has been a recent rise in
the medicalization of FGM, with the procedure taking
place in hospitals with sterile equipment and anesthesia. However, FGM is still often performed by a local
nonmedical practitioner under nonsterile conditions
and using basic instruments. Such FGM is often
greater in extent, with more scarring and risk of
infection.
• Any physical sequelae?
• How does she/the family feel about the practice?
You may be able to offer support to families traumatized by the events, or identify children at risk in
families who still support the practice.

Questions about perineal pain, dysuria, and dysmenorrhea may be relevant.

With the girl's/family's consent, you may need to
identify which type of FGM the girl has had, as this
may not be known. Physical exam will determine
whether or not the clitoris and labia minora and
majora are present. If she has had type III FGM, this
exam will be difficult, although this is the most identifiable type. Examination of the perineum and rectum
for possible fistula, scarring, and other wounds may
also be relevant.

Management

Support and education are vital. This may involve supplying contact details of charities that can provide information, counseling or, for some, you alone can provide the answers and support they need.

> **✋ Patient/parent advice**
>
> • It may be important to counsel the girl and her family about potential risks in the future, e.g. if she has had type III FGM, she may encounter difficulties with menstruation, sexual intercourse, conceiving, and labor later in life.
> • Girls have died from FGM, but many families are unaware of the risks, and their encounter with you may be the first time they hear of the risks.

For those who have had FGM type III, there is the possibility of deinfibulation, where the labia can be reopened under local or general anesthesia. Many women are not prepared for how different their genitals feel and appear after this procedure and will need appropriate support and counseling.

> **✋ Caution**
>
> Deinfibulation itself may also provoke traumatic memories of the initial FGM.

Further reading

Female Genital Cutting Fact Sheet at www.womenshealth.gov/publication/our-publication/fact-sheet/female-genital-cutting.cfm#b

FORWARD at www.forwarduk.org.uk

McCafferty C, Davis K, Momoh C. *Female Genital Mutilation*. Oxford: Radcliffe Publishing, 2005.

World Health Organization at www.who.int/topics/female_genital_mutilation/en

14 Normal puberty

Jennifer C. Kelley[1] and Frank M. Biro[2]

[1]Children's Hospital of Philadelphia, Philadelphia, PA, USA
[2]Cincinnati Children's Hospital Medical Center, Cincinnati, OH, USA

Puberty is the stage of development through which a child transitions into a sexually mature young adult, and involves both physical and psychosocial changes. The biologic milestones in puberty are characterized by the reactivation of the hypothalamic–pituitary–ovarian (HPO) axis and thus secretion of gonadal hormones, maturation of gametogenesis, and the development of secondary sexual characteristics and fertility. The term adolescence is often used interchangeably with puberty; however, adolescence encompasses the cognitive, emotional, and psychosocial changes that are associated temporally with pubertal development.

Puberty involves the separate processes of adrenarche and gonadarche. With the onset of adrenarche, just prior to the onset of puberty, the zona reticularis of the adrenal gland produces the adrenal androgens found to be elevated in puberty. In gonadarche, the gonads become functional and begin to produce sex hormones responsible for the development of secondary sex characteristics. In females, further pubertal milestones include thelarche and menarche. Thelarche refers to the onset of breast development, and menarche to the onset of menses, which is the response of the endometrial lining to elevated estrogen levels. Pubarche refers to the development of sexual pubic hair in response to elevated androgen levels.

The hypothalamic–pituitary–ovarian axis

The HPO axis is first activated during fetal and neonatal growth, and is responsible for gonadal development and sexual dimorphism. During this period, the hypothalamus releases gonadotropin-releasing hormone (GnRH), which acts at the anterior pituitary to stimulate the release of the gonadotropins follicle-stimulating hormone (FSH) and luteinizing hormone (LH). In females, FSH and LH then act at the ovaries to stimulate gametogenesis and the formation of estradiol, respectively. During the fetal and neonatal stages, the HPO axis functions at pubertal levels, but after the neonatal period it becomes increasingly sensitive to negative feedback from the sex hormones. During childhood, trace levels of sex steroids are adequate for inhibition of the HPO axis, and GnRH release is minimal.

In the late prepubertal stage of childhood, through mechanisms that are not fully understood, the HPO axis gradually becomes less sensitive to negative feedback on the hypothalamus from the sex hormones. This decreased inhibition of the HPO axis results in an increase in the pulsatile release of GnRH, and the HPO axis once again becomes active and results in pubertal and, eventually, adult levels of circulating gonadotropins. One of the initial hormonal changes

Practical Pediatric and Adolescent Gynecology, First Edition. Edited by Paula J. Adams Hillard.
© 2013 John Wiley & Sons, Ltd. Published 2013 by John Wiley & Sons, Ltd.

resulting from the maturation of the HPO axis, and the hallmark of early puberty, is a sleep-related increase in LH release. This creates a notable diurnal variation of gonadotropin levels that persists during puberty until adulthood, when the diurnal variation becomes less pronounced. FSH is released in tandem but is less responsive to GnRH; thus there is an increase in the LH:FSH ratio.

The adrenal cortex and adrenarche

In a separate and independent stage of development that begins approximately 1–2 years before the maturation of the HPO axis, adrenarche involves the reactivation of adrenal androgen release following a regression after the fetal stage. During mid-childhood, the zona reticularis of the adrenal cortex begins to develop and respond to adrenocorticotropic hormone (ACTH) released by the anterior pituitary. The major hormone released by the pathways in the zona reticularis is dehydroepiandrosterone sulfate (DHEAS), the primary marker of adrenarche, and dehydroepiandrosterone (DHEA). The levels of DHEAS gradually rise during late childhood and throughout puberty, and reach a level sufficient for pubic hair development in early puberty.

Timing and progression of puberty

The initiating factor for puberty is not entirely known, but there is not likely one single mechanism that triggers the start of puberty. There are several biologic factors that are probably responsible for the changes noted during puberty. The onset and timing of puberty is thought to be determined by genetics, including race and ethnicity, which may account for at least half of the variability in the progression of puberty. Other determinants include general health, nutrition, skeletal maturation, and the effects of growth hormone (GH), insulin-like growth factors (IGFs), and hormonally active chemicals found in the environment, known as endocrine disruptors. Of these factors, nutrition appears to be a key determinant and improved nutrition a reason for the earlier age at onset of puberty that has been seen in females in the US. A critical level of body fat appears to be essential for the onset of puberty and adequate

nutrition is required for normal reproductive function.

> ### ⚗ Science revisited
>
> - Recent studies have shown that leptin, a hormone released from adipose cells, and kisspeptin, a hormone found within the hypothalamus, signal pubertal development.
> - In childhood and late prepuberty, leptin concentrations rise and provide feedback to the hypothalamus about the energy state of the body and its readiness for pubertal maturation.
> - Leptin specifically appears to increase the expression of the *KiSS-1* gene in the hypothalamus and therefore promotes the production of kisspeptin.
> - Kisspeptin, in turn, acts as a neuropeptide signaler to the HPO axis and stimulates GnRH release.

In general, onset of puberty is considered to occur between the ages of 7 and 13 years in females. Ethnic and environmental differences may account for variations in this range. Further, recent studies have shown that age of onset of puberty appears to be decreasing in the general population.

For the majority of females, the stages in puberty often follow a predictable course and usually occur over 4–5 years (Figure 14.1). The initial stage of puberty is usually thelarche, with the development of sexual pubic hair within the following year. Menarche typically occurs 2.5 years following thelarche, though the normal range is 0.5–3.0 years later.

There are several normal clinical variations to the typical progression of puberty. Thelarche may be associated with asymmetrical breast tissue development. Pubarche may also occur before or along with thelarche. In addition, the usual age ranges for pubertal development have been shown to differ by race and ethnicity. In the US, non-Hispanic African-American girls may experience thelarche approximately 1 year earlier than their non-Hispanic white counterparts, and thus start breast development at 7 years of age.

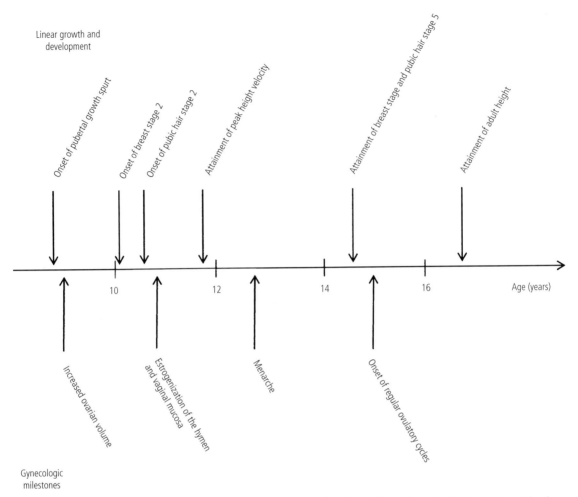

Linear growth and development

Onset of pubertal growth spurt

Onset of breast stage 2

Onset of pubic hair stage 2

Attainment of peak height velocity

Attainment of breast stage and pubic hair stage 5

Attainment of adult height

10   12   14   16   Age (years)

Increased ovarian volume

Estrogenization of the hymen and vaginal mucosa

Menarche

Onset of regular ovulatory cycles

Gynecologic milestones

Figure 14.1 Timing of pubertal events in non-Hispanic white girls in the US. (timing of events in African-American girls is 0.4–0.6 years earlier).

Based on data collected from the National Heart, Blood, and Lung Institute Growth Study. Reproduced from Biro FM, Huang B, Crawford PB, *et al.* Pubertal correlates in black and white girls. *J Pediatr* 2006;148:234–240. Elsevier.

✋ **Patient/parent advice**

• The onset of breast development may be unilateral and is considered a normal variant.

• Each breast may develop at a separate rate, which may occasionally lead to asymmetric breast size as an adult, but this is not a sign of underlying pathology.

Stages of puberty

Puberty may be evaluated clinically through determining the stages of pubertal development, commonly referred to as Tanner staging or sexual maturity rating. In females, separate sets of ratings exist for the evaluation of breast and pubic hair development, both of which consist of five stages of maturity (Figures 14.2 and 14.3; see also Appendix 1.9.4).

The average age of menarche is between 12 and 13 years, but varies by race, with Caucasian girls reaching menarche later than African-American girls.

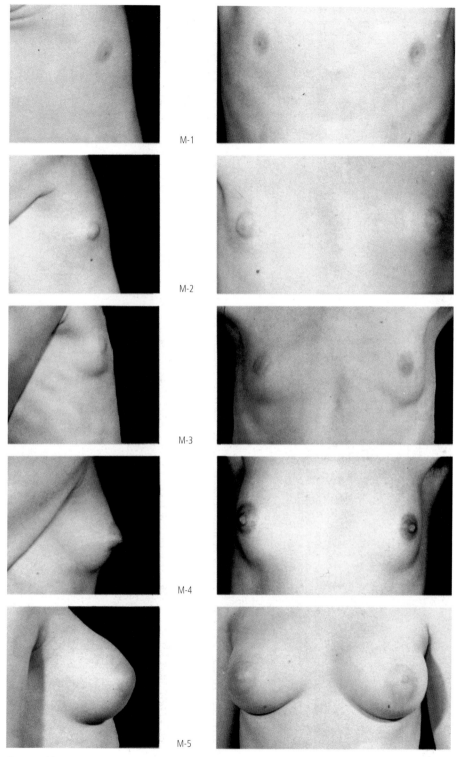

Figure 14.2 Stages of breast development in girls. Stage 1: prepubertal, with no palpable breast tissue. Stage 2: Breast bud; elevation of the papilla and enlargement of areolar diameter. Stage 3: Enlargement of the breast, without separation of areolar contour from the breast. Stage 4: Formation of secondary mound above breast, from projection of areola and papilla. Stage 5: Recession of areola to contour of breast; papilla beyond contour of areola and breast.

Reproduced from Roede MJ, van Wieringen JC. Growth diagrams 1980: Netherlands third nation-wide survey. *Tijdschr Soc Gezondheids* 1985;63(Suppl):1–34.

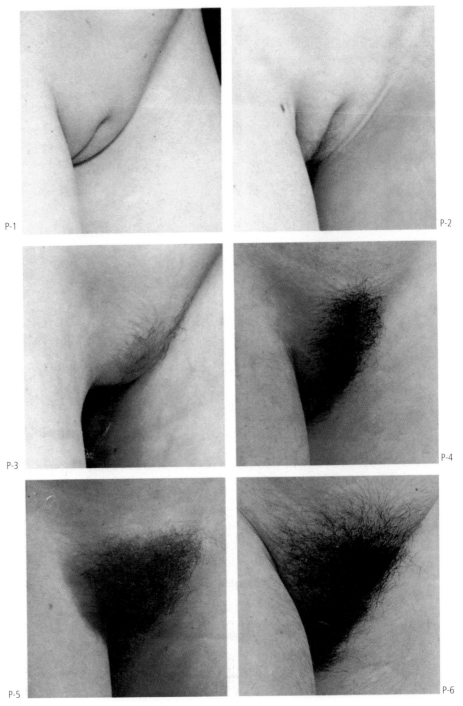

Figure 14.3 Stages of pubic hair development in girls. Stage 1: prepubertal with no pubic hair. Stage 2: sparse, straight hair along the lateral vulva. Stage 3: hair is darker, coarser, and curlier, extending over the mid-pubis. Stage 4: hair is adult-like in appearance, but does not extend to the thighs. Stage 5: hair is adult-like in appearance, extending from thigh to thigh.
Reproduced from Roede MJ, van Wieringen JC. Growth diagrams 1980: Netherlands third nation-wide survey. *Tijdschr Soc Gezondheids* 1985;63(Suppl):1–34.

Tips and tricks

⭐ **Tips and tricks**

- When determining puberty stage during the physical exam, it is important to both inspect and palpate the breasts.
- Breast development may be inaccurately assessed due to adipose tissue deposition in the chest. Thus, when palpating the breast, it is important to differentiate adipose from mammary gland tissue.
- An extra light source may be helpful in differentiating the short, light hairs of PH1 from PH2.
- Axillary hair, while a sign of increasing androgen hormones, is not reliable for staging pubertal development.
- On average, axillary hair development follows that of pubic hair by 1 year.

During puberty, the HPO axis is still maturing and approximately 50% of menstrual cycles are anovulatory in the first 2 years following menarche. This often produces more cycle irregularity and intermenstrual variability. On average, regular ovulatory cycles are not seen until approximately 2 years following menarche.

Growth and puberty

Besides the development of secondary sexual characteristics and reproductive development, puberty is also marked by a significant linear growth spurt, called the pubertal growth spurt. In females, the pubertal growth spurt usually begins shortly before B2 and the peak height velocity (PHV) is usually reached within the following 2 years. PHV is notable for an increase, on average, of 7–9 cm per year in height. Menarche usually occurs about 6–12 months following PHV. The growth spurt is a result of the synergistic effects of both the release of sex hormones and a rise in GH, which is secreted from the anterior pituitary. The release of GH is promoted by the increasing level of sex steroids and results in an increase in IGF-1 release during this period of growth (levels are higher than those found in adults and peak

in the later stages of puberty). Estrogens and androgens also directly stimulate growth at the epiphysis. Estradiol and estrone in particular are responsible for eventual closure at the epiphyses. The pubertal growth spurt usually occurs over a period of 2–3 years, with adult height achieved after the full maturation of secondary sexual characteristics.

Effects of puberty on the body

Aside from the linear growth spurt observed during puberty, there is also a distinct change in body composition and body mass index (BMI) during this period. During puberty, females increase lean body mass; they acquire more adipose tissue as compared to males, with a larger percentage of fat cells deposited in the lower portion of the body such as the hips and thighs. In addition to the changes in body composition, reproductive function, and secondary sex characteristics, the elevated levels of sex steroids also have effects on other body systems. For example, hemoglobin concentration rises and red blood cell mass increases. Estrogen and progesterone also appear to decrease the level of inflammatory response cells and, in the cardiovascular system, may stabilize the endothelium. Notably, lipid levels change during puberty, with total cholesterol peaking in early puberty and low-density lipoprotein (LDL) levels peaking in later puberty. High-density lipoprotein (HDL) levels tend to remain constant throughout puberty in girls and triglycerides show a slight rise. In accordance with pubertal gain in height, blood pressure also gradually increases. In addition, the effects of elevated androgen levels promote growth and function of the apocrine glands and odor production, while androgenic stimulation of the sebaceous gland can lead to acne. Girls with moderate acne in early puberty typically will develop severe acne by mid to late puberty.

Puberty and adolescence

Puberty plays a key role in the developmental milestones of adolescence. Besides the physiologic changes established by puberty, adolescence is defined by behavioral, psychosocial, and sexual maturation. Cognitive development in particular undergoes a significant shift in early adolescence, with maturation of concrete thought processes of childhood into abstract thought (see Chapter 20; Appendix 1.9.2). Throughout the course of adolescence, the frontal and prefrontal cortex undergo neurodevelopmental changes and ultimately, in those with normal cognitive abilities, transition to abstract thought content, the progression of moral development, and decreased emotional lability. Further, it is during this time that adolescents develop a further understanding of their body and its physiologic processes, and have a deeper grasp of the concept of illness.

Adolescence also involves the attainment of a personal adult identity. This is a time of sexual exploration and experimentation, and when a person begins to establish an adult self-image. Further, an adolescent's relationships with her peers and family may undergo significant changes through separation and individuation from parents, with increased peer identification, as she experiences the world during this intense period of change.

The onset and relative timing of puberty can be extremely important in adolescent development. Several studies have shown that girls who mature relatively early often have a more negative self-image.

The rates of depression, anxiety, disordered eating, and risk behaviors, including substance use and unsafe sexual practices, are higher in females who enter puberty at an earlier age than their peers. As a clinician, it is important to understand and appreciate the effects of puberty across the entire context of adolescent development.

Further reading

Biro FM, Huang B, Crawford RB, *et al*. Pubertal correlates in black and white girls. *J Pediatr* 2006;148:234–240.

Bordini B, Rosenfield R. Normal pubertal development: Part I: The endocrine basis of puberty. *Pediatr Rev* 2011;32; 223–229.

Roede MJ, van Wieringen JC. Growth diagrams 1980: Netherlands third nation-wide survey. *Tijdschr Soc Gezondheids* 1985;63(Suppl):1–34.

Acknowledgements

Supported in part by the Breast Cancer and the Environment Research Centers grant numbers U01 ES/CA12770 and U01 ES/CA019453.

15 Precocious puberty

Paul B. Kaplowitz

Children's National Medical Center and George Washington University School of Medicine and Health Sciences, Washington, DC, USA

Early pubertal maturation in girls is a common concern in pediatric offices, and while most such patients are seen by pediatric endocrinologists, it is important for primary clinicians to be aware of the major diagnoses encountered, including and perhaps especially, the benign normal variations which require no intervention. Central precocious puberty (CPP), which starts early enough and progresses rapidly enough to merit treatment, is present in only a minority of cases. It is suggested that most cases can be diagnosed accurately based on the history and physical exam, and that hormone levels and X-ray and ultrasound imaging are helpful only in selected cases. Less common problems include ovarian cysts and tumors, and a puzzling condition called premature menarche.

The traditional definition of precocious puberty is the appearance of breast or pubic hair development in girls prior to 8 years of age. Recent studies confirm that the appearance of breasts and pubic hair in girls prior to age 8 years has become increasingly common. African-American girls have an earlier onset of pubertal signs than do white girls, with Hispanic girls being intermediate in their age of pubertal onset. Approximately 15–20% of African-American girls and 5–10% of white girls have been found to have either breast or pubic hair development by age 7–8

years. It may be concluded from this that many of the girls labeled as having precocious puberty are in fact normal girls at the lower end of the new normal range. It appears that girls may be starting puberty earlier now but are progressing to menarche more slowly than in the past, as there has been only a slight decline in age of menarche over time.

> ### ⚙ Science revisited
>
> **Why are girls starting puberty earlier than in the past?**
> • Higher BMI is correlated with earlier onset of breast and pubic hair development, and menarche. This may be due to higher levels of leptin, derived from fat cells.
> • Chemicals in the environment with weak estrogen-like properties, including pesticides, phthalates, bisphenol A, and plant-derived phytoestrogens, or low levels of estrogens in the food supply have been blamed, although scientific evidence for this is sparse.

There are two common and benign scenarios: premature adrenarche and premature thelarche.

Practical Pediatric and Adolescent Gynecology, First Edition. Edited by Paula J. Adams Hillard.
© 2013 John Wiley & Sons, Ltd. Published 2013 by John Wiley & Sons, Ltd.

Premature adrenarche

The great majority of girls who present with the early appearance of pubic and/or axillary hair, usually accompanied by axillary odor, have premature adrenarche, a benign normal variation, due to an earlier than normal increase in adrenal androgen secretion. It can be seen as early as age 3–4 years and occasionally earlier, and is more common in black than white girls. In typical cases, extensive hormonal testing and adrenal and/or ovarian imaging are not indicated. The only hormonal abnormality generally seen is an increase in dehydroepiandrosterone sulfate (DHEAS). No treatment is needed, but parents may be advised that these girls, particularly those who are overweight, have an increased risk of developing polycystic ovary syndrome in their teenage years.

Early pubic hair is rarely seen in girls with virilizing adrenal or ovarian tumors, but such girls will generally have clitoral enlargement, a pronounced growth spurt, and often acne as well. A small proportion of girls have mild nonclassical congenital adrenal hyperplasia (CAH) with elevated levels of 17-hydroxyprogesterone. There is no consensus, however, that girls with mild nonclassical CAH need to be treated with glucocorticoids to suppress the adrenal glands.

Premature thelarche

Breast development starting before age 3 years may be worrisome to parents and pediatricians, but is nearly always due to premature thelarche. During follow-up over a period of 6–12 months, the size of the breast tissue increases little if at all, but it may persist for years or fluctuate in size over weeks to months. Unilateral breast enlargement is not a pathologic process, and there is no need for ultrasound or biopsy, provided the breast is nontender and feels like normal glandular tissue.

The etiology is unclear, but some studies have found that small ovarian cysts are common in this condition, suggesting estrogen stimulation from a cyst that then regresses. In typical cases, hormonal testing is not needed. LH is invariably in the prepubertal range, and FSH and estradiol do not reliably distinguish prepubertal from early pubertal girls.

When should true precocious puberty be suspected?

Progressive enlargement of glandular breast tissue (which needs to be distinguished from adipose tissue in chubby girls by careful palpation) starting before age 8 years and accompanied by accelerated growth is suggestive of true or central precocious puberty (CPP). This condition is uncommon before age 6 years but has become increasingly common in 6–8-year-old girls, probably because the onset of breast development in the general population has shifted to younger ages. Many girls with early breast development have a nonprogressive or slowly progressive form of precocious puberty, so if at the initial encounter breasts are at Tanner stage 2 (see Appendix 1.9.4 and Figure 14.2), a 4–6-month period of observation is suggested to make sure that puberty is advancing; if breasts are at stage 3 at the initial visit, this period of observation is not needed.

Diagnosis

Laboratory evaluation of precocious puberty should be kept simple:
• Random LH is the most useful test to discriminate prepubertal from pubertal girls: a random LH greater than 0.3 U/L is diagnostic of CPP; most prepubertal girls have a LH of less than 0.1 U/L.
• An estradiol level of greater than 20 pg/mL supports a diagnosis of CPP.
• Measuring adrenal steroids in girls with both early breast and pubic hair development is not helpful.
• Thyroid testing is rarely necessary as long-standing primary hypothyroidism is associated with large multicystic ovaries; there are obvious signs and symptoms of hypothyroidism, and growth is slowed instead of accelerated.

If results are unclear, the girl should be referred to a pediatric endocrinologist for additional dynamic testing [measurement of LH after administration of a gonadotropin-releasing hormone (GnRH) analog].

There is controversy as to whether all girls with CPP need to have a brain MRI to rule out tumors or the non-neoplastic hypothalamic hamartoma. One large study of over 200 girls found that the incidence of central nervous system (CNS) findings in girls with onset before age 6 years is about 20%, but only 2% for girls with onset between the ages of 6 and 8 years. Unless there is unusually rapid progression or worrisome CNS symptoms, such as headache or alterations in vision, many endocrinologists elect not to order a brain MRI in girls with onset of puberty between the ages 6 and 8 years.

The value of pelvic ultrasound in the evaluation of early breast development is also debatable. Several studies have shown that while the ovaries and uterus are enlarged relative to age-matched controls, there is overlap between measurements in prepubertal and early pubertal girls. For early-maturing girls who are mid–late pubertal, ultrasound is likely to show bilateral ovarian enlargement, but in such cases, physical exam and hormone testing are generally diagnostic. One situation where ultrasound is essential is in the girl with rapidly progressing breast enlargement whose screening lab results show a very elevated estradiol (>50–100 pg/mL) combined with a suppressed LH of less than 0.1 U/L, findings suggestive of an ovarian tumor or large ovarian cyst. Ovarian tumors in young girls are quite rare, but the most common, the granulosa cell tumor (see Chapter 48.2), has low malignant potential, typically following a benign course, with only a small percentage showing aggressive behavior. Primary treatment is surgical, with a unilateral salpingo-oophorectomy.

A more challenging scenario is the girl with similar clinical and lab findings as above but the pelvic ultrasound shows a large ovarian cyst (see Chapter 48.1). Most clinicians cite cases where large solitary cysts have regressed without intervention and argue for conservative management. One diagnosis which needs to be considered is McCune–Albright syndrome. Findings in classic cases include rapid breast development with typically a single large ovarian cyst, irregular large café-au-lait pigmentation which does not cross the midline, and cystic bone lesions called polyostotic fibrous dysplasia. However, only two of the three findings are present in a high proportion of cases. It is important to make this diagnosis, as GnRH analogs, which are effective in treating CPP, are of no benefit in this and other forms of gonadotropin-*independent* precocious puberty.

Management

GnRH analog therapy works in CPP to desensitize the pituitary gonadotropes by exposing them to continuous rather than pulsatile GnRH. The question of when and whether to use GnRH analog therapy is best left to pediatric endocrinologists with experience and expertise in this area. Treatment is expensive, with costs typically in the range of $10 000–15 000 per year.

The most compelling reason for treating CPP is to prevent compromise of adult stature due to early closure of the epiphyses. However, the majority of girls with CPP, particularly those with the slowly progressive form, achieve a normal adult height without treatment.

The greatest concern of most parents of girls with CPP is the negative psychological impact of early menses. Using a GnRH analog solely to delay menses or to alleviate the consequences of a girl being more physically developed than her peers has not been convincingly shown to improve psychological outcomes, though controlled studies addressing this issue are lacking. Girls who start puberty at age 8 years or later rarely attain menarche prior to age 10, and the author's experience is that few experience severe stress, particularly if a parent has prepared them ahead of time. However, girls who have progressive CPP starting at age 7 years often have menarche by age 9, which tends to worry parents greatly, and these girls may benefit psychologically from GnRH analog therapy to delay menarche until after age 10–11 years.

Premature menarche

A puzzling situation which can be easily confused with precocious puberty is the onset of vaginal bleeding in a girl who has not yet started to develop breast tissue. The differential diagnosis includes vaginal foreign body, vaginal tumors, and sexual abuse. If, after consideration of these conditions, no specific cause is found, the diagnosis of premature menarche can be made. While these episodes are quite worrisome for the family, they almost always resolve over a period of 1–4 months. Ultrasound or vaginoscopy may be considered in cases where the bleeding is heavy, the problem does not resolve quickly or there is considerable parental anxiety. There is still no satisfactory hormonal explanation for this paradoxical situation.

✋ Caution

Situations indicating need for rapid evaluation by a specialist (pediatric endocrinology or pediatric gynecology for vaginal bleeding) are:

- Early appearance of pubic hair:
  - If accompanied by growth acceleration (not just tall stature)
  - If accompanied by clitoral enlargement or severe acne.
- Early appearance of breast development:
  - If Tanner 3 or greater at the first visit
  - If the amount of breast tissue has increased significantly over a period of 4–6 months in a girl younger than 8 years old.
- Early onset of vaginal bleeding:
  - If there is no or very little breast development, the genital exam is normal, and bleeding persists or recurs for more than a month
  - If there is late pubertal breast development and the child is younger than 9 years old
  - If there are café-au-lait spots suggestive of McCune–Albright syndrome.

Further reading

Carel J-C, Eugster E, Rogol A, *et al.* Consensus statement on the use of gonadotropin-releasing hormone analogs in children. *Pediatrics* 2009;123(4):e752–762.

Kaplowitz PB. Link between body fat and the timing of puberty. *Pediatrics* 2008;121(2;Suppl 3):S208–217.

Kaplowitz PB, Oberfield SE. Reexamination of the age limit for defining when puberty is precocious in girls in the United States: implications for evaluation and treatment. *Pediatrics* 1999;104(4):936–941.

16 Delayed puberty

Sara E. Watson,[1] Peter A. Lee,[1,2] and Christopher P. Houk[3]

[1]Department of Pediatrics, Riley Hospital for Children, Indiana University School of Medicine, Indianapolis, IN, USA

[2]Department of Pediatrics, The Milton S. Hershey Medical Center, Penn State College of Medicine, Hershey, PA, USA

[3]Department of Pediatrics, Medical College of Georgia, Augusta, GA, USA

In a girl with pubertal delay, timely medical assessment is important as studies have shown that as many as half of these girls have an underlying pathology. Irrespective of the cause of pubertal delay, appropriate treatment, including estrogen therapy to stimulate pubertal development, may lessen the negative psychosocial impact and improve biologic factors such as bone density. When caused by a constitutional delay in normal growth and development, temporary treatment is needed and normal adult gonadal function is expected. When the delay is associated with a permanent dysfunction, hormone substitution is lifelong and the potential for fertility must be assessed.

The age of onset of puberty among girls is dependent upon racial/ethnic background. Generally the lack of breast development by age 12.8 years for Caucasian and Hispanic girls, and 12.4 years for Black girls is considered delayed. The lack of menarche by age 15 years in all ethnicities is considered delayed. Lack of pubertal progression at a reasonable rate, such as progression to the next Tanner stage within a year or lack of menarche within 3 years of breast development or by age 15 years, may also be considered delayed puberty.

To ascertain whether breast development has begun requires palpation. The appearance of a mound of tissue is insufficient to differentiate glandular breast tissue from an accumulation of fatty subcutaneous tissue. A disc of firmer, and often tender, tissue centered beneath the areolae is a sure sign that breast growth has begun. An area of less firm tissue directly beneath the nipple and areolae, the "donut sign," indicates that the visible mound is fatty tissue. In addition, an increasingly pigmented areola that is wider than 1.5 cm is consistent with the onset of puberty. Inverted nipples support a prepubertal state, while a protruding nipple with a diameter of greater than 3 mm suggests puberty.

The presence of breast tissue development indicates the onset of physical pubertal change, but does not necessarily indicate the onset of a pubertal hypothalamic–pituitary–ovarian (HPO) axis (see Chapter 14). Minimal breast tissue, particularly if present for some time without progression, may be the consequence of mild estrogen stimulation that is independent of the HPO axis.

The onset of pubic and other sexual hair growth does not indicate pubertal onset when it is not associated with estrogen-mediated physical changes. The adrenal cortex begins to secrete increased amounts of adrenal androgens (adrenarche) around the same time as typical puberty begins, and occurs both separately and independently of the activity of the HPO axis. These relatively weak androgens [dehydroepiandrosterone (DHEA) and androstenedione] stimulate the development of pubic hair development (pubarche), axillary hair, and adult-type body odor. Circulating levels of DHEA sulfate (DHEAS) are elevated in

Practical Pediatric and Adolescent Gynecology, First Edition. Edited by Paula J. Adams Hillard.
© 2013 John Wiley & Sons, Ltd. Published 2013 by John Wiley & Sons, Ltd.

adrenarche and can be measured as a marker of this physiologic event.

The onset of puberty among girls occurs concomitantly with an increased rate of linear growth and is followed by progression of pubertal changes. Hence, the girl with absent/minimal breast development that is slowly progressive – with or without pubic hair – and is not associated with growth acceleration is not in puberty.

Evidence at a glance

Delayed puberty includes:
- No breast development by age 12.8 years (Caucasians and Hispanics); 12.4 years (Blacks)
- No menarche by age 15 years
- No menarche by 3 years after onset of breast development
- Lack of progression to next Tanner stage in a year.

Clinical presentation

Patients may present with concerns of lack of breast development or of amenorrhea after their peers have had menarche. Those with lack of breast development may also be concerned about short stature. However, there is a wide variety of clinical presentation, making it important to evaluate the pubertal development of every adolescent.

Puberty is considered delayed when breast development has not begun within the normal range as outlined above, and when there is no accelerated growth rate. The development of pubic hair is not a convincing sign of pubertal onset and when it precedes breast development, generally results from adrenal activity and does not indicate ovarian activation.

Diagnosis

History should include recent changes in height and weight, sense of smell (Kallmann syndrome), systemic, endocrine, or gastrointestinal illnesses and their therapies (including radiation or chemotherapy), history of alcohol use, family history of infertility, and timing of pubertal development.

★ Tips and tricks

- Sexual hair onset does not necessarily mean the onset of puberty and may be due to adrenal androgen secretion.
- In addition to pubertal delay, an unusually slow tempo of pubertal development warrants evaluation to exclude pathology.
- Hypergonadotropic hypogonadism is always a pathologic state.
- The association of anosmia with pubertal delay is strongly suggestive of Kallmann syndrome.

The physical exam should verify height, weight, weight for height (BMI), upper segment/lower segment ratios (ratios <1 indicate prepubertal proportions, those approximating 1 are pubertal, while those greater than 1 are suggestive of hypogonadism), and arm span (arm span exceeding height by 5 cm or more suggests delayed epiphyseal closure resulting from delay in sex steroid exposure). A general exam should be done, noting midline facial defects and syndactyly, and a neurologic exam, including visual findings and sense of smell. Pubertal staging of breast development and pubic hair should be noted. The genital exam includes visualization of the vaginal opening and clitoris.

Evidence at a glance

Characteristics of Turner syndrome
- Characteristic facies
- Micrognathia
- Epicanthal folds
- Ptosis
- Low-set ears
- Low hairline
- High-arched palate
- Neck webbing
- Shield chest
- Hypoplastic nipples
- Cubitus valgus
- Pigmented nevi
- Short fourth metacarpals
- Spoon-shaped fingernails

Table 16.1 Relative frequency of categories of pubertal delay among girls

- Low gonadotropins:
  ○ Temporary delay with normal potential HPG function:
    – Constitutional delay   30%
    – Secondary to systemic disease   20%
  ○ Permanent defect:
    – Hypogonadotropic hypogonadism   20%
- Elevated gonadotropins:
  ○ Hypergonadotropic hypogonadism   25%
- Other   5%

Based on data from Sedlmeyer IL, Palmert MR. Delayed puberty: analysis of a large case series from an academic center. *J Clin Endocrinol Metab* 2002;87:1613–1620. The Endocrine Society.

Initial laboratory testing

Serum luteinizing hormone (LH) and follicle-stimulating hormone (FSH) levels need to be obtained to document or exclude a hypergonadotropic state. Hand and wrist X-rays are done to determine skeletal maturity (bone age), which documents "biologic age" and estimates growth potential. Based on these results, second-tier testing should be directed toward a specific diagnosis:
- If *elevated* gonadotropins: karyotype, pelvic/abdominal ultrasound
- If *low* gonadotropins: complete blood count (CBC), electrolytes, liver function tests (LFT), prolactin, insulin-like growth factor 1 (IGF-1), thyroid-stimulating hormone (TSH), free thyroxine (FT4), gonadotropin-releasing hormone (GnRH) stimulation, brain MRI, and pelvic/abdominal ultrasound.

Delayed puberty is classified based upon gonadotropin levels (Table 16.1).

Hypergonadotropic hypogonadism

The etiologies of high gonadotropin levels, which are always pathologic (Table 16.2) include:
- Injury from prior radiation or chemotherapy
- Primary ovarian insufficiency [POI; previously termed premature ovarian failure (POF)] as with Turner syndrome, autoimmune disease, or galactosemia

Table 16.2 Hypergonadotropic hypogonadism: elevated LH and FSH (always pathologic)

- Turner syndrome
- Autoimmune ovarian failure
- Previous radiation or chemotherapy (partial recovery may occur)
- Galactosemia
- Gonadal dysgenesis (XX or XY)
- Androgen insensitivity (androgen receptor defect in 46, XY)

Table 16.3 Temporary gonadotropin deficiency: low LH and FSH levels

- Constitutional delay
- Systemic disease:
  ○ Inflammatory disease
  ○ Hypercortisolism
  ○ Malnutrition/eating disorder
  ○ Excessive exercise (e.g. gymnastics)
  ○ Psychogenic or stress-related
  ○ Hypothyroidism
  ○ Prolactinoma
  ○ Brain tumor (e.g. craniopharyngioma)
  ○ Alcohol use/abuse

- Gonadal dysgenesis
- Androgen receptor defects.

Karyotype, ovarian antibodies, and pelvic ultrasound are indicated to assess for Turner syndrome, gonadal dysgenesis, androgen insensitivity, and autoimmune ovarian failure.

Hypogonadotropic hypogonadism

Etiologies associated with low gonadotropin levels include both temporary and permanent conditions (Table 16.3). Temporary conditions include constitutional delay, systemic disease, excessive physical activity, and malnutrition. Permanent conditions include estrogen biosynthetic defects, Kallmann syndrome, GnRH or GnRH receptor defects, and pituitary insufficiency. When hypogonadotropic hypogonadism is verified, other pituitary functions should be assessed.

Constitutional delay is the most common single cause of pubertal delay in girls (approximately 30%)

Table 16.4 Eugonadotropic hypogonadism (normal pubertal onset but lack of menarche)

• Chronic anovulation [polycystic ovary syndrome (PCOS)]
• Anatomic abnormality (Müllerian agenesis)
• Hypothalamic amenorrhea, excessive exercise, extreme weight loss, or psychogenic stress

and results from a delay of the pubertal amplification and frequency of GnRH release. There is often a family history of delayed puberty (approximately 40%). Significant delay is associated with skeletal age delay. At presentation, it can be very difficult or impossible to distinguish constitutional delay of growth and development from hypothalamic hypogonadism.

Systemic diseases and other chronic conditions may result in delayed puberty. These conditions are associated with immature or impaired GnRH pulsatile release. Delayed/arrested puberty may be the presenting complaint in girls with brain tumors, including craniopharyngiomas and prolactinomas, and may be associated with galactorrhea.

Eugonadotropic eugonadism

This category describes normal pubertal onset but lack of menarche (Table 16.4). It may be a consequence of chronic anovulation, including polycystic ovary syndrome; anatomic abnormalities, including Müllerian duct agenesis; or hypothalamic amenorrhea with onset after pubertal onset, which is associated with excessive exercise, extreme weight loss, or psychogenic stress. Pelvic exam and ultrasound evaluation is used to evaluate for vaginal abnormalities, absence of uterus, ovarian size and symmetry, and the presence of hematocolpos.

Management

While the outcome of hypergonadotropic hypogonadism is clearly lifelong, the functional outcome of girls with hypogonadotropic hypogonadism may not

---

⚛ Science revisited—

Causes of hypogonodotropism
• **PROP-1 defect:** PROP-1 is a transcription factor involved in pituitary development; most frequent gene defect in patients with combined pituitary hormone insufficiency.
• *DAX-1* **mutation:** nuclear receptor protein, primarily involved in steroidogenesis and reproductive development, results in hypogonadotropic hypogonadism and adrenal hypoplasia congenita (AHC).
• **Isolated defect in gonadotropin production:** result from defects in the production of GnRH (post-translational processing) that lead to decreased release of gonadotropins or GnRH receptor mutations.
• **Kallmann syndrome:** hypogonadotropic hypogonadism with anosmia from failure of differentiation or migration of the GnRH-releasing neurons; may be associated with facial midline defects and synkinesia (mirror image movements).
• **Leptin deficiency** is associated with early-onset obesity and delayed puberty.
• **Mutations in the *FSH-β* gene:** characterized by undetectable FSH and elevated LH.
• *GPR54* **mutations:** kisspeptin receptor that, together with kisspeptin, plays a role in the pubertal stimulation of GnRH secretion.

---

become clear for years. Thus, once a girl is verified to have delay of onset or progression of puberty and has been adequately assessed, it is appropriate to begin estrogen therapy to stimulate pubertal changes, even when a final diagnosis is not yet possible. Stimulating the development of pubertal changes and accelerated linear growth to help catch-up with peers is appropriate for psychosocial and physical reasons, including adult body composition and build, sexual maturity, and adult bone density. Therapy is discontinued in constitutional delay if endogenous ovarian function begins (as would occur in constitutional delay). Among patients with Turner syndrome, height and treatment with growth hormone are considered when deciding when to initiate sex steroid therapy, as prolonging the pubertal delay may allow more time to repair a height deficit.

Induction of puberty begins with the lowest available dosage, with gradual dosage increases to full replacement over 2–3 years. It may be that a transdermal form provides the lowest available dosage, using part of a patch if it can be cut to deliver 25 µg or less of estradiol daily. The lowest dosage of conjugated estrogens is 0.3 mg, which can be given daily or every other day. Patients may benefit from the addition of a progestational agent when breakthrough bleeding occurs or after 18 months of estrogen therapy. This is given for 10 days at the end of a 21-day cycle, followed by a week of no medication. Once sexual maturity is reached, the most convenient way to continue sex steroid replacement is to employ an oral contraceptive using an estrogen:progestin combination.

If the permanency of hypogonadotropism is unclear, therapy can be discontinued and the patient reassessed after 6 months. When an underlying condition is present, primary therapy is directed toward that etiology, although estrogen therapy can be used before this process is resolved to attempt to stimulate pubertal progression. When hyperprolactinemia is identified, hypothyroidism should be eliminated as a secondary cause and a magnetic resonance imaging scan (MRI) should be done and dopamine agonists can be used.

The potential for fertility depends upon whether ovaries containing ova are present, or in the case of *in vitro* fertilization using donated ova, whether a competent uterus is present. In a patient with Turner syndrome, it must be assessed whether the cardiovascular system is competent to support a pregnancy. For those with hypogonadotropism, GnRH, or recombinant FSH and LH, or human chorionic gonadotropin (hCG) and human menopausal gonadotropin (hMG) can be used to stimulate ovulation.

Throughout the process of assessment and therapy, the patient and her family should be provided with the background physiology and rationale for assessment and therapy. It is important for the patient to understand that her physical development will catchup and within a few years she will be physically, including sexually, similar to any other adult female, with a capacity for normal sexual function and responsiveness.

✋ Patient/parent advice

- No matter what the cause of pubertal delay, it is possible to stimulate physical pubertal development so the woman looks like a normal adult and can respond sexually as a normal adult.
- Whether fertility will be a problem depends upon the underlying cause of delay:
  ○ If the delay is temporary, fertility is likely possible.
  ○ If hormone substitution is needed, this can stimulate ovulation if eggs are present within the ovaries.
  ○ Other assisted fertility techniques are possible:
    – If eggs are present but hormones cannot stimulate ovulation, it may be possible to retrieve eggs for *in vitro* fertilization.
    – If a uterus is present but a uterus is not, donated eggs can be considered for fertilization and implantation in the uterus.
    – If eggs are present but a uterus is not, implantation of fertilized eggs in a surrogate mother can be considered.

Summary

Delayed puberty is the failure to begin breast development by age 13 years or failure to reach menarche by age 15 years. While constitutional growth delay is the most common etiology overall, about two-thirds of girls with delayed puberty have underlying pathology. The major diagnostic categories, based upon gonadotropin levels, are: hypergonadotropic hypogonadism, which is always pathologic, and hypogonadotropic hypogonadism, which may be temporary or permanent. Correction of the temporary forms accompanying underlying disorders generally allows normal pubertal development to resume. Therapy with sex steroid results in physical maturity while fertility potential depends upon multiple factors, including the presence of ova.

Further reading

Crowley WF, Pitteloud N. Diagnosis and treatment of delayed puberty. www.uptodate.com

Reindollar RH. Turner syndrome: contemporary thoughts and reproductive issues. *Semin Reprod Med* 2011;29: 342–352.

Sedlmeyer IL, Palmert MR. Delayed puberty: analysis of a large case series from an academic center. *J Clin Endocrinol Metab* 2002;87:1613–1620.

Adolescent girls

17 Initial assessment: consultation with an adolescent girl

Paula J. Adams Hillard

Department of Obstetrics and Gynecology, Stanford University School of Medicine, Stanford, CA, USA

The structure of an initial outpatient office visit with an adolescent who presents for clinical care may vary, depending on whether the visit is with a primary clinician to establish ongoing primary care, or with a gynecologist or specialist in adolescent medicine for a consultation regarding a specific problem. Ongoing care in a primary care setting for an adolescent may also be structured in a different manner. The clinician will need to establish the reason for the visit and to understand the expectations of the family in the context of the patient's primary and specialty healthcare. The gynecologist might assume responsibility for preventive care and screening related to reproductive healthcare needs on an ongoing basis, or serve as a consultant by establishing a diagnosis and recommending a management plan that might then be implemented by the patient's primary clinician.

> ### ✋ Patient/parent advice
>
> • The American College of Obstetricians and Gynecologists (ACOG) has recommended that the initial visit with a gynecologist for the provision of health guidance, screening, and preventive healthcare services should take place between the ages of 13 and 15 years.
>
>   This visit does not generally include a pelvic exam.

This chapter will describe one model for the structure of a gynecologic consultation visit that the author has developed over the last 30 year of providing gynecologic care to adolescents. The model acknowledges adolescents' need for confidential healthcare, preventive guidance, and screening; the context of adolescents' lives within a family; and parents' need for guidance and advice about adolescent health. The initial visit with an adolescent typically takes 45 minutes to an hour, and the visit should be scheduled accordingly. This model relies on principles of good communication; an ability to establish trust with an adolescent and her parent(s); an awareness of the critical importance of confidentiality in adolescent healthcare; knowledge of adolescent development in the realms of physical, cognitive, social, and psychosexual growth; and an ability to facilitate effective communication between and among family members. Clinical care for adolescents is based on specific knowledge about confidentiality (see Chapter 18), adolescent sexuality (see Chapter 20), legal considerations (see Chapter 19), screening for substance use and mood disorders (see Chapter 25), and the provision of preventive care for adolescents (see Chapter 21). While the model was developed to promote and uphold the practice of these principles of adolescent care, the principles are vitally important, even if the clinician chooses or circumstances dictate that the structure of the visit differs.

The Committee on Care of Adolescents in Private Practice of the Society for Adolescent Health and Medicine has described characteristics required for providing medical care to adolescents:

"The style and personality of the provider and his/her philosophy of medical care are particularly important in the medical care of adolescents. The provider should be mature and open-minded, and genuinely interested in teenagers as persons first, then in their problems, and also in their parents. He/she should not only like teenagers but must also feel comfortable with them. He/she should be able to communicate well with his/her patients and their parents. The provider should help enhance family communication while assuring confidentiality when requested around personal issues."

The model for the structure of an initial assessment of an adolescent is diagrammed in Figure 17.1. The visit begins by seeing the adolescent and her parent together. For gynecologic visits, the accompanying parent is usually the mother, but in certain circumstances or situations it may be the father (e.g. if the father is a single parent with custody) or a guardian or foster parent. It may be that two parents accompany the adolescent, particularly when there are serious health concerns. The clinician should introduce her/himself initially to the adolescent, ask the adolescent who is accompanying her, and then greet the accompanying adult(s).

The nature of the visit should be established – ascertaining whether this is a visit for preventive guidance, to diagnose and manage a specific concern, for a second opinion, etc.

The structure of the visit is briefly described to the family (Figure 17.1). The history of the present illness/complaint/concern is obtained initially; the clinician will often find that a better history (e.g. of irregular bleeding) can frequently be obtained from the adolescent with her mother's help than from the teen alone. In addition, the clinician can directly observe the dynamics of the relationship; e.g. the mother may attempt to answer all questions on behalf of her daughter, rather than allowing the adolescent to speak, or the daughter may insist on arguing about every aspect of the history. Past medical history is determined from both the teen and parent, as often the parent will be able to provide a better history of medical diagnoses and events from early childhood.

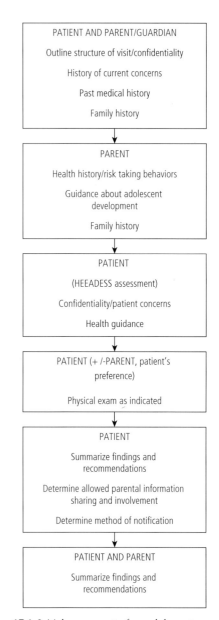

Figure 17.1 Initial assessment of an adolescent.

Family history is determined, with particular focus on conditions that are relevant to gynecologic conditions (Table 17.1). The mother's and daughter's memories may be complementary, and if the daughter is unaware of specific familial conditions, this can be educational for her.

Next, the parent is briefly seen alone while the adolescent waits in the waiting area. This provides

Table 17.1 Family history relevant to gynecologic conditions

- Mother's age of menarche
- Family history of "early menopause"
- Family history of irregular menses during adolescent or young adult years
- Gynecologic diagnoses in the family:
  - Irregular menses
  - Heavy menses
  - Dysmenorrhea
  - Polycystic ovary syndrome:
    - Irregular menses
    - Hirsutism
    - Obesity
    - Infertility (specifically anovulatory)
  - Uterine fibroids
  - Endometriosis
- Family history of malignancies:
  - Breast cancer
  - Ovarian cancer
  - Uterine cancer
  - Colon cancer
  - Cervical cancer
- Family history of venous thromboembolism:
  - Deep vein thrombosis, pulmonary embolism
  - Recurrent miscarriages
  - Specific thrombophilias (protein S, C, antithrombin III deficiency)
- Cardiovascular disease:
  - Diabetes
  - Hypertension
  - Hyperlipidemia
  - Sudden death
  - Stroke

the parent with the opportunity to express specific concerns, including concerns about the need for contraception, disordered eating or depression, or specific possible diagnoses. The parent's observations about risk-taking behaviors are ascertained, as well as general observations about school performance and social activities. The clinician can state that while they will always encourage an adolescent to talk with the parent, the clinician's policies include providing confidential answers to any specific questions that the adolescent may have.

Next, the adolescent is seen privately, after ushering the parent back to the waiting area (to assure that they are not hovering outside the exam room door, attempting to overhear the conversation).

★ Tips and tricks

Talking with parents
- Gain an understanding of the family structure (e.g. are parents divorced/separated; does the teen see her biologic father).
- Elicit the parent's concerns and questions about well-being, growth, and development.
- Provide preventive guidance (e.g. "It is reasonable to insist that you know where your daughter is going and with whom, and to set limits.")
- Provide information about normative behaviors, e.g. by stating, "many 14 year olds behave as if they are not listening to parental guidance."
- Encourage ongoing discussions about risky behaviors, sexuality, and responsibility.
- Encourage parents to discuss their own beliefs about issues such as responsible sexual decision-making, alcohol consumption, use of tobacco.

★ Tips and tricks

Talking with adolescents
- Begin by asking about home, school, friends, after school activities, or sports to facilitate rapport and to provide insights and understanding of the teen's life.
- Take a genuine interest in the teen's health and well-being.
- Be respectful and listen well.
- Listen more than you talk.
- Be nonjudgmental.
- Treat the adolescent's concerns seriously and with concern.
- Ascertain the teen's perspective on her illness, and determine what in particular it is that troubles or worries her about her symptoms.
- Explain and repeat policies about confidentiality.
- Normalize questions about risk taking; "I ask all the girls I see about..."
- Do not try to dress or talk like an adolescent.

In speaking with the patient privately, assurances of confidentiality are given, along with caveats about situations that would entail disclosure, such as abuse or self-harm. Further history is obtained, including psychosocial questions.

Evidence at a glance

Adolescent Psychosocial History and Risk Assessment (HEEADSSS) based on epidemiologic evidence of the major causes of morbidity and mortality in adolescents (see also Appendix 1.13):

H: Home
E: Education and employment
E: Eating
A: Activities with peers
D: Drugs
S: Sexual activity
S: Suicide and depression
S: Safety.

If a physical exam is deemed necessary, the nature of the exam is described to the adolescent: e.g. a "brief" exam similar to that previously performed by the primary physician, examination of the external genitalia, or a complete pelvic (or gynecologic) exam. The exam can be described in more detail if the teen desires (see Chapter 30.1). Regardless of the extent of the exam required, the adolescent should be given the opportunity to have whomever she chooses be with her during the exam or to have the exam done privately.

The adolescent should then be given a summary of the findings on exam and the overall assessment of the gynecologic problem. It may be helpful to suggest that further questions and more details can be provided, but that the parent will want to know about the findings. The extent of information sharing with the parent should be established. For example, even if the adolescent does not want it known that she has requested STD testing, the clinician can suggest that the parent would appreciate knowing that "the exam was normal," and ask permission to state this to the parent. It can be helpful to obtain a cell phone number for the confidential reporting of STD testing. It may be necessary to state caveats about lab testing, such

Table 17.2 Goals of gynecologic care of an adolescent

- Establishing a relationship of trust with a clinician
- Facilitating patient/parent communication
- Screening for risks:
  - Unprotected sexual activity (risks for unintended pregnancy, STIs)
  - Substance use and abuse (comorbidities associated with unprotected sexual activity)
  - Depression and suicidal ideation
- Screening for adolescent antecedents of adult diseases (osteoporosis, polycystic ovary syndrome, diabetes mellitus, cardiovascular disease)
- Preventing menstrual morbidities (quality of life)
- Facilitating healthy psychosexual development
- Modeling appropriate health-seeking behaviors and development of self-efficacy
- Facilitating empowerment to learn about and care for her own body (first pelvic exam)
- Providing preventive guidance to patient and parent

as the fact that an insurance explanation of benefits (EOB) may or may not state the nature of specific testing, and to offer options such as referral to clinics that provide confidential free or sliding scale care. Counseling regarding risk-taking behaviors, need for contraception, and recommended lifestyle changes may be based on an awareness of the stages of change model to help patients change behaviors. Techniques of motivational interviewing can be helpful.

Finally, a summary of findings, assessment, recommendations, and plans for follow-up are provided to the adolescent and her parent together.

The goals of the initial assessment and consultation with an adolescent girl and subsequent gynecologic care are described in Table 17.2.

Further reading

American College of Obstetricians and Gynecologists. Tool Kit for Teen Care. ACOG, 2010.

Rosenthal SL, Cohen SS, Burklow KA, *et al.* Family involvement in the gynecologic care of adolescents. *J Pediatr Adolesc Gynecol* 1996;9:59–65.

Woods ER, Neinstein LS. Office visit, interview techniques, and recommendations to parents, In: Neinstein LS, ed. *Adolescent Healthcare: A Practical Guide*, 5th edn, 2008, Wolters Kluwer, 2008.

18 Confidentiality

Janice Bacon[1] and Jennifer A. Greene[2]

[1]Lexington Medical Center, Women's Health & Diagnostic Center, West Columbia, SC, USA
[2]Department of Obstetrics and Gynecology, University of South Carolina School of Medicine, Columbia, SC, USA

Adolescence is a time of considerable change. The individual will experience mental, physical, and physiologic evolution during this tumultuous period. There may be a shift in healthcare provider during this time, from a single, well-known and trusted pediatrician or family practitioner, to general care continued by a primary care provider, often with the addition of a gynecologist. The clinician who cares for adolescents will be of paramount importance in helping the adolescent navigate the changes expected with menarche, discovery of sexual identity, and commencement of sexual activity. A new responsibility will be placed on the adolescent, with a changed expectation – that she actively participates in the healthcare process, compared to the passive role she took previously. There will also be an important change in the focus of healthcare; this population is generally unburdened by serious health conditions, and instead is at much greater risk of morbidity and mortality due to high-risk behaviors and their consequences.

The establishment of trust is pivotal when caring for the adolescent patient. Confidentiality is central to attaining patient trust and creating a relaxed, secure forum for education, discussions, and questions related to the confusing subjects of sex, contraception, STIs, and sexuality. In addition, this forum will provide a venue for discussion of health maintenance and behaviors that will continue the patient on the road to lifelong health.

The opening discussion during an initial adolescent visit should focus on establishing the framework of

Evidence at a glance

- Data conclusively support the benefits of education and counseling to prevent unintended pregnancy and sexually-transmitted infections (STIs; acquisition, transmission, and treatment).
- The ultimate goal of these measures is the prevention of long-term health complications by providing education and healthcare in a confidential manner.

☆ Tips and tricks

Providing information about policies of confidentiality

- A booklet can be included in the new patient information packet sent prior to the visit.
- Additional pamphlets and posters can be displayed in the office reception area to reintroduce the subject matter from reliable sources.
- Office forms can specifically outline the adolescent confidentiality policy of the medical office.
- All office staff should be well informed about such policies to ensure that the patient's confidentiality is appropriately guarded.
- Patients and their family members should be educated regarding their rights.

Practical Pediatric and Adolescent Gynecology, First Edition. Edited by Paula J. Adams Hillard.
© 2013 John Wiley & Sons, Ltd. Published 2013 by John Wiley & Sons, Ltd.

confidentiality for both the patient and, if present, the parent or guardian (see also Chapter 17). Both parties should be assured jointly and separately that the information volunteered will be confidential within the constraints of the law. They then should be informed of the legal exceptions to confidentiality in your state law (see Chapter 19) and questions from both parties should be addressed to ensure understanding, as these will likely be novel concepts. An understanding of the office policies and the state law will facilitate disclosure and thus permit more comprehensive patient care.

Some clinicians structure visits such that first the parent is spoken to privately, after asking the teen to wait in the waiting area. This is done to assess the parent's perspective and elicits any particular concerns that they have. If the clinician chooses to speak privately with the parent, it should always be done *prior* to speaking with the adolescent; if the teen is seen alone prior to the clinician speaking privately to the parent, she may have concerns that her confidentiality is being breached.

The adolescent is then seen privately so full confidential disclosure can occur. The next portion of the encounter may consist of the examination, which can be performed with or without the parent or guardian present as the patient chooses. A discussion of the results should then follow between patient and provider initially; a clear understanding should be reached with the patient regarding pathology, recommended therapy, and follow-up, as well as what information the patient desires be kept confidential and what the physician is able to keep confidential given ethical and legal guidelines (see Chapter 19). The patient's wishes should be clearly documented in the patient record and referred to before any future disclosure of patient clinical data; if paper records rather than electronic medical records are kept, it can be noted in a different section or on paper of a different color.

The final portion of the visit should include all parties, and provides an opportunity for the practitioner to discuss findings within the constraints of the adolescent's preferences, and permits reinforcement of the proposed plan. The provider should encourage open communication between the parent and adolescent, as well as introduce health maintenance topics.

Further resources for developing office policy

Professional organizations, including the American College of Obstetricians and Gynecologists (ACOG), the American Academy of Pediatrics (AAP), the American Academy of Family Physicians (AAFP), the North American Society for Pediatric and Adolescent Gynecology (NASPAG), the American Medical Association (AMA), and the Society for Adolescent Health and Medicine (SAHM), recognize the tremendous necessity adolescents have for confidential medical care. These organizations act as patient and physician advocates, working to bring these issues to light, assisting in the development of policies, and lobbying for legal statutes to lessen barriers and improve access to these much needed services (Table 18.1). In

Table 18.1 Educational resources

American College of Obstetricians and Gynecologists: Confidentiality in Adolescent Healthcare – Toolkit for

www.acog.org

American Medical Association: Confidential care for minors

www.ama-assn.org

American Academy of Pediatrics: Confidentiality in adolescent healthcare

www.aap.org

American Academy of Family Physicians: Adolescent healthcare, confidentiality

www.aafp.org

The Society for Adolescent Medicine: Position Paper on Confidentiality

www.adolescenthealth.org

North American Society for Pediatric and Adolescent Gynecology: Tips for protecting youth confidentiality and Letter to Parents

www.naspag.org

Center for Adolescent Health and the Law: State minor consent laws

www.cahl.org

National Center for Youth Law

www.teenhealthlaw.org

Guttmacher Institute

www.guttmacher.org

Table 18.2 Minors' consent laws

State	Contraceptive Services	STI Services	Prenatal Care	Adoption	Medical Care For Minor's Child	Abortion Services
Alabama	All[b]	All[a]	All	All	All	Parental Consent
Alaska	All	All	All		All	Parental Notice
Arizona	All	All		All		Parental Consent
Arkansa	All	All[a]	All		All	Parental Consent
California	All	All	All	All		▼ (Parental Consent)
Colorado	All	All	All	All	All	Parental Notice
Connecticut	Some	All		Legal counsel	All	All
Delaware	All[a]	All[a]	All[a]	All	All	Parental Notice[c]
Dist. of Columbia	All	All	All	All	All	All
Florida	Some	All	All		All	Parental Notice
Georgia	All	All[a]	All	All	All	Parental Notice
Hawaii	All[a, b]	All[a, b]	All[a, b]	All		
Idaho	All	All[b]	All	All	All	Parental Consent
Illinois	Some	All[a]	All	All	All	▼ (Parental Notice)
Indiana	Some	All		All		Parental Consent
Iowa	All	All				Parental Notice
Kansas	Some	All[a]	Some	All	All	Parental Consent
Kentucky	All[a]	All[a]	All[a]	Legal counsel	All	Parental Consent
Louisiana	Some	All[a]		Parental consent	All	Parental Consent
Maine	Some	All[a]				All
Maryland	All[a]	All[a]	All[a]	All	All	Parental Notice
Massachusetts	All	All	All		All	Parental Consent
Michigan	Some	All[a]	All[a]	Parental consent	All	Parental Consent
Minnesota	All[a]	All[a]	All[a]	Parental consent	All	Parental Notice
Mississippi	Some	All	All	All	All	Parental Consent
Missouri	Some	All[a]	All[a]	Legal counsel	All	Parental Consent
Montana	All[a]	All[a]	All[a]	Legal counsel	All	Parental Notice
Nebraska	Some	All				Parental Consent
Nevada	Some	All	Some	All	All	▼ (Parental Notice)
New Hampshire	Some	All[b]	Some	All[d]		Parental Notice

(Continued)

Table 18.2 (*Continued*)

State	Contraceptive Services	STI Services	Prenatal Care	Adoption	Medical Care For Minor's Child	Abortion Services
New Jersey	Some	All[a]	All[a]	All	All	▼ (Parental Notice)
New Mexico	All	All	All	All		▼ (Parental Consent)
New York	All	All	All	All	All	
North Carolina	All	All	All			Parental Consent
North Dakota		All[a, b]	ξ[a]	All		Parental Consent
Ohio		All		All		Parental Consent
Oklahoma	Some	All[a]	All[a]	All[b]	All	Parental Consent and Notice
Oregon	All[a]	All	All[a, c]			
Pennsylvania	All[b]	All	All	Parental notice	All	Parental Consent
Rhode Island		All		Parental consent	All	Parental Consent
South Carolina	All[e]	All[e]	All[e]	All	All	Parental Consent[c]
South Dakota	Some	All				Parental Notice
Tennessee	All	All	All	All	All	Parental Consent
Texas	Some	All[a]	All[a]			Parental Consent and Notice
Utah	Some	All	All	All	All	Parental Consent and Notice
Vermont	Some	All		All		
Virginia	All	All	All	All	All	Parental Consent and Notice
Washington	All	All[b]	All	Legal counsel		
West Virginia	Some	All	Some	All		Parental Notice
Wisconsin		All				Parental Consent
Wyoming	All	All		All		Parental Consent and Notice
TOTAL	26+DC	50+DC	32+DC	28+DC	30+DC	2+DC

Notes: "All" applies to those 17 and younger or to minors of at least a specified age such as 12 or 14. "Some" applies to specified categories of minors (those who have a health issue, or are married, pregnant, mature, etc.) The totals include only those states that allow all minors to consent.

▼ Enforcement permanently or temporarily enjoined by a court order; policy not in effect.

[a] Physicians may, but are not required to, inform the minor's parents.

[b] Applies to minors 14 and older.

[c] Delaware's abortion law applies to women younger than 16. Oregon's prenatal care law applies to women at least 15 years old. South Carolina's abortion law applies to those younger than 17.

[d] A court may require parental consent.

ξ A minor may consent to prenatal care during the 1st trimester and for the first visit after the 1st trimester. Parental consent is required for all other visits during the 2nd and 3rd trimesters.

[e] Applies to mature minors 15 and younger and to all minors 16 and older.

Source: Guttmacher Institute, State Policies In Brief, New York: Guttmacher, 2013, http://www.guttmacher.org/statecenter/spibs/spib_OMCL.pdf, accessed 8th January 2013.

Table 18.3 Promoting confidential care in the office

- Familiarize all office staff with state statutes
- Provide confidentiality rights information [Health Insurance Portability and Accountability Act (HIPAA)] to the patient
- Invite and address questions regarding rights and HIPAA
- Offer reliable educational references and resources
- Discuss confidentiality at each visit
- Provide "time alone" with an adolescent
- Offer a gender-matched provider if desired; when available
- Limit exposure to multiple providers
- Limit visibility during encounters:
  - Private areas for questions
  - Patient gowns
  - Doors not exposing examination tables

the experience of many "seasoned clinicians," most parents are supportive of confidentiality protection that encourages the adolescent to communicate freely with the clinician, especially clinicians with whom there is an established relationship.

In developing office policy, providers also need to be familiar with their state consent and confidentiality laws. Most states have statutes that allow minors to consent to certain ob/gyn care, but the scope of those statutes and the services vary by state (see Table 18.2). Most clinicians and parents agree that parental involvement in minors' healthcare is desirable; however, the reality is that many adolescents will not seek care for some reproductive health services if they are required to inform and involve their parents. In recognition of this, many states explicitly permit all or some minors to obtain contraception, prenatal care, and STI services without parental involvement. Currently the majority of states require parental involvement (notification and/or consent) in a minor's abortion, unless the minor goes through a judicial bypass process. U.S. Supreme Court precedent requires states to have a judicial bypass option (or something analogous) if they require parent involvement for abortion.

Conclusion

As care providers to adolescents, we are obligated to provide a confidential forum that will help the patient and parent feel that their confidences are safeguarded, that their healthcare needs are being met, and that they have been made aware of their right to confidentiality (Table 18.3). Education, reinforcement, and involvement of the patient, her family, and the healthcare team will facilitate this process. Establishing a relationship with an adolescent that fosters confidence and honesty will offer the best setting for total, relevant disclosure, and subsequently permit care that will aid the adolescent and her family in navigating this turbulent time.

Further reading

American College of Obstetricians and Gynecologists Committee on Adolescent Health Care. *Guidelines for Adolescent Health Care*, 2nd edn. ACOG, 2011.

Berlan E, Bravender T. Confidentiality, consent and caring for the adolescent patient. *Curr Opin Pediatr* 2009;21: 450–456.

Boonstra H, Nash E. Minors and the rights to consent to health care. *Issues Brief (Alan Guttmacher Inst)* 2000; 2:1–6.

English, A. *State Minor Consent Law, A Summary*. 3rd edn. individual states available from www.cahl.org

Acknowledgment

The editor would like to thank Rebecca Gudeman and Abigail English for their review of this chapter for consistency with Chapter 19, Legal Issues.

19 Legal issues

Rebecca Gudeman[1] and Abigail English[2]

[1]National Center for Youth Law, Oakland, CA, USA
[2]Center for Adolescent Health & the Law, Chapel Hill, NC, USA

Law affects the delivery of healthcare in many ways. This chapter reviews legal issues related to consent, confidentiality, and payment. Ethical principles are also of critical importance in the delivery of healthcare, but are beyond the scope of this chapter. Much law is specific to particular states and practice situations. Therefore, it is important to consult individual counsel for legal advice.

Consent to treatment

Healthcare professionals generally must obtain *consent* before they provide healthcare to a patient. Providing care before obtaining consent may put a healthcare professional at risk of an assault or battery charge, among other liability concerns. Typically, a patient aged 18 years or older – an *adult* – consents for her own care. Thus, "adolescents" in their late teens or early 20s generally provide consent for themselves. When an adolescent patient is a *minor* – typically under age 18 years – there are several persons who may be able or required to consent for the patient's treatment:

• **Parental consent.** A parent or legal guardian normally provides consent for a minor's healthcare. However, there are many exceptions to this general rule that allow minors or others to consent, particularly when minors seek obstetric or gynecologic care. These exceptions are described below.

• **Third party consent.** In some situations, particularly if a minor is not living with her parents or is in state custody, state law allows other people to consent for the minor's care. Depending on state law, consent may be provided by a court, a social worker, a probation officer, or an adult caregiver, such as a foster parent or relative with whom the minor is living.

• **Minor consent.** Every state has laws that allow minors to consent to their own healthcare based on the status of the minor patient and on the type of care or treatment being sought (see later). In addition, there are federal rules that enable minors to consent for family planning services, which apply when those services are funded by certain federal programs.

• **Emergencies.** While the general rule is that a healthcare professional must have consent before treating a patient, an important exception is emergencies. If a healthcare professional cannot obtain consent in a timely manner, the professional may proceed without consent in emergency situations. Often state law provides specific guidance on what medical conditions qualify as emergencies, usually based on the level of risk to the patient if treatment is foregone or delayed. The setting in which a patient seeks treatment is not determinative. Some patients seeking care in an emergency department may not have an "emergency" for consent purposes and some

---

Practical Pediatric and Adolescent Gynecology, First Edition. Edited by Paula J. Adams Hillard.
© 2013 John Wiley & Sons, Ltd. Published 2013 by John Wiley & Sons, Ltd.

seeking care in a doctor's office may be facing a situation that qualifies as an emergency. Healthcare professionals should be familiar with their state law for emergency care.

- **Abortion and consent.** In some states, minors may consent to abortion on a confidential basis, but in the majority of states, state law requires parental consent or notification before a minor may obtain an abortion. States that require parental consent or notification, however, also must provide an alternative procedure, often called *judicial bypass*, that allows a minor to obtain an abortion on a confidential basis. Judicial bypass allows a minor to ask a court for an order that either allows her to consent for the abortion herself, or approves the abortion as in her best interests, in either case without involving her parents. The specific process and legal standard used by the court to determine whether to grant the order is prescribed by state law, as is the parental notification and consent process. These laws are frequently changed or challenged in court. Professionals who provide abortion care should assure they understand their current state law.

Minor consent

Consent based on status
In every state, minors are able to consent to their own healthcare if they meet certain *status* exceptions. In most states, if a minor has been *emancipated by a court* or is *married*, the minor may consent to his or her own general healthcare as would an adult. Depending on the state, minors also may be able to consent to their own care if they are *pregnant; parenting; homeless, or living on their own and financially independent from their parents; in the armed forces; or considered "mature" enough to consent.* These

exceptions are defined by state law and differ from state to state. Healthcare professionals should be familiar with their state's status and emancipation laws.

Consent based on services
In every state, minors are able to consent to certain obstetric and gynecologic care for themselves. Depending on the state, this may include the right to consent to *contraception services; prenatal care; childbirth delivery services; abortion; and diagnosis, treatment and preventive care related to sexually-transmitted infections* (see Table 18.2). In addition to consent for OB/GYN-related care, most states have laws that allow minors to consent to at least some other healthcare services on their own behalf. For example, in some states, minors also may consent to *care related to the prevention, diagnosis and treatment of reportable communicable diseases; mental health counseling; and substance abuse treatment.* Some, but not all, state consent laws contain age restrictions that only allow minors above a certain age to consent to their own care. Healthcare professionals should be familiar with their own state minor consent laws.

Consent based on funding source
A few public funding programs require that services be provided based on minor consent. For example, when healthcare services are funded in full or in part by the federal Title X Family Planning Program [Title X], federal regulations specify that services must be available to minors as well as adults and that services must be confidential. Title X is part of the federal Public Health Service Act, and is one of the largest public funders of family planning in the US.

✋ Caution

Pregnancy and parenting status "emancipates" minors for the purpose of consenting to healthcare in *some*, but not all, states. Healthcare professionals should know what their state law says regarding emancipation, pregnancy, and parenting status, and the rights of minors to consent to treatment.

⚙ Law revisited

Minors must be allowed to consent to their own family planning services when those services are funded by the federal Title X Family Planning Program. This federal regulation supersedes any state law that otherwise requires parental consent or notification. Title X-funded family planning services are available in approximately 75% of all US counties.

★ Tips and tricks

What to look for in your state's minor consent laws
- Scope of status exceptions.
- Scope of services covered, [e.g. Does the law allow minors to consent to prevention of sexually-transmitted infections (STIs) or just diagnosis and treatment of STIs?].
- Age limits.
- Language regarding the right of a minor to refuse treatment.
- Abortion consent or notification laws.

Confidentiality

Both federal and state laws protect the confidentiality of medical information and medical records. Generally, these laws prevent the release of personally identifiable information without written permission, but most also include exceptions that allow or require healthcare professionals to release protected information without authorization in certain circumstances.

Laws

There are confidentiality laws at the federal and state level that restrict disclosure of individual health information. At the federal level, regulations implementing the Privacy Rule under the Health Insurance Portability and Accountability Act (HIPAA) protect the confidentiality of and limit disclosure of individually identifiable health information held by most healthcare professionals. States often have their own laws that apply in addition to HIPAA. There also are laws that apply based on other variables, such as funding source. The applicable laws and policies may depend on funding, service setting, and type of service provided. Healthcare professionals should be familiar with the laws that apply to their particular practice.

⚖ Law revisited

Confidentiality laws and policies determine:
- When health information *may not* be released.
- When health information *may* be released.
- When health information *must* be released.

HIPAA
The HIPAA Privacy Rule generally requires the authorization of the "individual" for release of protected health information. The "individual" in this case is typically the patient's legal representative (i.e. parent or guardian) when the patient is a minor. However, when a minor is allowed to consent for her own care, she is considered the "individual" for the purposes of HIPAA and her authorization, rather than that of her legal representative, is required for release of her protected health information. There are exceptions in HIPAA that allow or require health care providers to release protected health information without this authorization at times (see later).

For minors who are considered "individuals" under HIPAA, the question of whether their parents have access to their protected health information depends on "state or other applicable law." Thus the other federal and state confidentiality laws are critically important in determining when parents have access to confidential information for minors who have consented to their own care.

State laws
State laws that affect the confidentiality of medical information include state laws implementing the HIPAA Privacy Rule, medical record laws, professional licensing laws, evidentiary privileges (e.g. the physician–patient privilege), and funding program requirements. In addition, many of the state minor consent laws also contain confidentiality requirements.

Funding programs

Two federal programs provide the bulk of public family planning funding – Title X and Medicaid. Both programs assure the confidentiality of family planning services for minors as well as adults, and this assurance has been affirmed by several courts.

Title X
Federal regulations require that all personal information provided during provision of Title X-funded care be kept confidential. The federal regulations strictly limit when this information may be disclosed. This requirement applies to minors as well as adults.

Medicaid

Medicaid law contains a confidentiality requirement. Medicaid also requires that family planning services be provided to eligible beneficiaries, including adolescents who are sexually active. Some states have expanded the eligibility requirements for family planning services in Medicaid to include women and adolescents up to higher income levels than required by federal law.

⚖ Law revisited

Parents and legal guardians typically have a right to review medical information regarding their child; however, this general rule often does not apply when minors obtain obstetric and gynecologic care. Whether parents legally can obtain information regarding their child's obstetric and gynecologic care will vary depending on the funding for the service, the type of service provided (e.g. abortion versus contraceptive counseling), and the service setting, as well as state law. As a result, there may be times that healthcare professionals have to share confidential information with parents, despite objections to disclosure by the minor. There also may be times that the professionals are legally prohibited from sharing information with parents, even when they believe disclosure is in the patient's best interest. Healthcare professionals should be familiar and comfortable with the applicable rules before they begin practicing with minors.

Allowable and required disclosures

Exceptions in HIPAA and other laws sometimes allow or require disclosures even when there is no written authorization for the release. These include various reporting requirements under state law, as well as situations requiring healthcare professionals to exercise discretion to protect the patient or others. Here are a few examples:

• **Child abuse reporting.** Every state has laws requiring healthcare professionals to report child abuse to law enforcement and/or child welfare authorities.

This reporting generally results in a loss of confidentiality for the patient. The definitions of sexual abuse and sexual assault vary from state to state but these laws all include some forms of sexual abuse or sexual assault among the types of abuse that must be reported. Sometimes the definitions are broad enough to include sexual activity that healthcare professionals may consider voluntary and not abusive. It is important to be familiar with the specifics of the state reporting laws and which requirements are mandatory or discretionary.

• **Reporting certain violence.** Most states require or allow the reporting of certain types of injuries and wounds to law enforcement. This may include reporting injuries that result from domestic violence at times. It is important to be familiar with the specifics of the state reporting laws and which requirements are mandatory or discretionary.

• **Reportable diseases/public health.** Every state requires that certain diseases, including several sexually-transmitted diseases, be reported to public health authorities. These laws provide confidentiality protections as part of the reporting process, but may result in confidential communications by public health personnel with a patient's sexual contacts.

• **Danger to self or others.** Medical and mental health professionals have a legal obligation to disclose confidential information when a patient poses a danger to herself or others. In some instances, when the patient has expressed an explicit threat against an identified individual, there may be a duty to warn or take other preventive measures.

• **Payment, treatment, and healthcare operations.** The HIPAA Privacy Rule allows disclosure without authorization for purposes of treatment, payment, and healthcare operations. These terms are specifically defined. State law may include similar types of exceptions that further define these terms.

Payment and insurance

Responsibility for payment

Typically, parents and legal guardians are financially responsible for health services provided to their children. Some minor consent laws specify that when a minor consents to healthcare, she is responsible for payment and the parent is not. However, with the high cost of medical services, it is rare that minors

> ### ★ Tips and tricks
>
> **What your applicable confidentiality laws may tell you**
> - Who has a right to sign an authorization to release information.
> - When you are *required to disclose* information (e.g. child abuse reporting).
> - When you are *allowed to disclose* information without an authorization.
> - When you are *prohibited from disclosing* information.
> - Whether parents have a right to information about their minor child.

can afford to pay out of pocket for their own care. Thus insurance issues are of great importance.

Insurance

The majority of adolescents do have health insurance coverage, either through private health insurance, Medicaid, or the Children's Health Insurance Program (CHIP). With the exception of abortion, which remains controversial and in flux as a legal matter, increasingly most OB/GYN services are covered by public and private insurance.

When fully implemented, the Affordable Care Act (ACA), the federal health insurance law enacted in 2010, will both expand the number of adolescents who will have private health insurance coverage or Medicaid as well as improve financial access to some OB/GYN services. For example, private health insurance plans will have to make contraceptive services available without a copayment once ACA is implemented.

Other funding

Federally-funded Title X clinics provides family planning services based on a sliding fee scale. Only the income of the adolescent patient, not her family, is considered.

Some states have funding programs that can be used to pay for healthcare services to adolescents. However, these funds are limited and programs do not exist in all states. One important source of health-

care for adolescents is school-based health centers, which are generally funded through a combination of public funds, private donations, and insurance payments.

Payment and confidentiality

Many elements of the billing and insurance claims process result in a loss of confidentiality for patients. The HIPAA Privacy Rule allows disclosure without authorization for purposes of treatment and payment. Also, patients are routinely asked to sign authorizations to allow healthcare professionals to disclose information for the purpose of filing insurance claims and billing. Beyond that, once insurance claims are filed, some insurance companies routinely send Explanations of Benefits (EOBs) to policyholders. For a young person enrolled in her parents' insurance plan, this means parents receive EOBs with information regarding the youth's care. This issue is complex and in flux, so healthcare professionals should be aware of the implications of billing and insurance claims for confidentiality. At minimum, for ethical reasons, patients should be alerted to the potential for loss of confidentiality when insurance claims are filed.

> ### ✋ Caution
>
> - Billing and insurance claims may result in unexpected loss of confidentiality, particularly when adolescents are covered under their parents' insurance.
> - Patients should be alerted to the potential for disclosure.
> - If patients are concerned about disclosure, alternative funding or service settings should be discussed.

Conclusion

Laws are an important source of authority on consent for healthcare, confidentiality protections, and responsibility for payment. There are federal laws that apply in every state, but many important issues are controlled by state law and vary. Laws also change and evolve over time. Healthcare professionals should seek guidance and regular updates on the laws in their own states and the relevant federal laws.

Further reading

English A, *et al. State Minor Consent Laws: A Summary*, 3rd edn. Chapel Hill, NC: Center for Adolescent Health & the Law, 2010. www.cahl.org

Guttmacher Institute. State Policies in Brief: State Level Adolescent Resources. http://www.guttmacher.org/statecenter/adolescents/html

National Center for Youth Law. Teen Health Law website. http://www.teenhealthlaw.org

20 Adolescent sexuality

Linda M. Kollar

Cincinnati Children's Hospital Medical Center, Cincinnati, OH, USA

Sexuality during adolescence is a fluid concept, subject to change as the teenager completes the developmental task of acquiring a mature sense of sexual identity. One challenge for adults in their lives is to help them develop positive feelings about sex and engage in healthy decision-making within a mature consensual relationship. Sexuality evolves within the context of relationships and interaction with the social environment. However, it is usually reported and researched in terms of number of sexually-transmitted infections, unplanned pregnancies, and incidence of unprotected sexual intercourse.

Adolescence spans the second decade of life and is traditionally broken down into three stages: early adolescence (10–14 years) middle adolescence (15–17 years), and late adolescence (18–21 years). The variance in adolescence is related to a combination of maturation level, personal experiences, and cultural environment. Some of the characteristics of adolescents at each developmental level are outlined in Table 20.1.

During adolescence, the young person experiences a complete restructuring of her biologic, cognitive, and emotional functioning with the goal to emerge as a socially functioning adult. The biologic changes include the physical changes of puberty, including growth in stature and the development of secondary sexual characteristics. The physical changes of puberty have a more negative impact on girls than boys. Girls experience higher rates of depression and lower self-esteem during the adolescent transition. Girls who mature early are at higher risk for low self-esteem and body dissatisfaction when compared to late-maturing girls.

Cognitively, the adolescent moves from concrete thinking to the ability to understand and think abstractly. The ability to see shades of gray allows the adolescent to interpret and think about the world and the environment in new ways. This can result in many questions and sometimes conflicts with adults as they begin to question and push back against parental rules and boundaries.

> ### ☆ Tips and tricks
>
> - During times of stress, adolescents will regress into concrete thinking.
> - The healthcare visit is often stressful for the adolescent.
> - Utilize concrete explanations, assess understanding, and present information in a variety of formats to enhance comprehension.

Cognitive development and abstract thinking allow the adolescent to reason and consider possibilities; these skills are essential for decision-making,

---

Practical Pediatric and Adolescent Gynecology, First Edition. Edited by Paula J. Adams Hillard.
© 2013 John Wiley & Sons, Ltd. Published 2013 by John Wiley & Sons, Ltd.

Table 20.1 Adolescent developmental changes

	Body image	Cognitive	Family	Peer group	Sexuality
Early adolescent (10–14 years)	Onset of puberty Preoccupation with pubertal changes Self-conscious	Concrete thinking Daydreaming Mood swings Idealistic vocational goals	Less interest in family activities Anti-adult: appear to prefer friends to family Parents are a source of embarrassment	Same sex friendships Best friend Opposite sex interactions in school and large group activities Difficulty negotiating peer relationships, loneliness common	Physical attractiveness of partner most important; date in groups or non face-to-face "dating" (text, internet) Masturbation begins Gay/lesbian/bisexual/ transgender/questioning (GLBTQ): realize aroused by same gender, identity confusion in a heterosexist world
Middle adolescent (15–17 years)	General acceptance of body Concerns over making herself more attractive	Some abstract thinking; fall back to concrete thinking in times of stress Creativity Risk taking behavior and feelings of omnipotence, invulnerability, and immortality	Begin to question family rules/values Parental concern and conflict peaks More time away from family	Mixed gender peer group, more time with peers Conformity with peer values	Intense, short-term romantic relationships. More concerned with herself in a relationship than she is about her partner Partner usually 2 years older Looking for image of ideal romantic partner Increased sexual activity and experimentation GLBTQ: Begins to think of herself as lesbian/ transgender and aligns with others
Late adolescent (18 years and older)	Acceptance of body	Adult reasoning skills Realistic vocational goals	Move toward adult relationship with parents	Peer group values less important Friendships based on similar interests/ activities	Long-term committed relationships Reciprocity in the relationship GLBTQ: Integration of homosexual identity into life

especially during emotionally-charged moments. Adolescents thrive when given developmentally appropriate opportunities for autonomy and independent decision-making. When adolescents make decisions that are counter to family rules and values, the parents must impose consequences as well as offer increased independence as the adolescent demonstrates the ability to negotiate relationships and social situations safely.

Science revisited

- The prefrontal cortex assists with brain executive functions, including planning ahead, considering consequences, and managing impulses.
- This part of the brain is not fully developed until the end of adolescence.

It is developmentally appropriate for adolescents to begin to explore sexual feelings and behaviors. These behaviors/sexual activities may range from kissing, to touching, to oral sex, to vaginal or anal intercourse. By the end of high school the majority of adolescents have engaged in some type of sexual behavior. Most adolescents have sexual intercourse within a romantic relationship and many use protection from sexually-transmitted diseases (STDs) and pregnancy. Unfortunately, a minority of adolescents engage in risky sexual behavior with multiple partners and many fail to use effective contraception or condoms. Earlier sexual initiation is associated with higher risk, including a greater number of lifetime partners, abusive relationships, increased risk of STDs and pregnancy.

Caution

- Many healthcare providers make the false assumption that young people with mental retardation or physical disabilities are asexual.
- The development of a sexual identity and the need for support and education is equally important for adolescents with mental retardation and those with physical disabilities (see Chapter 28).

The quality of the parent–adolescent relationship is influential in promoting healthy sexual development and expression of sexuality. When the parent–adolescent relationship includes open communication with clear expectations, the adolescent is more likely to delay initiation of sexual intercourse, and when sexually active is more likely to utilize effective contraception and protect herself from STDs. During the health visit with a teenager, you should provide some education for the parent and adolescent simultaneously and spend some time targeting the relationship between the parent and the adolescent.

Parent advice

- Parental monitoring is essential for risk reduction.
- Parents should know their teen's friends, teachers, and school environment.
- Parents should also know their teen's itinerary when out with friends, with the expectation that they will be kept up to date with changes.

Parents maintain the greatest influence on adolescents, but the peer group also has some pull. Adolescents move from spending most of their time within the family environment to interacting and socializing with their friends. The peer group is an important source of information for the teen about social norms of all types of behavior. They provide additional feedback about skills and personality traits which is less biased than the information they receive from their families. The peer group is also influential in the age of initiation of sexual intercourse. Adolescents with a peer group that is supportive of sexual activity are more likely to initiate sexual intercourse.

Tips and tricks

- The adolescent's perception of peer norms for sexual behavior is an important indicator of risk for sexual initiation.
- During the sexual history, ask about her perception of sexual activity within her peer group: "Are any of your friends having sex yet? What do you think about that?"

Connectedness is a key protective factor in the development of a healthy sexual identity; it decreases sexual risk taking. Resilience is enhanced when young people have interpersonal connections to both adults and peers. The quantity of interactions is not as important as the quality of the bonds to family, peers, school, and community. Teenagers should be able to identify at least one trusted adult whom they can confide in and seek out in times of stress. The identified adult is usually one or both parents.

Social media provide an electronic space for adolescents to "hang out" with friends and acquaintances. The electronic medium is another place to develop and define their sexual identity by posting their interests, reading about the interests of others, practicing flirting, and using sexualized language. Teens may be less inhibited when communicating electronically; this allows them to say things they would not say in real life. One of the risks of social media is easy access to unwanted sexual materials that they have not learned how to filter. There also may be painful learning curves about how much personal information and conversations to post on social media sites. Most teens never have an opportunity to watch parents or other supportive adults negotiate websites and social media. Interacting electronically is a normalized behavior for most adolescents; questions about social media use are an important part of obtaining a social history with an adolescent. Those at high risk in other areas of their life are probably taking risks online as well.

Sexual behaviors usually occur within romantic relationships. Dating relationships are an additional part of the social world for many adolescents. The relationships are often brief, and the intensity and characteristics of the relationship are different at each of the developmental stages (Table 20.1). These partnerships provide additional opportunities for adolescents to learn about negotiation and compromise. They also provide opportunities to learn about rejection and heart break.

During adolescence, young people become aware of their attractions to the opposite sex, same sex or both sexes. GLBTQ (gay, lesbian, bisexual, transgender, and questioning) adolescents have the additional burden of trying to understand their identity and sexuality in an environment that at best sends mixed messages and at worst may be hostile or dangerous. The process of coming out or identifying oneself as gay, lesbian or bisexual generally begins in adolescence. Sexual identification begins with the recognition that they are aroused by people of the same gender; this may cause confusion in a heterosexist society. The young person eventually begins to identify herself as gay, lesbian, bisexual or transgender. At this time she may align herself with others in the gay, lesbian or bisexual community. The final stage is integration of a lesbian or bisexual identity into her life. Not everyone completes all of these stages during adolescence. Girls often identify themselves as lesbian before ever engaging in sex; young men usually have same-sex sexual encounters prior to identification as gay. The coming out process can lead to family conflicts; adolescents benefit from supportive guidance to figure out whether or not to disclose their sexual identity and the best method to do so.

On an individual level, the social stigma against homosexuality can have negative consequences, especially if lesbian, gay, and bisexual people attempt to conceal or deny their sexual orientation. GLBTQ youth are at higher risk for victimization, high-risk sexual behavior, substance abuse, and suicide (see Chapter 27). In addition to needing comprehensive screening for sexually transmitted infections, healthcare providers should also provide comprehensive mental health screening and appropriate treatment and referrals for these high-risk young people.

✋ Parent advice

Encourage parents to monitor their adolescent's social media usage, e.g.parents should not hesitate to require their child to "friend" them on Facebook.

⚙ Tips and tricks

• When obtaining a sexual history, ask about sexual attractions and behaviors rather than sexual identity. "Are you attracted to men, women or both?"
• This will provide more insight into sexual development, level of risk, and sexual orientation.

Parents play the main role in assisting the adolescent in her transition into adulthood. Healthcare providers need to empower parents to influence and guide their child's sexual development. Parents are a source of sexual information and role modeling beyond the traditional "sex talk" about reproduction and anatomy. Healthcare providers should encourage parents to take available opportunities to share their values related to sexuality and sexual decision-making, discuss healthy relationships, review expectations for achievement, and monitor adolescent behavior. The absence of family conflict and a sense of family warmth, closeness, and support are associated with a more positive transition into adulthood.

The expression of adolescent sexuality evokes strong emotions and opinions among the adults that interact with them. The decision to initiate sexual activity as a teen, adolescent pregnancy, and even sexual expression through clothing choices can be "hot button" issues for adults working with teens. Failure of healthcare providers to recognize their own biases may impede the development of effective relationships with adolescent patients. Open discussion about sexual feelings and healthy romantic relationships between adolescents and their healthcare providers can help teens safely negotiate the transition into adulthood.

Further reading

American College of Obstetricians and Gynecologists. *Tool Kit for Teen Care*, 2nd edition. ACOG, 2009.

Levine SB. Facilitating parent–child communication about sexuality. *Pediatr Rev* 2011;32(3):129–130.

Short MB, Rosenthal SR. Psychosocial development and puberty. *Ann NY Acad Sci* 2008;1135:36–42.

21 Adolescent preventive care for healthy teens

Kristin L. Kaltenstadler[1] and Corinne Lehmann[2]

[1]Suburban Pediatrics Associates, Cincinnati, OH, USA
[2]Department of Pediatrics, Division of Adolescent Medicine, Cincinnati Children's Hospital Medical Center, Cincinnati, OH, USA

Confidentiality

Adolescent healthcare *must* include confidential care. Adolescents are more likely to engage in care and discuss sensitive health-related behaviors if confidentiality is assured. Given that the majority of morbidity and mortality that occurs during adolescence is related to risk behaviors and mental health problems, making the adolescent feel comfortable to disclose potential risk behaviors or other concerns is imperative (see Chapter 18). Laws regarding delivery of confidential care to adolescents are state dependent (see Chapter 19). The American Medical Association (AMA), the American Academy of Pediatrics (AAP), and the American College of Obstetricians and Gynecologists (ACOG), among other professional organizations, all support confidential care for adolescents.

✋ Patient/parent advice

Adolescent patients and parents should be informed about confidential care practices at the start of each visit, and the clinician should strive to involve the parent when possible and to encourage patient –parent communication.

☆ Tips and tricks

Learn more about your state's minor consent statutes at The Guttmacher Institute (www.guttmacher.org) or The Center for Adolescent Health & the Law (www.cahl.org).

Assessment priorities and challenges throughout the stages of adolescence

During all stages of adolescence, recommended priority issues should be addressed at the initial and subsequent annual primary care visits, including physical growth and development, social and academic competence, emotional well-being, risk reduction, and violence and injury prevention. Table 21.1 illustrates the various challenges and features of the three stages of adolescence. Understanding the challenges encountered at each adolescent stage is crucial so as to appropriately address each priority issue (see also Chapter 17).

Social history

An essential portion of any initial assessment of an adolescent girl must include a thorough psychosocial

Practical Pediatric and Adolescent Gynecology, First Edition. Edited by Paula J. Adams Hillard.
© 2013 John Wiley & Sons, Ltd. Published 2013 by John Wiley & Sons, Ltd.

Table 21.1 Stages of adolescence

Early adolescence (11–14 years)	Middle adolescence (15–17 years)	Late adolescence (18–21 years)
• Transition to middle school (e.g. multiple teachers, harder course work, higher expectations) • Increased logical, abstract, and idealistic thinking • Desire to belong to a peer group • Increased time without adult supervision • Changes to family relationships (adolescent striving for greater independence)	• School and associated activities become central focus of life • May receive driving permit/license • Peers' importance as sources of information • Increased interest in interpersonal relationships (e.g. dating, sexual activity) • Developmental period with highest risk for mental health disorders	• May be entering college, starting first job, becoming a parent, or serving in the military • Cognitive development still ongoing • May live in a variety of settings • Legally allowed to vote, smoke, or drink • Self-identity, rational and realistic conscience developed • Moral, religious, and sexual values refined • Decreased participation in health supervision visits

history. The U.S. Preventive Services Task Force has recommended that this history be a component of all new adolescent encounters. A helpful framework for approaching the psychosocial history is the HEEADSSS interview, which is best performed with the parent out of the room after a discussion of confidentiality with both the patient and the parent (Table 21.2). Most parents will accept that this is routine, particularly if the format of the visit is described at the beginning of the visit. If the parent refuses to leave the room or the patient requests that the parent stay in the room, this fact should be documented.

Examination and history

A thorough physical exam should be conducted at the initial primary care visit and annually thereafter. Special areas for attention include the following:
• **Blood pressure (BP).** Measurement at the initial visit and annually thereafter is recommended. BP values for girls younger than 18 years should be assessed using standardized charts for age, gender, and height percentage; BP values for women older than 18 years may be assessed using adult guidelines (Table 21.3). Pediatric BP charts may be found on the National Heart, Lung, and Blood Institute website (http://www.nhlbi.nih.gov/guidelines/hypertension/child_tbl.pdf). Apps are also available for mobile devices (such as Stat Growthcharts).
• **Growth.** At the initial visit and annually thereafter, the adolescent's height and weight should be meas-

ured and plotted on growth charts. Body mass index (BMI) should be calculated and also plotted on the correct growth chart. Growth charts for adolescent girls can be found on the Centers for Disease Control and Prevention (CDC) website (http://www.cdc.gov/growthcharts). It is important to note that definitions of overweight and obese vary by age category. For girls and young women younger than 18 years, overweight is defined as greater than the 85th percentile for BMI for age, and obese is defined as greater than the 95th percentile for BMI for age. For women aged 18 years or older, the definition of overweight is a BMI greater than $25\,kg/m^2$, and of obese is a BMI greater than $30\,kg/m^2$. Mobile device apps are available (Stat Growthchart).
• **Menstrual history.** Now considered a vital sign, it is imperative to elicit the date of the patient's last menstrual period. Concurrently, it is important to obtain a menstrual history. If the patient is postmenarchal, the provider should ascertain the age at menarche, regularity of periods, presence and severity of dysmenorrhea, and quality of menstrual flow (i.e. light, moderate, or heavy).
• **Breast exam.** At initial visits with adolescent girls and annually thereafter, breast development should be assessed using Tanner staging (see Appendix 1.9.4). Clinical breast exams as a screening tool for breast cancer detection are not indicated until an adolescent reaches the age of 18–20 years (see Chapter 29.2).
• **Genitourinary.** At the initial visit for an adolescent girl, an external genitourinary exam should be

Table 21.2 HEEADSSS(S) screening questions

	Category	Sample questions
H	Home	Who do you live with at home? How do you get along with people at home? Do you feel safe at home?
E	Education/ employment	What school do you go to? What grade are you in? What types of grades do you usually make? What do you want to do after you finish school? Do you work? What type of work do you do, and how many hours a week do you work?
E	Eating	How do you feel about your body? What changes would you want to make to your weight or body? What do you usually eat? What are you doing to change your weight?
A	Activities	What do you like to do for fun? What do you do with your friends?
D	Drugs	Have you ever tried smoking cigarettes or marijuana or drinking alcohol? How often are you using? What do you think about quitting? What problems have you had because of using?
S	Sexuality	Are you attracted to males, females, or both? Are you in a relationship now? Have you ever had sex? How old were you when you first had sex? How often are you using condoms? Are you on any type of contraception or interested in it? Have you ever had a sexually-transmitted illness? Have you ever been pregnant?
S	Suicidality/depression	How would you describe your mood? Do you have trouble sleeping? Have you ever had any thoughts of or tried anything to hurt or kill yourself?
S	Safety	Has anyone been hurting you physically, emotionally, or sexually? Have you been bullied?
(S)	Spirituality	What do you consider to be your religion or spiritual background? How do your religious beliefs impact how you make decisions for your health?

Table 21.3 Blood pressure levels for girls by age and height percentile.

Age (Year)	BP Percentile ↓	Systolic BP (mmHg) ←Percentile of Height→							Diastolic BP (mmHg) ←Percentile of Height→						
		5th	10th	25th	50th	75th	90th	95th	5th	10th	25th	50th	75th	90th	95th
11	50th	100	101	102	103	105	106	107	60	60	60	61	62	63	63
	90th	114	114	116	117	118	119	120	74	74	74	75	76	77	77
	95th	118	118	119	121	122	123	124	78	78	78	79	80	81	81
	99th	125	125	126	128	129	130	131	85	85	86	87	87	88	89
12	50th	102	103	104	105	107	108	109	61	61	61	62	63	64	64
	90th	116	116	117	119	120	121	122	75	75	75	76	77	78	78
	95th	119	120	121	123	124	125	126	79	79	79	80	81	82	82
	99th	127	127	128	130	131	132	133	86	86	87	88	88	89	90
13	50th	104	105	106	107	109	110	110	62	62	62	63	64	65	65
	90th	117	118	119	121	122	123	124	76	76	76	77	78	79	79
	95th	121	122	123	124	126	127	128	80	80	80	81	82	83	83
	99th	128	129	130	132	133	134	135	87	87	88	89	89	90	91
14	50th	106	106	107	109	110	111	112	63	63	63	64	65	66	66
	90th	119	120	121	122	124	125	125	77	77	77	78	79	80	80
	95th	123	123	125	126	127	129	129	81	81	81	82	83	84	84
	99th	130	131	132	133	135	136	136	88	88	89	90	90	91	92
15	50th	107	108	109	110	111	113	113	64	64	64	65	66	67	67
	90th	120	121	122	123	125	126	127	78	78	78	79	80	81	81
	95th	124	125	126	127	129	130	131	82	82	82	83	84	85	85
	99th	131	132	133	134	136	137	138	89	89	90	91	91	92	93
16	50th	108	108	110	111	112	114	114	64	64	65	66	66	67	68
	90th	121	122	123	124	126	127	128	78	78	79	80	81	81	82
	95th	125	126	127	128	130	131	132	82	82	83	84	85	85	86
	99th	132	133	134	135	137	138	139	90	90	90	91	92	93	93
17	50th	108	109	110	111	113	114	115	64	65	65	66	67	67	68
	90th	122	122	123	125	126	127	128	78	79	79	80	81	81	82
	95th	125	126	127	129	130	131	132	82	83	83	84	85	85	86
	99th	133	133	134	136	137	138	139	90	90	91	91	92	93	93

Reproduced from Blood pressure guidelines by age and height percentiles for adolescent females. From http://www.nhlbi.nih .gov/guidelines/hypertension/child_tbl.pdf Source: National Heart, Lung, and Blood Institute; National Institutes of Health; U.S. Department of Health and Human Services. NHLBI.

performed to assess for development using Tanner staging and to look for any lesions or abnormal findings. If the patient discloses that she is sexually active and is experiencing symptoms, such as vaginal discharge, a pelvic exam is recommended (see Chapter 30.1). Per the 2009 ACOG guidelines, Pap smear tests are not recommended until the adolescent reaches 21 years of age (see Chapter 30.2).

✋ Caution

- While electronic medical records are gaining in popularity and ease of use, it is important to remember that their normative values (including those for BMI and BP) are not always pediatric or adolescent specific!
- Make sure to use appropriate growth charts and normative scales for girls under 18 years of age.

Screening recommendations

The following should be performed at the initial primary care visit or at specific time points during adolescence:

- **Vision.** At the initial visit with an adolescent girl, vision should be screened. Vision screening should occur at least once during each stage of adolescence and if the patient is reporting any visual difficulties.
- **Hearing.** If the adolescent reports difficulty hearing, screening tests should be performed and a referral provided if appropriate.
- **Lipid panel.** New guidelines released in 2011 by an expert panel appointed by the National Heart, Lung, and Blood Institute (and endorsed by the AAP) call for all adolescents, regardless of risk factors, to have their lipid panel checked between the ages of 9 and 11 years, with another full lipid screen performed between the ages of 18 and 21 years. Either a nonfasting total cholesterol screen or a fasting full lipid panel can be obtained.
- **Complete blood count (CBC).** If the patient reports a history of heavy menstrual bleeding, consider ordering a CBC at any stage of adolescence for evaluation of potential anemia. With normal test results, there is no need for annual screening unless the patient becomes symptomatic.

- **Sexually-transmitted infection (STI) screening.** If an adolescent is sexually active, routine STI screening should be conducted at her initial visit, with annual chlamydia screening (CDC guidelines). Consider testing for gonorrhea, trichomoniasis, human immunodeficiency virus (HIV), and syphilis.
- **Human chorionic gonadotropin (hCG) testing of urine.** This test should be performed for any postmenarchal girl who is sexually active and not on contraception or for any postmenarchal girl with irregular bleeding.
- **Tuberculosis screening.** Consider a tuberculin skin test (TST) or an interferon-gamma release assay (IGRA) blood test only if the adolescent has risk factors for tuberculosis exposure. A good resource for this topic is the "Red Book" published by the AAP (aapredbook.aappublications.org).

★ Tips and tricks

- Routine urinalysis is no longer recommended screening for adolescents.
- Consider urinalysis if a girl complains of urinary symptoms.
- A urine specimen (nonclean catch) can be sent for gonorrhea and chlamydia testing.

Vaccinations

At the initial visit, the immunization record of the patient should be reviewed and vaccines administered per the Advisory Committee on Immunization Practices (ACIP) schedule. This schedule may be viewed on the CDC website (http://www.cdc.gov/Vaccines/recs/schedules/child-schedule.htm). Remember that any visit with an adolescent patient should be considered a potential opportunity to "catch up" on immunizations (see Chapter 24). It is not uncommon to encounter an adolescent patient with incomplete vaccination records because many parents have elected to refuse vaccines for a myriad of reasons. It is important to continue to stress the importance of vaccination and to offer applicable vaccines to these patients. Human papillomavirus (HPV) vaccination in particular may have been deferred due to parental concerns about safety or lack of necessity.

♀ Pearls

- Remember that different ages represent different stages of adolescence; each is associated with particular features and challenges.
- Social history is best obtained using the HEEADDSSS format. Make all attempts to obtain this history while alone with the patient after a discussion of confidentiality.
- When evaluating BP and BMI for girls under the age of 18 years, make sure to refer to appropriate limits using normative charts.
- Universally recommended screenings for adolescent girls include vision, lipids (at 9–11 and 18–21 years of age), and STIs (if sexually active).

Further reading

Delisi K, Gold MA. The initial adolescent preventive care visit. *Clin Obstet Gynecol* 2008;51:190–204.

Goldenring JM, Rosen DS. Getting into adolescent heads: An essential update. *Contemp Pediatr* 2004;21:64–90.

Hagan JF, Shaw JS, Duncan P M (eds). *Bright Futures: Guidelines for Health Supervision of Infants, Children, and Adolescents*, 3rd edn.. Elk Grove Village, IL: American Academy of Pediatrics, 2008.

22.1 Overweight and obesity and gynecologic conditions

Stephanie Crewe[1] and Maria Trent[2]

[1]Division of Adolescent Medicine, Virginia Commonwealth University Medical Center, Richmond, VA, USA

[2]Department of Pediatrics, Johns Hopkins School of Medicine, Baltimore, MD, USA

Obesity among adolescents has reached epidemic proportions in the US and addressing obesity is a national health priority. Obesity is a well known risk factor in the development of medical and psychological consequences, including metabolic derangements, degenerative abnormalities, and adverse social–emotional outcomes. Reproductive health-related concerns and complications of obesity pose a unique challenge to providers of obstetric and gynecologic care. Identifying obesity as a related clinical issue and helping patients understand its relationship to basic reproductive health outcomes is an essential aspect of ongoing care.

Body mass index (BMI), a calculation based on the ratio of weight to height squared [weight (kg)/height $(m)^2$], is used to assess weight status because it is relatively easy to determine and has been shown to correlate with adiposity. In children and adolescents, obesity is defined as a BMI greater than or equal to the 95th percentile for age and overweight is defined as a BMI greater than or equal to the 85th percentile for age, but less than the 95th percentile (Table 22.1.1). Age and sex are considered when interpreting BMI percentiles in adolescents since the amount of body fat changes with age and also differs between males and females. Adults and adolescents over age 18 with a BMI of $25\,\text{kg/m}^2$ or greater are overweight, of $30\,\text{kg/m}^2$ or greater are obese, and of $40\,\text{kg/m}^2$ or greater are considered severely obese.

Evidence at a glance

- According to National Health and Nutrition Examination Survey (NHANES) 2007–2008 data, 17% of adolescents females aged 12–19 are obese, approximately three times the 5% of adolescents who were considered obese in the NHANES study conducted between 1976 and 1980.
- There are significant racial and ethnic differences in obesity prevalence among adolescent females:
  - Non-Hispanic black females (29.2%)
  - Non-Hispanic white Americans (14.5%)
  - Mexican-American females (17.4%).

Impact on health

The importance of identifying obese adolescent girls in clinical practice cannot be overemphasized because of its association with a number of adverse health consequences. It has been well documented that obese adolescents have a significant risk of becoming severely obese adults, thus increasing the likelihood of being diagnosed with potentially life-threatening conditions.

Practical Pediatric and Adolescent Gynecology, First Edition. Edited by Paula J. Adams Hillard.
© 2013 John Wiley & Sons, Ltd. Published 2013 by John Wiley & Sons, Ltd.

Table 22.1.1 Estimated BMI percentiles for adolescent and young adult females by age (12–20 years)

Age (years)	5th percentile	50th percentile	85th percentile	95th percentile
12	14.79	18.05	22.90	25.17
13	15.31	18.74	23.88	26.30
14	15.81	19.35	24.71	27.26
15	16.31	19.93	25.46	28.12
16	16.75	20.45	26.13	28.91
17	17.21	20.90	26.72	29.63
18	17.55	21.28	27.25	30.33
19	17.77	21.55	27.76	31.03
20	17.43	21.72	28.26	31.80

Adapted from Centers for Disease Control and Prevention, National Center for Health Statistics, CDC, http://www.cdc.gov/growthcharts/html_charts/bmiagerev.htm#females

Evidenced at a glance

Associations with obesity

- Chronic diseases:
  - Noninsulin dependent diabetes mellitus
  - Hypertension
  - Dyslipidemias
  - Nonalcoholic fatty liver disease
  - Orthopedic complications
  - Sleep abnormalities
- Reproductive health-related disorders:
  - Polycystic ovary syndrome
  - Menstrual disturbances
  - Infertility
  - Pregnancy-related complications
- Sociodemographic outcomes for obese adolescents as adults, compared to women who were not obese as adolescents:
  - Lower household incomes
  - Lower levels of education
  - Lower rates of marriage

Gynecologic and obstetric associations

Clinical and diagnostic assessments

The clinical assessment of an obese adolescent female can be potentially challenging based on the amount of abdominal adipose tissue. Abdominal or adnexal masses may be under-diagnosed and the determination of an acute abdomen may prove to be very difficult. Visualization of the cervix during a speculum exam may also be problematic among obese patients

✮ Tips and tricks

Caring for the obese patient

- Prepare office staff to manage overweight and obese patients in a sensitive manner from registration to the clinical examination.
- Make the office space easily accessible, waiting rooms comfortable, and triage areas private.
- Provide clinical staff with equipment that can reliably measure clinical parameters and perform examination:
  - Large adult and thigh blood pressure cuffs
  - Scales that accurately weighs patients over 300 lbs
  - Sufficiently large specula for pelvic examinations
  - Exam tables and gowns that are sufficiently sized for use by obese patients
- Promote clinician proficiency in skilled maneuvers to maximize successful and gentle pelvic examinations of patients (e.g. raising the legs with increased hip flexion for better view of the cervix).

because of vaginal sidewall prolapse, and may lead to discomfort, anxiety, and negative feelings about future pelvic examination and care-seeking behavior. Furthermore, transabdominal ultrasound evaluation may be extremely limited for the obese female, leading to inadequate visualization of pelvic structures. Transvaginal ultrasound can be effectively used to better visualize structures in patients who are able to tolerate the ultrasound probe and require additional imaging.

Menstrual disturbances

Obese adolescent girls may commonly present to their reproductive healthcare provider with abnormal menstrual cycles as their chief complaint and sole reason for the visit. Anovulation and menstrual cycle disturbances have been observed in patients with higher BMI but no other signs suggestive of polycystic ovary syndrome.

Polycystic ovary syndrome

Polycystic ovary syndrome (PCOS) is a common, heterogeneous reproductive endocrine disorder that is characterized by menstrual irregularities and hyperandrogenism, and typically presents during adolescence (Table 22.1.2). Although insulin resistance is not one of the diagnostic criteria for the disorder, it is a common feature of PCOS. Many adolescents with PCOS are obese or overweight and have an increased incidence of dyslipidemias, diabetes, and hypertension compared to normal-weight females with PCOS (see Chapter 50).

While the use of both combination hormonal contraceptives and antiandrogens such as spironolactone will regulate menses and reduce the clinical effects of acne and hirsutism, weight loss in obese patients with

PCOS often results in significant improvement in menstrual function and fertility.

Contraceptive conundrums

Nearly two-thirds of births to females younger than 18 and more than half among 18–19 year olds are unintended. For adolescent females, the lack of consistent contraceptive use as well as contraceptive failure rates account for the majority of these unplanned pregnancies. While obesity is not considered a contraindication for any method, obesity may result in lower contraceptive efficacy for some methods. It is important to screen for possible comorbidities (e.g. hypertension) and to use the U.S. Medical Eligibility for Contraceptive guidelines (http://www.cdc.gov/mmwr/pdf/rr/rr59e0528.pdf) to counsel young women on the benefits of contraception in the context of obesity.

Pregnancy-related complications

Among adolescent and adult females, maternal obesity has been linked to an increased risk for many pregnancy-related complications, including gestational diabetes, hypertensive complications, prematurity, stillbirth, postpartum hemorrhage, and increased cesarean delivery rates. Childbearing among adolescent females, particularly obese teens, presents additional challenges and increases the risks of adverse maternal and fetal outcomes, such as preterm birth, low birth weight, pre-eclampsia, and cesarean delivery. The Institute of Medicine has recently published recommendations for maternal weight gain during pregnancy designed to both ensure healthy development of the fetus as well as prevention of adverse maternal–fetal outcomes (Table 22.1.3).

Table 22.1.2 Diagnostic criteria for polycystic ovary syndrome*

- Menstrual irregularity (e.g. anovulation/oligo-ovulation)
- Clinical or laboratory evidence of androgen excess
- Polycystic ovaries on ultrasound

*After ruling out other causes of androgen excess, two of the three clinical criteria must be met.

Table 22.1.3 Recommendations for total weight gain during pregnancy based on prepregnancy BMI

Prepregnancy BMI	Total weight gain (lbs)
Underweight (<18.5 kg/m^2)	28–40
Normal weight (18.5–24.9 kg/m^2)	25–35
Overweight (25.0–29.9 kg/m^2)	15–25
Obese (≥30 kg/m^2)	11–20

Surgical considerations

Preoperative evaluation should be used to determine potential risks that might complicate a gynecologic procedure. Obesity increases patient risk for having comorbid conditions such as cardiovascular disease, diabetes mellitus, and obstructive sleep apnea. It also increases a patient's risk for poor wound healing and deep venous thromboses in the postoperative period. It is important to identify all comorbid conditions in the preoperative assessment, and ensure venous access can be obtained, the risks of DVTs minimized, and an adequate airway can be maintained. A careful discussion that includes the risks of complications should take place prior to gynecologic procedures, and close follow-up is warranted to assess wound healing and recovery.

Screening

As part of each annual visit, weight and height should be assessed and BMI should be calculated. These measurements should subsequently be compared to appropriate age and gender normative values. Normative measures, growth charts, and patient handouts can be found on the Centers for Disease Control and Prevention website (http://www.cdc.gov/growthcharts/). If it is determined that an adolescent is overweight or obese, a dietary and general health assessment, including past medical and family history, should be obtained to identify the presence of and risk for chronic medical problems, and medication use or behaviors that are influencing weight status. The HEADDSSS assessment can be a useful approach to the social history (see Chapter 21).

Clinical examination should focus on the chief complaint, but also identify clinical signs of obesity-associated comorbidities (Table 22.1.4). Clinical history and examination should guide screening for reproductive endocrine disorders (e.g. PCOS, thyroid disease) beyond recommendations for routine screening laboratories. Screening for coexisting or evolving psychologic issues will be helpful in determining a strategic approach to clinical management and counseling.

Management

Obesity among adolescent females is a multifactorial problem which requires treatment strategies that utilize a multifaceted approach to achieve successful short- and long-term outcomes. Once patients are

Table 22.1.4 Conditions to screen for during routine care of the overweight or obese adolescent

Condition	Assessment	Abnormal finding
Hypertension	Blood pressure measurement	95% Female sitting BP by age:
		12 years 126/82 mmHg
		13 years 128/83 mmHg
		14 years 129/85 mmHg
		15 years 130/86 mmHg
		16 years 131/85 mmHg
		17 years 132/84 mmHg
		18 years 132/84 mmHg
		If elevated, arrange repeat on three separate visits
Diabetes/glucose intolerance	Skin examination	Acanthosis nigricans (insulin resistance)
	Random glucose	≥200 mg/dL
	Fasting glucose	≥126 mg/dL
	2-hour glucose tolerance	>140 mg/dL (glucose intolerance)
		>200 mg/dL (diabetes)
Hyperlipidemia	Total cholesterol	>180–200 mg/dL
		If abnormal repeat fasting level

identified as overweight or obese, practitioners have an inherent challenge to provide developmentally appropriate, culturally sensitive, and pragmatic guidance that is achievable and unique to the individual patient. Current clinical management strategies for the treatment of adolescent obesity primarily include dietary modification and behavioral change therapies involving physical activity. The first step for the development of a behavior plan is to identify the adolescent's stage of change (Table 22.1.5) so that the recommendations match the behaviors to which the patient is capable of adhering. Pharmacologic therapy and surgical interventions have been identified as potential alternatives, but are considered secondary and tertiary options after failure of intensive lifestyle modification and if significant comorbidities persist.

Dietary interventions/physical activity

Therapeutic lifestyle change (TLC) is the foundation for treatment of obese adolescent females. TLC focuses on adopting healthy eating practices, increasing aerobic physical activity, as well as minimizing sedentary activities, such as prolonged TV viewing and excessive computer use. Dietary interventions should promote the consumption of fiber-rich food sources, emphasize the reduction of high fat foods and sugar-sweetened beverages, and endorse portion control. Patients should be encouraged to choose aerobic activities that are enjoyable and should participate in these activities for at least 1 hour per day on most days of the week.

Table 22.1.5 Stages of behavioral change

Precontemplation	No interest in weight loss
Contemplation	Ambivalent about weight loss – weigh the benefits versus barriers
Preparation	Begin to prepare for weight loss activities. May make small changes (switch from sugared beverages to water or zero-calorie sweeteners; research prices and classes at local gym)
Action	Actively engaged in weight loss behaviors (e.g. regular exercise, dietary changes)
Maintenance	Keep up behaviors initiated during the action phase
Relapse	Patient engages in unhealthy behaviors. Feels demoralized. Supportive measures such as motivational interviewing that allow the patient to acknowledge the period of success are important for moving them back through stages of change

---

🔬 Science revisited

Pharmacologic therapy of obesity

- Two drugs, sibutramine and orlistat, have been studied in adolescents for weight loss.
- Sibutramine, an FDA-approved medication permitted in adolescents over the age of 16 years, functions to promote satiety and enhances energy expenditure by inhibiting the reuptake of norepinephrine and serotonin.
   - Major side effects include elevated blood pressure, palpitations, and headaches.
- Orlistat, an FDA-approved medication permitted in adolescents over the age of 12 years, is not systemically absorbed and blocks fat absorption by inhibiting intestinal lipase.
   - Malabsorption of fat soluble vitamins and oily stools are untoward side effects associated with its use.
   - An over-the-counter formulation of orlistat can be purchased by patients without a prescription.
   - It is recommended that patients consult a physician prior to initiating any therapeutic agent for obesity management.
- Based on the known side effect profiles, medication use is not considered first line therapy in weight reduction management plans for obese adolescent females.

Surgical interventions

Surgery is not considered a primary treatment option for adolescent obesity. Consideration for surgical intervention (e.g. laparoscopic banding, gastric bypass) is suggested for severely obese adolescents whose BMI is greater than 50 or greater than 40 with comorbidities, and the potential candidate has failed a structured lifestyle modification program. Cognitive maturity and emotional stability of the adolescent are considered additional requirements when this option is considered as patients will still need to be sufficiently motivated to maintain a healthy lifestyle that incorporates dietary restrictions following surgical intervention.

✋ Patient/parent advice

Useful advice can be found at:
• American Academy of Pediatrics, Changing Your Role: Helping Your Overweight Adolescents. http://www.healthychildren.org/English/health-issues/conditions/obesity/pages/Your-Changing-Role-Helping-Your-Overweight-Teen.aspx
• Centers for Disease Control and Prevention, Healthy Weight – It's not a diet, it's a lifestyle! http://www.cdc.gov/healthyweight/assessing/bmi/childrens_bmi/about_childrens_bmi.html
• Polycystic Ovary Syndrome (PCOS): A Guide for Teens; Center for Young Women's Health, Boston Children's Hospital. http://www.youngwomenshealth.org/pcosinfo.html

Summary

Providers of reproductive health services are in a unique position to advise adolescent girls and young adult women on healthy weight behaviors in the context of ongoing care. As such, they must be cognizant of the distinct developmental stages and supportive needs of this population of patients. Screening for obesity and associated comorbidities, promoting weight control, healthy eating, and physical activity in adolescent girls is a key first step in obesity prevention. Weight loss is a long process that is fraught with everyday struggles to prevent relapse; however, small changes in lifestyle and weight (5–10 lbs) can have positive life-altering effects. Patients will need to partner with health providers in a variety of settings to achieve these modest goals.

Further reading

ACOG Committee on Adolescent Health Care. The overweight adolescent: prevention, treatment and obstetric-gynecologic implications. ACOG Committee Opinion No. 351, American College of Obstetricians and Gynecologists. *Obstet Gynecol* 2006;108(5):1337–1348.

Bruni V, Dei M, Peruzzi E, Seravalli V. The anorectic and obese adolescent. *Best Pract Res Clin Obstet Gynaecol* 2010;24:243–258.

Haeri, S, Guichard I, Baker AM, Saddlemire S, Boggess KA. The effect of teenage maternal obesity on perinatal outcomes. *Obstet Gynecol* 2009;113(2):300–308.

Rasmussen KM, Yaktine AL, the Committee to Re-Examine IOM Pregnancy Weight Guidelines, Weight Gain during Pregnancy: Re-Examining the Guidelines. National Academy of Sciences, 2009. Available at www.nap.edu

22.2 Eating disorders

Anne Hsii and Neville H. Golden

Department of Pediatrics, Division of Adolescent Medicine, Stanford University School of Medicine, Stanford, CA, USA

Eating disorders are prevalent in adolescent females, and may present to the gynecologist or primary clinician with menstrual irregularities and not necessarily with weight concerns. A thorough medical evaluation is warranted, and an eating disorder should be considered in the differential diagnosis.

☆ Tips and tricks

In an adolescent presenting with amenorrhea or menstrual irregularities, consider an underlying eating disorder.

This chapter will describe the diagnostic criteria, signs and symptoms, medical assessment, and treatment of eating disorders in adolescents.

☋ Science revisited

There are three major groups of eating disorders, as outlined in the Diagnostic and Statistical Manual of Mental Disorders, Fourth Edition, Text Revision (DSM-IV-TR)*:

- Anorexia nervosa (AN)
- Bulimia nervosa (BN)
- Eating disorder not otherwise specified (EDNOS).

*Proposed changes for DSM-5 are available at www.dsm5.org

Evidence at a glance

- Anorexia nervosa:
  - Point prevalence in adolescent females is estimated to be 0.1–0.4%
  - Lifetime prevalence 0.5–1%
  - Genetic predisposition: 9:1 female predominance
  - Onset in early to mid adolescence
- Bulimia nervosa:
  - Higher point prevalence than AN, estimated to be 0.4–4%
  - In contrast to AN, onset is in older adolescents

Anorexia nervosa

Features of AN include (see also Table 22.2.1):
- Refusal to maintain a weight at or above the minimally normal weight for age and height
- An intense fear of weight gain even though the person is underweight
- Body image distortion
- Amenorrhea.

AN is associated with serious medical and psychiatric morbidity and a mortality of 2–8%, six times that of the general population. Approximately 50% of deaths are due to complications of AN, 25% to suicide, and 25% to unrelated causes. Up to 80% of

Practical Pediatric and Adolescent Gynecology, First Edition. Edited by Paula J. Adams Hillard.
© 2013 John Wiley & Sons, Ltd. Published 2013 by John Wiley & Sons, Ltd.

Table 22.2.1 DSM-IV-TR Criteria for eating disorders

Anorexia nervosa

A. Refusal to maintain body weight at or above minimally normal weight for age and height (e.g. weight loss leading to maintenance of body weight less than 85% of that expected; or failure to make expected weight gain during period of growth, leading to body weight less than 85% of that expected)

B. Intense fear of gaining weight or becoming fat, even though underweight

C. Disturbance in the way in which one's body weight or shape is experienced, undue influence of body weight or shape on self-evaluation, or denial of the seriousness of the current low body weight

D. In postmenarcheal females, amenorrhea, i.e. the absence of at least three consecutive menstrual cycles. (A woman is considered to have amenorrhea if her periods occur only following hormone, e.g. estrogen administration)

Specify type:

Restricting type: during the current episodes of anorexia nervosa, the person has not regularly engaged in binge-eating or purging behavior (i.e. self-induced vomiting or the misuse of laxatives, diuretics, or enemas)

Binge-eating/purging type: during the current episode of anorexia nervosa, the person has regularly engaged in binge-eating or purging behavior (i.e. self-induced vomiting or the misuse of laxatives, diuretics, or enemas)

Bulimia nervosa

A. Recurrent episodes of binge eating. An episode of binge eating is characterized by both of the following:

    1. Eating, in a discrete period of time (e.g. within any 2-hour period), an amount of food that is definitely larger than most people would eat during a similar period of time and under similar circumstances

    2. A sense of lack of control over eating during the episode (e.g. a feeling that one cannot stop eating or control what or how much one is eating)

B. Recurrent inappropriate compensatory behavior in order to prevent weight gain, such as self-induced vomiting; misuse of laxatives, diuretics, enemas, or other medications; fasting; or excessive exercise

C. The binge eating and inappropriate compensatory behaviors both occur, on average, at least twice a week for 3 months

D. Self-evaluation is unduly influenced by body shape and weight

E. The disturbance does not occur exclusively during episodes of anorexia nervosa

Specify type:

Purging type: during the current episode of bulimia nervosa, the person has regularly engaged in self-induced vomiting or the misuse of laxatives, diuretics, or enemas

Nonpurging type: during the current episode of bulimia nervosa, the person has used other inappropriate compensatory behaviors, such as fasting or excessive exercise, but has not regularly engaged in self-induced vomiting or the misuse of laxatives, diuretics, or enemas

Eating disorder not otherwise specified

The eating disorders not otherwise specified category is for disorders that do not meet the criteria for any specific eating disorder. Examples include:

1. For females, all of the criteria for anorexia nervosa are met except that the individual has regular menses

2. All of the criteria for anorexia nervosa are met except that, despite significant weight loss, the individual's current weight is in the normal range

3. All of the criteria for bulimia nervosa are met except that the binge eating and inappropriate compensatory mechanisms occur at a frequency of less than twice a week or for a duration of less than 3 months

4. The regular use of inappropriate compensatory behavior by an individual of normal body weight after eating small amounts of food (e.g. self-induced vomiting after the consumption of two cookies)

5. Repeatedly chewing and spitting out, but not swallowing, large amounts of food

6. Binge-eating disorder: recurrent episodes of binge eating in the absence of the regular use of inappropriate compensatory behaviors characteristic of bulimia nervosa

---

patients with AN also have comorbid psychiatric disorders, especially depression and anxiety disorders [including social phobia and obsessive–compulsive disorder (OCD)].

Bulimia nervosa

Features of BN include (see also Table 22.2.1):
• Binge eating
• Inappropriate compensatory methods to prevent weight gain
• Preoccupation with body shape and weight.

Mortality is rare in BN, but BN is still associated with major medical and psychiatric morbidity. Like patients with AN, up to 83% of patients with BN have comorbid psychiatric disorders, including mood disorders (>50%) and substance use disorders (25%).

Eating disorder not otherwise specified

This category describes eating disorders that do not meet all criteria for AN or BN and encompasses a wide spectrum of conditions, including binge eating disorder and the female athlete triad. Patients with EDNOS may also have serious medical and psychiatric morbidity.

The female athlete triad (see Chapter 23) is comprised of three components:
• Energy deficit
• Low bone mineral density (BMD) for age
• Menstrual disturbances, including amenorrhea.

In these patients, caloric intake is insufficient for energy expenditure. Some of these athletes may be eating normally for a nonathlete, but are not eating enough to meet their energy needs as an athlete. Such patients will respond well to nutritional intervention and do not have an eating disorder; others, especially those resistant to caloric increases, may have an underlying eating disorder. Those at greatest risk for the female athlete triad are elite athletes in aesthetic sports (e.g. gymnastics, ice skating) or in sports that have a weight class (e.g. wrestling, judo), but the triad can also occur in recreational athletes.

Presenting signs and symptoms

Clinical presentation depends on degree of weight loss and/or behaviors related to weight control.

Menstrual irregularities include primary amenorrhea, oligomenorrhea, and secondary amenorrhea. Amenorrhea usually follows weight loss in AN, but up to 20% of patients may present with amenorrhea before significant weight loss. Additional clinical signs and symptoms of AN and BN are listed in Table 22.2.2.

Medical assessment

Adolescents presenting with menstrual irregularities should be asked about dietary intake, exercise, and body image concerns (Table 22.2.3). Physical findings, including vital sign abnormalities, may also support the possibility of an eating disorder (Table 22.2.2). Accurate height and weight should be measured, and body mass index (BMI) calculated [weight in kg/(height in meters)^2]. These measurements should be plotted on the CDC growth charts (available at www.cdc.gov/growthcharts) to assess appropriateness for age and height.

★ **Tips and tricks**

Ask screening questions and if you suspect an eating disorder, obtain appropriate referral.

Baseline laboratory tests are recommended to exclude infectious, inflammatory, and malignant causes of weight loss and amenorrhea/irregular menses (Table 22.2.4). The medical assessment may raise concerns that broaden the differential diagnosis of weight loss and menstrual issues and may warrant additional tests, such as an upper gastrointestinal/small bowel series, celiac screen, or MRI of the head. Baseline laboratory tests may identify electrolyte disturbances (hypokalemia, hypophosphatemia, hypomagnesemia), anemia, leukopenia, thrombocytopenia, elevated liver function tests, elevated amylase, low T3 syndrome, and evidence of hypothalamic amenorrhea [suppressed luteinizing hormone, follicle-stimulating hormone, and estradiol levels). An electrocardiogram may reveal bradycardia, prolonged QTc, and other arrhythmias. Medical complications include pubertal delay and growth retardation in AN, esophagitis in BN, and cortical brain atrophy seen on

Table 22.2.2 Clinical signs and symptoms of eating disorders

	Anorexia nervosa	Bulimia nervosa
Weight	Low	Marked fluctuation Usually normal, may be high or low
Menses	Amenorrhea (primary or secondary)	Usually regular, may be irregular
General	Cold intolerance Hypothermia Fatigue Dizziness Weakness Syncope	Dizziness Syncope
Oral		Dental enamel erosion Palatal petechiae Parotid hypertrophy
Cardiorespiratory	Bradycardia Hypotension Orthostasis Edema	Chest pain Palpitations Orthostasis Edema
Gastrointestinal	Early satiety Abdominal discomfort/pain Bloating Constipation	Gastroesophageal reflux disease Hematemesis
Endocrine	Short stature Pubertal delay Loss of libido Infertility	
Dermatologic	Lanugo Dry skin Hair loss Brittle hair and nails Acrocyanosis Hypercarotenemia Poor wound healing	Calluses on knuckles or back of hand due to self-induced vomiting (Russell sign)
Musculoskeletal	Proximal muscle wasting Fractures	
Neuropsychiatric	Seizures Poor concentration Irritability Depression Anxiety Obsessive–compulsive disorder Self-harm Suicidal ideation/attempt	Seizures Irritability Self-harm Suicidal ideation/attempt

Table 22.2.3 Screening questions for eating disorders

Weight and body image
- What was your highest weight at your current height? When was that?
- What was your lowest weight at your current height? When was that?
- What weight change (loss/gain) have you had over what time period?
- How do you think about your current weight (underweight, normal, overweight)?
- What would you like to weigh?
- What are your thoughts about gaining weight?
- Are there body parts you are unhappy with and would like to change? What parts?

Nutrition
- Tell me what you have eaten in the last 24 hours (food items, quantities).
- Have you stopped eating certain foods that you used to eat?
- Do you count calories/carbohydrates/fats?
- Do you drink caffeine? How much? How often?
- Do you take any nutritional supplements or multivitamins?

Exercise
- Do you exercise? If so, what type of exercise do you do?
- How long do you exercise each time (minutes/day)?
- How often do you exercise (days/week)?
- How intense is your exercise (e.g. recreational vs organized sport; level of sport)?
- Do you feel stressed if you miss exercising?

Behaviors
- Have you tried to control or lose weight by using: laxatives, diuretics, diet pills, ipecac, self-induced vomiting?
- Do you feel out of control when you eat? If you do, what do you eat and how much? How often does this happen? What do you do to compensate?

Menstrual history
- When was the onset of breast development?
- When did you have your first menstrual period?
- What is the frequency and duration of menses?
- When was your last normal menstrual period?

Family history
Medical and psychiatric (including eating disorders; mental illnesses, especially anxiety, depression, obsessive compulsive disorder; substance use/abuse)

Table 22.2.4 Recommended baseline tests

Laboratory tests
- CBC, ESR
- Chemistries, including electrolytes, BUN/creatinine, calcium, phosphorus, magnesium, LFTs, albumin
- TFTs: free T4, TSH, and total T3
- 25-OH vitamin D
- Serum amylase (if purging)
- LH, FSH, estradiol, prolactin (if amenorrheic)

Other tests
- EKG
- Urinalysis: specific gravity and pH
- DXA (if amenorrheic >6 months)

MRI in patients with AN. Indications of medical instability warranting inpatient hospitalization are listed in Table 22.2.5.

A bone densitometry (DXA) scan is recommended in patients with amenorrhea for more than 6 months or a history of recurrent or low impact fractures. In adolescents who may not yet have achieved peak bone mass, Z-scores (SD below age-matched norms) should be used in preference to T-scores (young adult norms) to assess bone mass and fracture risk.

Management

A patient suspected of having an eating disorder should be referred for evaluation and treatment to specialists experienced in the management of eating disorders. The interdisciplinary team typically consists of a physician, dietician, therapist, and psychiatrist as indicated. Medical goals of treatment are to reverse medical complications, maintain medical stability, restore weight, resume regular menses, and eliminate eating disorder behaviors. A therapist works with the adolescent and family through family-based or individual therapy. The Maudsley family-based therapy, in which parents oversee their adolescent's nutritional decisions and intake, and gradually allow their teenager to resume nutritional responsibilities with the guidance of a therapist and dietician, has been shown to be very effective in adolescents with eating disorders. In BN, cognitive-behavioral therapy is the modality most frequently used. The dietician monitors macro- and micro-

Table 22.2.5 Indications for hospitalization in an adolescent with an eating disorder

One or more of the following justify hospitalization:
• Severe malnutrition (weight <75% average body weight for age, sex, and height)
• Dehydration
• Electrolyte disturbances (hypokalemia, hyponatremia, hypophosphatemia)
• Cardiac dysrhythmia
• Physiologic instability:
  ○ Severe bradycardia (pulse <50 beats/min in daytime, <45 beats/min at night)
  ○ Hypotension (<80/50 mmHg)
  ○ Hypothermia (body temperature < 96 °F)
  ○ Orthostatic changes in pulse (>20 beats/min) or blood pressure (>10 mmHg)
• Arrested growth and development
• Failure of outpatient treatment
• Acute food refusal
• Uncontrollable binging and purging
• Acute medical complications of malnutrition (e.g. syncope, seizures, cardiac failure, pancreatitis, etc.)
• Acute psychiatric emergencies (e.g. suicidal ideation, acute psychosis)
• Comorbid diagnosis that interferes with the treatment of the eating disorder (e.g. severe depression, obsessive–compulsive disorder, severe family dysfunction)

Reproduced from Golden NH, Katzman DK, Kreipe RE, *et al.* Eating disorders in adolescents. Position paper of the Society for Adolescent Medicine. *J Adolesc Health* 2003;33:496, with permission from Elsevier.

nutrient intake and guides the patient towards intuitive eating.

Resumption of menses occurs with weight restoration, usually when weight reaches approximately 90% of median body weight (MBW) and the estradiol level is greater than 30 pg/mL. Continued weight gain may be necessary in those who have achieved a weight greater than 90% MBW but have not yet resumed menses. An estradiol level greater than 30 pg/mL is predictive of resumption of menses within 3–6 months in 90% of patients. Oral contraceptives have not been demonstrated to improve BMD in patients with AN and should not be prescribed for this purpose alone. It also often gives patients a false sense that they are at a healthy weight. Oral contraceptives can be used for other reasons, such as pregnancy prevention.

> ✋ **Caution**
>
> Oral contraceptives should not be used solely for regulation of menses or improvement of bone mineral density in patients with anorexia nervosa.

For those who fail outpatient treatment, higher levels of care are available. Intensive outpatient programs (IOPs), partial hospitalization programs (PHPs), and residential programs provide intensive therapy and nutritional counseling. IOPs and PHPs allow patients to continue living at home, and generally require medical follow-up with their regular physician. Residential programs require patients to live in housing provided by the program, and have medical, dietary, and therapy components in place.

Psychotropic medications are not effective for promoting weight gain in AN. Fluoxetine has been shown to be helpful in BN, reducing binge eating and purging behaviors. Psychotropics may be indicated for the treatment of comorbid anxiety, depression, or OCD. A psychiatric consult is advisable to help with management of psychotropic medications.

Prognosis

Recovery rates vary widely, depending on treatment course, behaviors, and other comorbid disorders. It is estimated that in adults with AN, approximately one-third achieve full recovery, one-third partial recovery with relapses, and one-third do not recover. Recovery rates in adolescents are much higher: 50–78% fully recover, 20% partially recover, and 10–20% do not recover. Adolescents receiving the Maudsley family-based therapy method have better recovery rates, with approximately 75% achieving full recovery. Early intervention is associated with improved outcomes. Recovery rates for those with BN vary from 35% to 85%, but it is estimated that one-third relapse within 1–2 years of recovery.

✋ Patient/parent advice

The following are useful resources for parents:

National Eating Disorders Association (NEDA): www.nationaleatingdisorders.org

National Institute of Mental Health (NIMH): www.nimh.nih.gov/health/topics/eating-disorders/index.shtml

Something Fishy, Website on Eating Disorders: www.something-fishy.org

Lock J, Le Grange D. *Help Your Teenager Beat An Eating Disorder.* New York: The Guilford Press, 2005.

Zucker N. *Off the C.U.F.F: A Parent Skills Book for the Management of Disordered Eating.* Duke University Medical Center, 2006.

Further reading

Academy for Eating Disorders. *Eating Disorders: Critical Points for Early Recognition and Medical Risk Management in the Care of Individuals with Eating Disorders.* 2011. www.aedweb.org/AM/Template.cfm?Section=Resources_for_Professionals&Template=/CM/ContentDisplay.cfm&ContentID=2779

Golden NH, Katzman DK, Kreipe RE, *et al.* Eating disorders in adolescents. Position paper of the Society for Adolescent Medicine. *J Adolesc Health* 2003;33:496.

Rosen DS, Committee on Adolescence. Clinical Report: Identification and management of eating disorder in children and adolescents. *Pediatrics* 2010;126:1240.

23 The female athlete

James R. Ebert

Departments of Pediatrics and Community Health, Wright State University Boonshoft School of Medicine, Dayton, OH, USA

Athletic participation is typically a health-enhancing behavior, with positive effects physically, socially, and emotionally. However, sports may also result in adverse consequences involving the breast and the uterus, as well as orthopedic issues that are unique to women. The breasts are affected primarily through mechanical events. The uterine manifestations of athletics may include oligomenorrhea or amenorrhea. These alterations in the menstrual cycle result from hormonal and metabolic changes associated with the exercise, as well as changes in dietary patterns. Young female athletes are at increased risk for certain lower extremity musculoskeletal syndromes. A full discussion of these orthopedic issues is beyond the scope of this chapter, but such issues may surface during a gynecologic encounter with an athlete and warrant further evaluation. Bone health, important for young athletes, is linked to the issues of dietary choices, exercise intensity, and the hormonal alterations that present clinically as reduction in frequency or flow of menses. Collaboration with other professionals may be required for optimal care of athletes.

The breasts

The breasts may be subjected to direct blunt trauma during contact sports. Soft tissue injury may result, accompanied by ecchymoses of the overlying skin and localized tenderness and swelling. Painful ecchymosis may indicate the presence of a hematoma, which can be localized and drained with ultrasonography, resulting in relief of pain and more rapid resolution. Traumatic fat necrosis may also occur, which can result in findings on palpation and images on mammography that are difficult to distinguish from carcinoma. Such lesions tend to regress over time. Serial examination is sufficient management in the majority of cases.

The nipples are susceptible to abrasion in athletes. Friction with the athletic jersey or undergarment is the usual cause, and the risk is related to the extent of the contact. So-called "runner's nipples" can be prevented by the wearing of a compressive athletic bra or by the application of adhesive bandage strips over the nipples during activity.

> ### ✋ Patient/parent advice
>
> A compressive athletic bra will prevent most breast problems associated with sports requiring running and jumping.

Musculoskeletal injuries

Growing adolescents are susceptible to a variety of musculoskeletal injures, both acute and chronic, that are the result of open growth plates, a thicker

---

periosteum, less mineralization compared to adults, and a greater tendency to develop chondral or osteochondral fragmentation from overuse. The geometric alignment of the female pelvis and lower extremities makes knee pain syndromes more common in female athletes. Any report of bone or joint pain related to sports activity in an adolescent female athlete warrants further evaluation by a sports medicine or orthopedic specialist.

Sports and training activity should be quantified accurately, including hours of participation daily, miles run or laps swum, changes in intensity, and rest days taken. Musculoskeletal pain may be caused by an overly aggressive training regimen, and may indicate the presence of an overuse injury such as a stress fracture. Referral to an orthopedic surgeon or sports medicine physician is recommended. An elite athlete may benefit from consulting a certified athletic trainer for a comprehensive evaluation of her training and conditioning program even in the absence of musculoskeletal symptoms.

★ Tips and tricks

- Athletes are highly driven individuals who understand the importance of teamwork.
- Know her goals when formulating recommendations.
- Use team-oriented language in making referrals in order to improve adherence.

Osteoporosis, defined as bone mineral density (BMD) less than 2.5 standard deviations (SD) below peak bone mass in adults, and osteopenia, defined as BMD greater than 1 and less than 2.5 SD below peak bone mass, are best evaluated with dual beam X-ray absorptiometry (DXA) but may present clinically with bone pain and the finding of stress fracture by routine X-ray or bone scan. Risk factors include amenorrhea, family history of osteoporosis, Caucasian race, lean body habitus, glucocorticoid use, anticonvulsant use, or the presence of conditions such as thyroid disorder or diabetes. Smoking and alcohol consumption are also risk factors, but are less commonly associated with competitive female athletes.

Prevention of osteopenia and osteoporosis requires close attention to dietary history. Inadequate intake of calcium and vitamin D are common findings on nutritional screening. Calcium excretion is promoted by the consumption of carbonated and caffeinated beverages, as well as the high-protein dietary supplements that are actively marketed to young athletes. Daily calcium intake for adolescent female athletes should be at least 1300 mg. Vitamin D intake should be at least 400 mg daily. Numerous over-the-counter and prescription products are available at low cost, including combinations of calcium and vitamin D.

Management of stress fractures and other manifestations of diminished BMD include restoration of normal menses through use of oral contraceptive pills or other physiologic hormone replacement methods, adequate calcium intake, elimination of modifiable risk factors, and temporary reduction in the intensity of training.

The uterus

Exercise-associated amenorrhea (EAA) occurs in as many as 66% of athletes, and has been reported in women participating in nearly all sports. The cause is believed to be hypothalamic, involving the suppression of gonadotropic-releasing hormones. Associated predisposing factors include the onset of competitive training prior to menarche, delayed menarche, inadequate caloric intake, intensity of training regimen, low body weight, adolescent or young adult, and demonstrated hormone changes with exercise. EAA is a diagnosis of exclusion. In addition to the guidance in evaluating amenorrhea provided in Chapter 40, you should obtain a history of athletic training, including onset, duration, intensity, and frequency. Any history of stress fractures or other injuries is important, as is any history of disordered eating. Amenorrhea is a defining component of the female athlete triad, a syndrome described in physically active women which also includes osteoporosis and disordered eating.

Nutrition and eating disorders

The disordered eating of the female athlete triad may not completely fulfill the DSM-IV criteria for either anorexia nervosa or bulimia nervosa (see Table 22.2.1), but commonly includes such behaviors as

⚛ Science revisited

- Exercise associated amenorrhea (EAA) is most commonly associated with low gonadotropins and hypoestrogenism resulting from disturbance of the hypothalamic–pituitary–ovarian axis. There is suppression of the pulsatile release of gonadotropin-releasing hormone (GnRH), which occurs less often than the normal 60–90-minute pattern.
- GnRH suppression reduces pituitary secretion of luteinizing hormone (LH), which reduces the ovarian production of estradiol.
- This profile is most common in sports where low body weight is desired or encouraged, and caloric intake may be restricted (gymnastics, ballet, running).
- Women participating in sports where the emphasis is on strength and endurance (swimmers, racquet sports) may have hormone profiles showing elevated LH:FSH ratios, normal estrogens, and higher androgens, resembling polycystic ovary syndrome. This constellation in amenorrheic athletes is less common and not as well studied as the EAA associated with thinness.
- Ongoing research may establish a clearer role for leptin, secreted by adipocytes, which appears to influence bone metabolism, regulate the basal metabolic rate, and interact with receptors in the hypothalamus that regulate GnRH secretion.

self-induced vomiting, chewing and spitting out without swallowing food, recurrent binging, fasting, and the use of diuretics, laxatives, or enemas.

Female athletes are under significant pressure to achieve a low percentage of body fat. Cultural expectations, peer pressure, commercial marketing and advertising, and even some misguided coaches and trainers are to blame. The optimal percentage of body fat typically falls in a range determined by individual performance and nutrition needs. The beliefs that "every sport has an ideal body weight" or "the thinner, the better" should be rejected. Rather than prescribing a specific weight, a range should be provided to the athlete, accompanied by proper nutritional guidance to prevent deficiencies in essential

nutrients. Consultation with a registered dietician should be considered if weight reduction recommendations are to be made, or if there has been a recent change in weight of 5% or more.

⚛ Caution

- There is a widespread false belief that the leaner the athlete, the better her performance in sport.
- Extremes in dieting and training may result in nutritional compromise, and increase the risk of developing an eating disorder.
- Monitor the athlete closely for weight loss of more than 5%, or unrealistic expectations regarding reduction in weight or body fat percentage.

Nutritional myths are rampant among athletes of both sexes. The sale of nutritional adjuncts is a multimillion dollar industry, and young athletes are the prime target. Protein supplements, mostly whey or soy-based, may replace meat products in the diet, resulting in a deficiency of iron and subsequent hypochromic, microcytic anemia. Overemphasis on protein intake combined with caloric restriction to achieve weight loss can increase calcium excretion, even in the face of adequate calcium intake. Replacement of conventional meals, including the universally recommended five daily servings of fruits and vegetables, with athletic beverages, powder additives, shakes, energy bars, and other commercially prepared foods may result in vitamin, mineral, and trace element deficiencies. Such products are characteristically low in fiber, predisposing to other gastrointestinal disorders when consumed in place of conventional meals and healthy snacks.

The evaluation of menstrual disorders in adolescent athletes needs to include an assessment of her beliefs about ideal body weight, and explore her physical self-perception. If the interview suggests an eating disorder, referral to a mental health provider or an eating disorder specialist is indicated. A dietary history is essential, and should include a 24-hour recall of all food and beverage intake. The involvement of a registered dietician for assessment and teaching is the logical next step, especially if the patient's nutritional practices are significantly aberrant. Elite athletes or athletes in whom a weight change is desired will also benefit greatly from professional dietary consultation.

Evidence at a glance

Epidemiology of female athletic triad
- Even if you have not seen it, it has probably seen you!
- Disordered eating among female athletes ranges from 15–62%.
- Amenorrhea among athletes can be as high as 66%, compared to 2–5% in the general population.
- In the presence of amenorrhea, diminished bone density can be found in up to 50% of athletes.

Conclusion

Nutrition, exercise physiology, bone health, and mental health are closely intertwined in the gynecologic health of the adolescent athlete. The scope of care provided to the adolescent athlete in a women's health setting will vary depending upon the resources available in the practice. A team approach is best,

with the woman's health provider collaborating with a registered dietician, a certified athletic trainer, a mental health specialist, or a sports medicine specialist depending on the athlete's clinical needs.

Pearls

- The female athlete triad consists of amenorrhea, osteoporosis, and disordered eating.
- When one component of the triad is found in a female athlete, be on the lookout for the other two.
- Imbalance between energy intake and expenditure is the root cause.

Further reading

Ireland ML, Nattiv A. *The Female Athlete*. Philadelphia: Saunders, 2002.
Salis RE, Massimino F. *Essentials of Sports Medicine*. St Louis: Mosby, 1996.
Waldrop J. Early identification and interventions for female athlete triad. *J Pediatr Health Care* 2005;19(4):213–220.

Acknowledgements

With thanks to Leah Sabato RD, LD, MPH and Marietta Orlowski PhD for reviewing the chapter.

24 Immunizations

Amy B. Middleman

Baylor College of Medicine, Houston, TX, USA

Immunizations were once an area of medicine relegated only to pediatricians. As more vaccines are recommended for adolescents and adults, the scope of providers needed to make sure youth and adults are optimally protected against vaccine-preventable diseases has expanded. Although the influenza vaccine and hepatitis B vaccine have been recommended during pregnancy for many years, it is really the universal recommendation in 2006 for the human papillomavirus (HPV) vaccine among girls aged 11–12 years that has placed gynecologists among the top providers with the greatest opportunity to immunize adolescents.

Recommended vaccines (Table 24.1)

Vaccine recommendations for youth change with each advance in knowledge (up to date vaccine recommendations can be accessed online at the Centers for Disease Control and Prevention website; http://www.cdc.gov/vaccines/recs/schedules/default.htm). National immunization recommendations are created and vetted by the Advisory Committee for Immunization Practices and are formally approved and published by the CDC.

Current routinely recommended vaccines for adolescents include:

- **Meningococcal vaccine (MCV4).** The MCV4 was first recommended for adolescents in 2005. There is an increase in rates of meningococcal disease during the middle adolescent years through the early 20s. While meningococcal disease is relatively rare in the US, especially in recent years, the disease in its early stages is difficult to differentiate from more common viral illnesses and it causes morbidity/mortality within a very short period of time (often 24 hours). Adolescents are more likely than younger children to die from meningococcal disease. The vaccine is routinely recommended for those aged 11–12 years with a booster dose at age 16 years.
- **Tetanus toxoid, diphtheria toxoid, and acellular pertussis vaccines (Tdap).** In the early 1990s, it was noted that pertussis – or whooping cough – was on the rise again, primarily among early and middle adolescents. Immunity was found to wane approximately 5–8 years after vaccination or natural disease. Once coughing has begun, there is no effective treatment. To control the spread of disease, the Td booster vaccine recommended for adolescents was replaced by Tdap, which includes a pertussis component. Tdap is universally recommended for 11–12 year olds.
- **HPV vaccine.** In 2006, the HPV vaccine was universally recommended for females aged 11–12 years; in 2011, the recommendation was expanded to

Practical Pediatric and Adolescent Gynecology, First Edition. Edited by Paula J. Adams Hillard.
© 2013 John Wiley & Sons, Ltd. Published 2013 by John Wiley & Sons, Ltd.

Table 24.1 Recommended vaccinations

Products for adolescents	Manufacturer	Dose/route
Meningococcal vaccine		
MCV4-D (Menactra)	Sanofi-Pasteur	0.5 mL/IM
MCV4-CRM (Menveo)	Novartis	0.5 mL/IM
Tdap vaccine		
Tdap (Adacel)	Sanofi-Pasteur	0.5 mL/IM
Tdap (Boostrix)	GlaxoSmithKline	0.5 mL/IM
HPV vaccine		
HPV4 (Gardasil) (addresses HPV 6,11,16,18)	Merck	0.5 mL/IM
HPV2 (Cervarix) (addresses HPV 16,18)	GlaxoSmithKline	0.5 mL/IM

include males. Universal catch-up is recommended through age 26 years for females and 21 years for males; different recommendations are based on the impact of different disease epidemiology on cost effectiveness for each gender. HPV is associated with cervical, vaginal, vulvar, penile, anal, and oropharyngeal cancers (high-risk viral genotypes including genotypes 16, 18), as well as genital warts (low-risk genotypes 6,11) and recurrent respiratory papillomatosis. The HPV vaccine is now the second routinely recommended vaccine in the US that prevents cancer; hepatitis B vaccine was the first. Currently, two products are available; products addressing more genotypes are currently in development.

• **Influenza vaccine.** Over the past decade, recommendations for influenza vaccines have evolved to an annual universal recommendation for all persons over 6 months of age. Multiple products are available, including the live attenuated influenza vaccine (LAIV) administered to healthy, nonpregnant 2–49 year olds intranasally and a new product for those over 18 years of age that is administered intradermally. Delivery methods for this product are evolving quickly. Multiple products are available for varying patient ages (see www.cdc.gov).

• **Assorted other vaccines.** Catch-up is recommended for all vaccines not previously received. The catch-up immunization schedule is available at http://www.cdc.gov/vaccines/schedules/index.html

There are multiple mechanisms in place to track vaccine safety. The Vaccine Adverse Event Reporting System (VAERS) is most commonly referenced in the media. This is a *passive* surveillance system; anyone

⚗ Science revisited

• The meningococcal vaccine addresses four of the most common serogroups of *Neisseria meningitidis* affecting humans: A, C, W-135, and Y;
• These bacteria cause bacterial meningitis and meningococcal sepsis which carry mortality rates of approximately 10% and 40%, respectively.
• In the US, there is currently no vaccine against serogroup B which causes the majority of disease among infants and very young children; several are in development.

✻ Tips and tricks

Pregnancy testing
• Routinely recommended vaccines do not require pregnancy testing prior to administration. Due to a theoretical risk to a fetus resulting from live vaccines, asking a patient if she might be pregnant or planning a pregnancy in the next 4 weeks is recommended prior to administering varicella and/or measles, mumps, rubella (MMR) vaccines.

can report an "adverse event" associated with a vaccine. For example, if a neighbor overhears a conversation regarding a young woman harmed by her MCV4 vaccine 3 weeks ago, she can report this to

VAERS and it is documented. It is only after a report is received (and posted publically) that work is initiated to *validate* an alleged event. This open system allows the CDC to establish any potential adverse events associated with vaccines, but even after validation, it only allows the establishment of temporal – not causal – associations. Two other systems have been put in place to establish hypothesis-driven associations: Data Safety Link and Clinical Immunization Safety Assessment. Nearly all media reports pertaining to vaccine safety come from unsubstantiated VAERS reports; the investigation results rarely, if ever, receive media attention. It is critical that parents understand this when browsing the internet.

✋ Caution

Vaccine safety
- The internet abounds with misinformation about vaccines.
- It is very important that providers understand the source of safety data and address this with parents.
- The most critical concern of parents pertaining to vaccines is safety.

With the recommendation for the HPV vaccine, mode of disease transmission has become a topic of discussion for parents. This is despite the fact that the hepatitis B vaccine, for which there has been a universal infant recommendation since 1991, also addresses a primarily sexually-transmitted infection. It cannot be stressed enough that vaccination equals prevention of cancer, period. Mode of disease transmission is rarely – if ever – discussed for other disease-preventing vaccines; it should be no different for HPV vaccine. Prevention rather than treatment of disease is always the best strategy for health.

Systems issues

When the opportunity arises to vaccinate a patient with one vaccine, it is critical to use the opportunity to screen for all needed vaccines. Giving all necessary

---

✋ Patient/parent advice

Getting the HPV vaccine on schedule
- Immune response is more vigorous among younger rather than older adolescents.
- The vaccine is only effective if given *before* exposure; studies support vaccination at 11–12 years of age.
- Transmission can occur in the course of non–intercourse-related experimentation.
- With over 35 million doses distributed, no serious adverse events have been associated with vaccine.
- Sometimes being exposed to disease is not the patient's choice; protect your child.
- This vaccine prevents *cancer*.
- HPV vaccine may serve as a great opportunity for families/providers to discuss sexual health in an age-appropriate way to help further enhance a child's wellness.

---

vaccines in one visit increases adherence to the immunization schedule and improves vaccination rates among all age groups.

⋆ Tips and tricks

Multiple vaccines
- More than one vaccine may be given in an extremity;
- A 1-inch distance between administration sites is recommended.
- A 1.5-inch needle is needed intramuscular injections in females weighting over 90 kg.

Immunization screening forms and sample standing orders – both of which improve practice immunization rates – are available on the Immunization Action Coalition website (www.imunize.org). In addition, use of immunization information systems (IIS; formerly known as registries) help patients and providers track which vaccines they have received/given and when; as more providers become involved in immunizing, participating in the state's IIS will help you help your patients and will optimize the use of health resources. It is also helpful to familiarize yourself with appropriate methods for storage and handling the various vaccines; you can access this information in the General Immunization Recommendations published on the CDC website (www.cdc.gov).

Provider recommendations

Research supports the idea that one of the key determinants in parents agreeing to vaccinate their children is the strength of the provider's recommendation. As providers, we know that timely vaccination is critical to eliminating disease and protecting our patients. Studies continue to show that diseases re-emerge in areas of the country with low vaccination rates due to personal belief exemptions among other causes. A critical part of protecting the public health is making sure our children and adolescents are protected against vaccine-preventable diseases in the most timely way. There is no form of prevention more effective than primary prevention.

Summary

Vaccines are listed as one of the most important public health advances both in this century and in the last. There is no better way to fight disease than by preventing it from occurring in the first place. As more vaccines are developed, a more varied group of providers will be called upon to optimize patient health. Providers must know where and how to access the most up-to-date information and most effective counseling strategies to address parent and patient concerns. The health of our youth depends upon it.

Further reading

Atkinson WL (ed). *Epidemiology and Prevention of Vaccine-Preventable Disease*, 12th edn. Atlanta, GA: Centers for Disease Control and Prevention, 2011.

Kroger AT, Sumaya CV, Pickering LK, Atkinson WL. General recommendations on immunizations. *MMWR* 2011;60(RR02):1–60.

Middleman AB. Coordinating the delivery of vaccinations and other preventive health care recommendations for adolescents. *Preventive Med* 2011;53:S22–S28.

25 Substance abuse: screening and brief intervention

Patricia Schram and Sharon Levy

Harvard Medical School, Boston Children's Hospital, Boston, MA, USA

Substance use and substance use disorders are arguably the largest health threat to US adolescents. Drinking and drug use are associated with each of the top four causes of mortality in this age group: motor vehicle accidents, other unintentional injuries, homicides, and suicides. Beyond the potential for acute morbidity and mortality, early initiation of substance use is also associated with increased risk of addiction, which is a complex, chronic brain disease with enormous and costly health and social consequences.

Physicians and other primary clinicians have an important role to play in identifying and discouraging substance use by adolescents and referring those who have developed substance use disorders.

> ### ⚗ Science revisited
>
> The Substance Abuse and Mental Health Services Administration (SAMHSA) has developed *Screening, Brief Intervention, Referral to Treatment*, or SBIRT, as a framework to guide clinicians. Several studies have demonstrated the efficacy of SBIRT in the adult setting, and emerging research is demonstrating its utility with adolescents.

Clinicians who provide reproductive health services have an important role in screening adolescents for drug and alcohol use because individuals who engage in one high-risk behavior often engage in others. Our group has found that adolescents presenting for evaluation of a medical complaint or treatment of a medical disorder have high rates of alcohol and drug use. Young women who engage in risky sexual practices may be more likely to see a gynecologist than any other physician, making these visits a valuable opportunity to screen.

Screening

Developmentally appropriate screening tools and intervention strategies have been designed specifically for use with adolescents and should always be selected when working with this age group. This chapter will describe a practical strategy for identifying substance use and making interventions in the context of clinical care for adolescents.

We recommend asking all adolescents whether they have used alcohol, marijuana or another drug in the past year using unambiguous questions. Adolescents who do not report past year use need no further screening and should be given positive reinforcement from the physician (Figure 25.1). Patients who answer

Practical Pediatric and Adolescent Gynecology, First Edition. Edited by Paula J. Adams Hillard.
© 2013 John Wiley & Sons, Ltd. Published 2013 by John Wiley & Sons, Ltd.

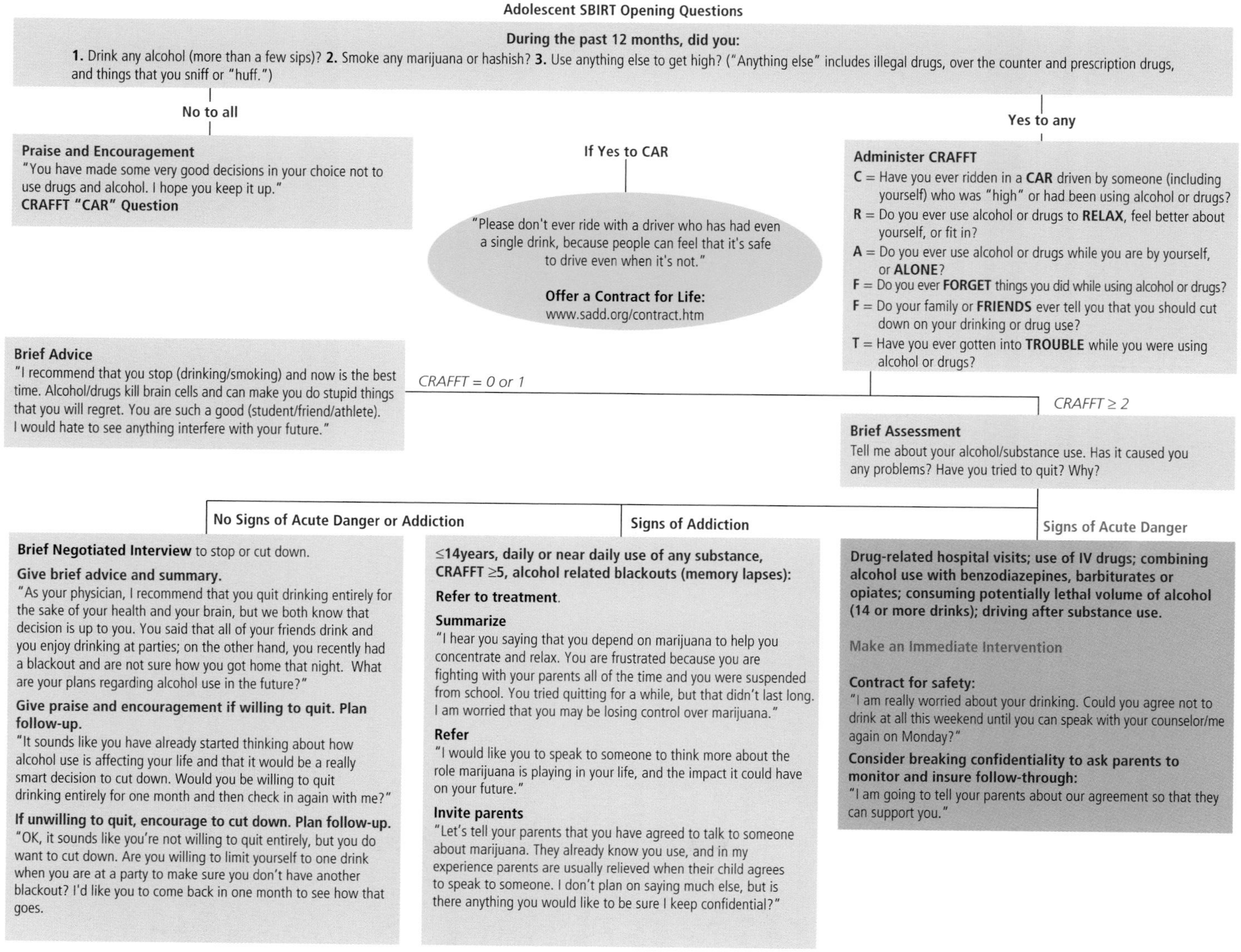

Adolescent SBIRT Opening Questions

During the past 12 months, did you:

1. Drink any alcohol (more than a few sips)? **2.** Smoke any marijuana or hashish? **3.** Use anything else to get high? ("Anything else" includes illegal drugs, over the counter and prescription drugs, and things that you sniff or "huff.")

No to all

Praise and Encouragement
"You have made some very good decisions in your choice not to use drugs and alcohol. I hope you keep it up."
CRAFFT "CAR" Question

Yes to any

Administer CRAFFT
C = Have you ever ridden in a **CAR** driven by someone (including yourself) who was "high" or had been using alcohol or drugs?
R = Do you ever use alcohol or drugs to **RELAX**, feel better about yourself, or fit in?
A = Do you ever use alcohol or drugs while you are by yourself, or **ALONE**?
F = Do you ever **FORGET** things you did while using alcohol or drugs?
F = Do your family or **FRIENDS** ever tell you that you should cut down on your drinking or drug use?
T = Have you ever gotten into **TROUBLE** while you were using alcohol or drugs?

If Yes to CAR

"Please don't ever ride with a driver who has had even a single drink, because people can feel that it's safe to drive even when it's not."

Offer a Contract for Life:
www.sadd.org/contract.htm

CRAFFT = 0 or 1

CRAFFT ≥ 2

Brief Assessment
Tell me about your alcohol/substance use. Has it caused you any problems? Have you tried to quit? Why?

Signs of Acute Danger

Drug-related hospital visits; use of IV drugs; combining alcohol use with benzodiazepines, barbiturates or opiates; consuming potentially lethal volume of alcohol (14 or more drinks); driving after substance use.

Make an Immediate Intervention

Contract for safety:
"I am really worried about your drinking. Could you agree not to drink at all this weekend until you can speak with your counselor/me again on Monday?"

Consider breaking confidentiality to ask parents to monitor and insure follow-through:
"I am going to tell your parents about our agreement so that they can support you."

No Signs of Acute Danger or Addiction

Brief Negotiated Interview to stop or cut down.
Give brief advice and summary.
"As your physician, I recommend that you quit drinking entirely for the sake of your health and your brain, but we both know that decision is up to you. You said that all of your friends drink and you enjoy drinking at parties; on the other hand, you recently had a blackout and are not sure how you got home that night. What are your plans regarding alcohol use in the future?"

Give praise and encouragement if willing to quit. Plan follow-up.
"It sounds like you have already started thinking about how alcohol use is affecting your life and that it would be a really smart decision to cut down. Would you be willing to quit drinking entirely and then check in again with me?"

If unwilling to quit, encourage to cut down. Plan follow-up.
"OK, it sounds like you're not willing to quit entirely, but you do want to cut down. Are you willing to limit yourself to one drink when you are at a party so you don't have another blackout? I'd like you to come back in one month to see how that goes.

Signs of Addiction

≤14years, daily or near daily use of any substance, CRAFFT ≥5, alcohol related blackouts (memory lapses):

Refer to treatment.

Summarize
"I hear you saying that you depend on marijuana to help you concentrate and relax. You are frustrated because you are fighting with your parents all of the time and you were suspended from school. You tried quitting for a while, but that didn't last long. I am worried that you may be losing control over marijuana."

Refer
"I would like you to speak to someone to think more about the role marijuana is playing in your life, and the impact it could have on your future."

Invite parents
"Let's tell your parents that you have agreed to talk to someone about marijuana. They already know you use, and in my experience parents are usually relieved when their child agrees to speak to someone. I don't plan on saying much else, but is there anything you would like to be sure I keep confidential?"

Brief Advice
"I recommend that you stop (drinking/smoking) and now is the best time. Alcohol/drugs kill brain cells and can make you do stupid things that you will regret. You are such a good (student/friend/athlete). I would hate to see anything interfere with your future."

Figure 25.1 Adolescent SBIRT algorithm. Reproduced from Boston Children's Hospital, 2011.

147

"yes" to one or more questions should be screened with a validated tool to determine the appropriate intervention.

A number of screening tools can be used effectively with adolescents. We use the CRAFFT (Figure 25.1) to screen for high-risk alcohol and drug use. It works equally well for alcohol and drugs, for younger and older adolescents, and for youth from diverse race/ethnicity backgrounds. The CRAFFT can be administered by a clinician or self-administered. A pocket card with the CRAFFT questions (in English, Portuguese, and Spanish) is available for clinical use at www.ceasar.org

Recently, the National Institute on Alcoholism and Alcohol Abuse developed an alcohol screening and brief intervention guide for use with adolescents (Alcohol Screening and Brief Intervention for Youth: A Practitioner's Guide; http://pubs.niaaa.nih.gov/publications/Practitioner/YouthGuide/YouthGuideOrderForm.htm). This brief, two-question screen may be particularly useful when time is too short for an entire psychosocial history, when screening younger adolescents (age 9–12 years), or when screening an adolescent who presents with a known history of alcohol use or alcohol-related problems. Recommendations for brief interventions are similar regardless of the screen chosen.

Brief intervention

Immediately following the screen, all adolescents should receive a brief intervention. Because all substance use by adolescents is risky, we encourage clinicians to encourage abstinence, even for adolescents whose screen results indicate that they are in a relatively low-risk group. These adolescents who have not yet experienced negative consequences related to alcohol or drug use may benefit from simple advice given by a trusted professional.

Adolescents who have not begun to use alcohol or drugs should get positive encouragement. Statements delivered by a physician, such as, "I see you have decided not to use alcohol or drugs – that is a smart decision and one of the best ways to protect your health," may reduce substance initiation rates.

Adolescents who report past year substance use but screen into the "lower risk" (i.e. CRAFFT negative or "low risk" on the NIAAA screen) should receive

clear advice to stop drugs and alcohol along with information about related health risks. For example, "I recommend that you stop drinking alcohol entirely. Young women are much more likely to have unprotected or unwanted sex after they drink alcohol". Brief advice from a reliable medical source seems to increase cessation rates among low risk adolescents.

★ Tips and tricks

- Use unambiguous questions.
- Give brief advice to quit that focuses on health.
- For patients who do not want to quit, encourage reduction and target high risk behaviors.
- Refer back to primary care to continue the conversation.

Adolescents who screen as "high risk"

Adolescents who screen as "high risk" should have a brief intervention with follow-up either by their primary care provider or a mental health professional. You should begin the brief intervention by asking a few questions to determine if substance use presents an acute safety risk or suggests addiction. Ask about problems associated with use, whether the adolescent has ever tried to quit, and if so, why. Asking about problems associated with use is a simple and effective motivational strategy.

★ Tips and tricks

Example scenario for an adolescent who screens at high risk
Screen: Mary is an 18-year-old high school senior who comes for emergency contraception. Before writing her prescription, you screen for alcohol use.

You: "In the *past year*, on how many days have you had more than a few sips of beer, wine, or any drink containing alcohol?" and: "If your friends drink, how many drinks do they usually drink on an occasion?"

Mary: "I drink two to three drinks at parties on weekends. My friends drink more than me."

You: "Have you ever ridden in a *car* driven by someone who had using alcohol and drugs?"

Mary: "No."

Brief intervention: "Good, please don't ever get in a car if the driver is not 100%."

Assessment:

You: "Did you ever have problems because of drinking?"

Mary: "I was suspended because I brought a bottle of vodka to a school football game last year. My parents were upset and grounded me but now they know I don't have an alcohol problem."

You: "Do you regret anything you did when you were drunk?"

Mary: "I was so drunk when I had sex 2 days ago. I don't know if I used contraception and now I regret the decision to have sex in the first place."

Brief intervention:

You: "It seems that drinking has gotten you into trouble. What would you like to do about it?"

Mary: "I don't think alcohol is a problem; I am not going to quit."

You: "OK. I *recommend* that you stop drinking entirely for the sake of your health, because people often make bad decisions when they drink. Of course only you can decide to stop. I hear that you are not interested in quitting right now, but you also don't want to have another black out. Can you try cutting back?"

Mary agrees and mentions that her parents know about her drinking but she does not want you to share any information with them. She does agree to follow up with her primary care physician in 1 month.

Encourage the adolescent to return to primary care for further assessment by expressing concerns in an empathetic fashion. We recommend starting the conversation by stating the concern, describing potential associated medical problems, and exploring the patient's own plans. For example, "I am concerned about your use of marijuana because it is bad for your health and can interfere with your grades. It sounds as if you feel that marijuana makes you "lazy," which is actually very common. You have the potential to be such a good student; I would hate to see anything interfere with your future. What you would like to do about it?" Reinforce any statements about reducing use and encourage the patient to continue the conversation with her primary physician.

★ Tips and tricks

Involvement of the parent

- Ask for permission to invite a parent into the conversation to help insure that the patient gets on-going care.
- In many instances parents are already aware of substance use and the patient will agree to include them.
- The clinician can create a positive interaction by focusing on positive steps that the patient has agreed to.
- For example, "Your daughter discussed her marijuana use with me, and she agreed both to start cutting back and also to continue the conversation with her primary care physician. Can you help arrange a follow up visit for her?"

✋ Caution

- Explain confidentiality to the adolescent and her parents.
- Always ask about substance use when you are alone with the patient.

Further reading

American Academy of Pediatrics. Substance use screening, brief intervention, and referral to treatment for pediatricians. *Pediatrics* 2011;128 (5):e1330–e1340. Available at: http://pediatrics.aappublications.org/content/early/2011/10/26/peds.2011-1754

Johnston LD, O'Malley PM, Bachman JG, Schulenberg JE. *Monitoring the Future National Results on Adolescent Drug Use: Overview of Key Findings*, 2010. Ann Arbor: Institute for Social Research, The University of Michigan 2011. Available at www.monitoringthefuture.org

National Institute on Alcohol Abuse and Alcoholism. *Alcohol Screening and Brief Intervention for Youth: A Practitioner's Guide*, 2011. Available at: http://pubs.niaaa.nih.gov/publications/Practitioner/YouthGuide/YouthGuide.pdf

Acknowledgements

We would like acknowledge Danielle J Murphy for her help in preparing this chapter.

26 Suicidal ideation and self-harm: screening

Matthew B. Wintersteen and Christopher V. Chambers

Thomas Jefferson University, Philadelphia, PA, USA

Adolescence is a period generally marked by good health. However, the rapid and often asynchronous changes in physical, cognitive, and emotional development during this period can be overwhelming to many teens (see Appendix 1.9.2). Sadly, suicide is the third leading cause of death among youth aged 10–24 years in the US and accounts for more deaths annually than the top seven non–injury-based medical conditions combined. Roughly, 20% of adolescents contemplate suicide, 10–12% make a plan for suicide, and 5–8% attempt suicide, resulting in over one million attempts each year.

Data show that puberty often has a negative impact on self-esteem, particularly among girls who develop early. Early puberty, which may result in a girl appearing physically like an adult while cognitively and emotionally still a child, a history of sexual abuse and a family history of mental illness are risk factors for psychological troubles that may contribute to suicidal thoughts and behavior. The loss of a friendship, school failure, or an awkward sexual interaction can trigger action.

Screening for risk

Most adolescents who have suicidal thoughts visit a physician at some point during their emotional distress but, as a rule, adolescents are unlikely to ask directly for help. For these reasons, it is widely recommended that physicians routinely screen adolescents for their emotional well-being at all office visits. A variety of simple screening tools are available and simple to implement. One is the HEEADSSS assessment (home, education/employment, eating, activities, drugs, sex, suicide/depression, and safety; see Appendix 1.13). Asking simple questions in each of these areas allows a physician to rapidly evaluate whether a teenage girl is functioning in the various domains of a typical adolescent's life. However, with experience, these content areas are often discussed organically. The "Tips and tricks" box provides an excellent outline for assessing risk factors associated with suicide, while addressing the recommended psychosocial elements offered by the American Academy of Pediatrics. Note that it is important to avoid asking about suicide at the beginning of the interview, as this may throw the patient off balance and lead to a rupture in the provider–patient relationship and less honest disclosure.

> ### ★ Tips and tricks
>
> Clinicians often find assessing for suicide risk challenging. The following psychosocial assessment is a useful guide to ease you into the topic:
> - "How is life going? How have things been going lately?"
>
> *(Continued)*

Practical Pediatric and Adolescent Gynecology, First Edition. Edited by Paula J. Adams Hillard.
© 2013 John Wiley & Sons, Ltd. Published 2013 by John Wiley & Sons, Ltd.

- "How are things at home? Work? School?"
- "How have you been getting along with family and friends?"
- "How has your mood been?"
- "Do you drink alcohol or use other drugs?"

Concerns with any response above should prompt:

- "Have things been going so badly that you think it'll never get any better?"
- "In the past week, including today, have you felt like life is not worth living?"
- "In the past week, including today, have you wanted to kill yourself?"
- "Have you ever made a plan about how you would kill yourself?"
- "Have you ever tried to kill yourself before? How many times?"

Do not forget to conclude with assessing protective factors to assist with treatment planning:

- "What keeps you alive right now? What are your reasons for living?"
- "Who do you talk to when you are having problems? Is it helpful?"

When approaching the topic of suicide, it is best to take a hierarchical approach to questioning. Normalizing distress and subjective experience through-out the process will reduce patient anxiety and shame, and increase the adolescent's willingness to disclose painful emotional experiences.

In addition to focusing directly on suicide risk, it is important to recognize the increasing prevalence of nonsuicidal self-injury in adolescents. While these behaviors may take many forms, cutting commonly occurs privately. In many adolescent girls, cutting occurs in areas not visible to others, including the ankles, lower abdomen, and groin.

The single most important variable to an accurate assessment is your ability to develop a collaborative relationship with the adolescent. Getting the patient to talk about her intense psychological pain and suffering is critical for providing the best healthcare possible. Remember to remain calm as you progress through the questioning. Beyond offering the always

⚖ Science revisited

- A common misconception in general medicine is that a patient must be depressed in order to feel suicidal.
- In fact, recent research by Nock *et al.* (2009) has found that anxiety, irritability/agitation, and substance abuse are stronger predictors of suicidal and self-injurious behaviors than depression.

✋ Caution

Differentiating between a suicide attempt and nonsuicidal self-injury can be challenging. The intent of the person is the key factor. Some questions that may be helpful in making this distinction are:

- "What did you hope would happen?"
- "How do your reasons for living compare to your reasons for dying?"
- "Would it have mattered to you if you had died as a result of your actions?"

When intent remains unclear after questioning, it is best to assume the behavior was a suicide attempt, since at least some intent for death was implied.

✋ Patient/parent advice

Suicide is a topic that is not frequently discussed. Many parents and youth want to learn more about risk factors and what they can do to help loved ones. The following are useful resources:

- American Association of Suicidology (www.suicidology.org)
- Suicide Prevention Resource Center (www.sprc.org)
- In an immediate crisis, you may call the National Suicide Prevention Lifeline at 1-800-273-TALK (8255). The Lifeline trains local crisis centers who will know the resources in your community.

helpful and caring ear, routinely screening adolescents for psychosocial problems, including suicide risk and nonsuicidal injury, can result in early identification of a youth at risk. Referrals to credentialed mental health professionals can result in improved physical and behavioral health outcomes.

Further reading

Bridge JA, Goldstein TR, Brent DA. Adolescent suicide and suicidal behavior. *J Child Psychol Psychiatry* 2006;47: 372–394.

McDowell AK, Lineberry TW, Bostwick JM. Practical suicide-risk management for the busy primary care clinician. *Mayo Clin Proc* 2011;86:792–800.

Nock MK, Hwang I, Sampson N, *et al*. Cross-national analysis of the associations among mental disorders and suicidal behaviors: Findings from the WHO world mental health surveys. *PLoS Med* 2009;6(e1000123):1–17.

27 Healthcare for lesbian, bisexual, and transgender adolescents

Elizabeth B. Erbaugh[1] and Margaret J. Blythe[2]

[1]Department of Sociology, Institute for Research on Social Issues, Indiana University-Purdue University Indianapolis, Indianapolis, IN, USA
[2]Indiana University School of Medicine, Indianapolis, IN, USA

Fear of discrimination and a limited number of providers well trained in the health needs of lesbian, gay, bisexual, transgender, queer and questioning (LGBTQ) individuals can limit the extent to which sexual minorities access health services. Understanding the experiences of LGBTQ adolescents seeking care and reviewing the health disparities encountered will enable healthcare environments to better respond to these inequities.

In providing care to adolescents it is important to avoid assumptions that an individual is heterosexual or identifies with the gender role traditionally associated with their biologic sex. The process of sexual development for adolescents leaves many unsure of their sexual orientation and/or gender identity, as gender, sexual identity, and the sex of sexual partners may change over time. With adolescents it is important to consider age and developmental stage in the ongoing process of gender and sexual identity development. Many teens are uncomfortable labeling themselves regarding gender identity and sexual orientation, or even discussing the sex of their sexual partners (see Chapter 20). Most adolescents though are able to understand and answer questions regarding sexual attractions (e.g. only attracted to females, mostly attracted to females, equally attracted to females and males, unsure).

Homophobia and social stigma contribute to an array of health issues, barriers to care, and risk behaviors among LGBTQ young people. Providing adolescents with health services that engage them and give them opportunities to discuss sensitive health issues is crucial. Providing "alone time" as well as the guarantee of privacy allows opportunities to discuss such topics as sexual orientation or gender identity.

> ## ✴ Tips and tricks
>
> **Creating a supportive clinical environment**
> - Offer LGBTQ-inclusive office materials such as magazines, posters, and brochures.
> - Train ancillary medical staff to be sensitive and nonjudgmental in response to adolescents' accounts of their sexual identities and behaviors.
> - Provide time for open, honest communication with providers.
> - Practice appropriate, sensitive documentation of sexual orientation and gender identity.

Health issues

Stress, victimization, and mental health

The association of a minority sexual orientation with stigma, victimization, and negative health-risk behaviors is well documented. Based on state and national data, an increased risk of suicidality and suicide

---

✋ Caution

Providing sensitive gynecologic care to transgender adolescents

• Based partly on research with female-to-male transgender adults, female-bodied adolescents with a masculine gender identity may have mixed or negative feelings about receiving gynecologic care.

• The experience of a gynecologic exam may heighten a sense of conflict between self-perception and physical anatomy.

• As with survivors of sexual violence (see Chapters 30.1 and 53) the vulnerability and physical touch involved in an exam may require special sensitivity and willingness to negotiate the terms and pace of the exam on the part of the clinician.

• With trust in the provider, over time, female-to-male transgender individuals may grow more comfortable obtaining regular gynecologic care.

attempts has been consistently reported by lesbian, gay, bisexual, and questioning youth (LGBQY) when compared to heterosexual youth. Researchers studying LGBQY often use the term "gay-related stress" to refer to stresses associated with coming out, being discovered, and being ridiculed. In addition, external stressors related to sexual orientation such as verbal insults, property damage, physical abuse and assault contribute to victimization. Such victimization has been found to mediate the association of sexual orientation and suicidality. Generally, the report of family rejection and/or homelessness in response to adolescent disclosure of homosexuality or bisexuality is associated with worse health and health-related outcomes.

Evidence at a glance

Threats to LGBTQ adolescent mental health

• Although research specifically focused on LGBTQ adolescents is limited, a survey of adults conducted by the CDC and Massachusetts' State Department of Health found that bisexual women were more likely than straight women to report tension and worry (37.2% vs 22.5%).

• Intent to commit suicide in the last year was reported at a rate almost ten times higher by bisexual women (27.5%) compared to heterosexual women (2.9%).

• A regional study of southern states found that lesbian women were more likely to report depression than women overall, both within and outside the South.

• A report recently released by The American College of Obstetricians and Gynecologists indicates that over half of transgender youth have attempted suicide.

Sexual experiences and victimization

Limited data exist comparing the sexual behaviors of heterosexual girls to bisexual and lesbian girls, but the available evidence indicates that LGBTQ adolescents may be at heightened risk for sexual health issues and victimization.

Evidence at a glance

Sexual experiences and victimization among LGBTQ adolescents

• There appear to be no significant differences in reports of sexual intercourse and age of first intercourse among bisexual, lesbian, and heterosexual girls.

• Based on available research, bisexual and lesbian girls are more than twice as likely to have reported pregnancy as heterosexual girls.

• Nonconsensual sexual contact was reported more often for bisexual and lesbian girls than for heterosexual girls.

• Parallel results have been found with adults; in the CDC–Massachusetts survey, sexual victimization was more likely to be reported by bisexual (57.3%) and lesbian women (34.5%) than by heterosexual women (18.1%).

Family and intimate partner violence

Public recognition of domestic violence as perpetrated mainly by men and the myth of the "lesbian utopia" lead many young LGBTQ people and their health-care providers to doubt that intimate partner violence occurs in lesbian relationships or that women can perpetrate dating violence.

✋ Caution

Violence and LGBTQ adolescents
- Young bisexual and lesbian women and female-to-male transgender people may be more likely than heterosexual adolescents to have experienced violence in their families of origin and in intimate relationships.
- Given that the gender of intimate partners may change over time, experiences of interpersonal violence may well figure in a LGBTQ adolescent's health history.

Risk behaviors

Overall, as a group LGBQY who have experienced high levels of victimization have been found likely to engage in substantially more health risk behaviors compared to heterosexual youth who have been similarly victimized.

- **Substance use.** National and state representative samples have consistently demonstrated higher rates of substance use among LGBTQ youth than heterosexual youth.

✋ Caution

Substance use among LGBTQ adolescents
- In comparison with adolescents who report only same-sex partnerships, self-identified bisexual adolescents and adolescents reporting both-sex partnerships are most consistently found to be at higher risk for substance use behaviors, including alcohol, tobacco, and other drug use, than heterosexual peers.
- Bisexual and lesbian women have been found to have higher rates of binge drinking and smoking than heterosexual women.

- **Eating disorders.** Research suggests that there are differences in risk for disordered eating between groups, with bisexual and lesbian girls reporting less body dissatisfaction when compared to heterosexual female adolescents. State and regional studies, as well as one study of college-age women, indicate that bisexual and lesbian women are more likely than their heterosexual peers to be overweight or obese.

Summary

Creating a welcoming environment, allowing LGBTQ adolescents to define their own gender and sexual identities, and being sensitive to the stressors and risks they face will aid clinicians in providing quality, supportive care to young LGBTQ women and transgender adolescents.

✋ Information for providers

Online resources can be found at:
American Academy of Pediatrics (AAP) http://pediatrics.aappublications.org/content/113/6/1827
American Academy of Family Practice (AAFP) http://www.annfammed.org/content/8/6/533
Gay and Lesbian Medical Association (GLMA) http://www.glma.org
Institute of Medicine http://books.nap.edu/openbook.php?record_id=13128
American College of Obstetrics and Gynecology (ACOG) http://www.acog.org
> Committee Opinion No. 512: Health Care for Transgender Individuals
> Transgender Health Resource Guide

✋ Patient/parent advice

Online resources can be found at:
American Academy of Child and Adolescent Psychiatry (AACAP) http://www.aacap.org/galleries/FactsForFamilies/63_gay_and_lesbian_adolescents.pdf
Centers for Disease Control (CDC) http://www.cdc.gov/lgbthealth/women.htm

American College of Obstetrics and Gynecology (ACOG) http://www.acog.org
   Tool Kit for Teen Care: Lesbian Teens
   Transgender Health Resource Guide

Further reading

Bontempo DE, D'Augelli AR. Effects of at-school victimization and sexual orientation on lesbian, gay, or bisexual youths' health risk behavior. *J Adolesc Health* 2002;30: 364–374.

Coker TR, Austin SB, Schuster MA. The health and health care of lesbian, gay and bisexual adolescents. *Ann Rev Public Health* 2010;31:457–477.

Dutton L, Koenig K, Fennie K. Gynecologic care of the female-to-male transgender man. *J Midwifery Womens Health* 2008;53:331–337.

28 Developmental delay

Lisa Allen[1] and Melanie Ornstein[2]

[1]Hospital for Sick Children, University of Toronto, ON, Canada
[2]Toronto East General Hospital, Toronto, ON, Canada

For individuals with developmental delay (DD) and their families, puberty offers unique challenges, and may create anxiety. Young women, their families, and caregivers may present to healthcare providers with questions around menstrual hygiene, menstrual dysfunction, behavioral issues, sexuality, vulnerability to abuse, and contraception; and how they relate to their disabilities. Many families present before onset of menarche, particularly when their daughter is more severely affected by DD or requires greater assistance with activities of daily living. The healthcare provider can take advantage of this early timing to provide anticipatory guidance and counseling regarding gynecologic concerns.

Young women with DD are a diverse population whose cognitive and physical impairments vary in severity, and in whom comorbidities are common. This translates into variable communication skills, wide variations in independence for activities of daily living, multiple prescription drugs, and differences in the ability to participate in informed consent. A comprehensive history from the individual adolescent and her family promotes understanding of complicated health concerns.

The developmentally challenged adolescent deserves reproductive healthcare following similar principles to those of their able bodied peers, i.e. care in their own best interest, in as confidential a manner and with as much assent or consent as is feasible within the capacity of their intellectual deficit.

It is important to involve the adolescent in her reproductive healthcare directly whenever possible. Young women with DD may have impairments in language abilities, speech, or hearing. They may face physical limitations, especially when wheelchair bound, providing accessibility concerns. Healthcare facilities can promote accessibility with appropriate architectural features. Healthcare visits should be structured with time to be flexible with communication styles and to tailor physical exams. Adolescents should be offered opportunities for private and confidential communication. For hearing-impaired adolescents, consider involving a sign language interpreter.

While involving the adolescent in her care is imperative, equally important is the recognition of the needs and stresses of caregivers. Cognitively and/or physically challenged individuals often have caregivers who have their own concerns, such as the capacity of the individual and caregivers to cope with menstrual hygiene, the inability to communicate pain, cyclic exacerbations of behavior, and concerns of pregnancy risk. Determination of all caregivers' roles in the home and school is important. Child behaviors and demands of caregiving negatively impact caregivers' physical and psychological health. Discussions of

Practical Pediatric and Adolescent Gynecology, First Edition. Edited by Paula J. Adams Hillard.
© 2013 John Wiley & Sons, Ltd. Published 2013 by John Wiley & Sons, Ltd.

social supports may reflect areas where family functioning could be enhanced.

Some caregivers may withdraw from personal hygiene requirements after onset of menses, placing more burden on others or requiring the adolescent to be withdrawn from activities. Menstrual calendars can be valuable, especially in environments where multiple caregivers are involved. Prospective charting may allow the anticipation of changes in behavior and behavioral modification. Calendars help distinguish physiologic menstrual symptoms from those suggesting pathology [secondary dysmenorrhea, premenstrual dysphoric disorder (PMDD)].

> ### ☆ Tips and tricks
>
> The onset of secondary sexual characteristics can serve as an excellent opportunity for healthcare providers to assess patients' and caregivers' understanding and fears related to sexual maturation, menarche, and the need for reproductive health care.

Physical exam

Indications to perform a pelvic exam do not differ in a disabled adolescent (see Appendix 1.7). Awareness of the young woman's physical disabilities (spasticity, muscle weakness, scoliosis, and contractures), can allow the healthcare provider to tailor the exam. The examination room should be sufficiently large to accommodate a wheelchair or mobility equipment. Transfer to an examination table can be aided by an assistant or a motorized examination bed. Transfers, dressing, and undressing may take additional time and appointments should account for this.

Modifications can be made to the lithotomy position: additional support for the extremities, avoiding foot stirrups (by using a support person to assist or knee-supported stirrups), and alternate positions, e.g. legs elevated without hip abduction, frog-legged or side-lying position with knees bent. Smaller, narrow specula may facilitate examination. If a speculum exam is not possible, passing a brush or Q-tip manually over a finger may allow collection of cervical cytology. Self-collected or healthcare-assisted vaginal swabs or first void urine specimens are an alternative

for sexually-transmitted infection (STI) testing. If a physical exam is not possible, and an exam is deemed essential, conscious sedation or general anesthesia can be considered.

> ### ☆ Tips and tricks
>
> • Spasticity can be increased when a young woman is speaking or if there is insufficient support for the lower extremities.
> • During pelvic exams reassure the patient verbally, avoid questions where a response is required, provide extra support to legs while abducted, or try alternate positions.

Consent

In providing care to young women with DD, capacity and consent are important. An individual must be able to understand the condition for which a treatment is proposed, as well as the purpose and the risks of undergoing or refusing treatment. Capacity to provide consent may vary depending on the seriousness of the condition and intervention. A young woman with DD may be able to consent to an exam, but not to surgery. If the adolescent is unable to provide consent, a legal guardian is appointed. The guardian makes decisions in the best interest of the individual. Even in situations where an adolescent with DD is not capable of providing consent, her assent should be obtained. Assent is particularly important when the young woman's participation in care is required, e.g. an intramuscular injection or a physical exam. A lack of assent may require an alteration of the care plan, e.g. different route for administration of menstrual suppression or imaging to replace a physical exam.

> ### ☆ Tips and tricks
>
> Capacity to provide consent varies with the treatment or intervention proposed and should be assessed on an ongoing basis during provision of healthcare.

Menstrual dysfunction and suppression

Families can be informed that the overall mean age of menarche for young women with DD is similar to healthy adolescents. Recent evidence suggests that woman with DD have similar experiences of dysmenorrhea, irregular menses, and heavy menstrual bleeding, and an appropriate evaluation is indicated.

Many young women with DD have medical comorbidities. Thyroid dysfunction, seizure disorders, psychiatric concerns, and malnutrition can impact menstruation and treatment options. Seizure disorders and valproic acid are associated with polycystic ovary syndrome (PCOS). Neuroleptics can lead to hyperprolactinemia and amenorrhea. Antibiotics may affect hormonal therapy efficacy. Malnutrition or G-tubes can impact route of drug administration and absorption. The differential diagnosis of irregular bleeding should include complications of sexual activity such as pregnancy or STIs.

When a family presents with menstrual concerns, defining both the patient's and the caregiver's reasons for intervention and the goals of treatment are important.

★ Tips and tricks

- Be aware that if an adolescent is unable to communicate dysmenorrhea, this may manifest as irritability, aggression, self-mutilation, and behavioral changes.
- Adequate analgesia may be all that is required. Nonsteroidal anti-inflammatory drugs, if there are no contraindications, are a good first-line therapy.

Hygiene during menses is often a major concern for caregivers. The physician can acknowledge this concern and provide tips, which may be as simple as suggesting the use of pads inside diapers of incontinent women, as pads are less expensive and may be changed more frequently than a diaper. Increased supervision or help within the school or work environment may be required.

In general, there is consensus that menstrual suppression therapy should not commence until menarche. Often, education and support of the normal progression through puberty and menarche are all that is required. Awaiting menarche confirms normal hormonal function and the absence of an obstructive anomaly. Once a decision is made to pursue treatment, interventions that are reversible, the least intrusive, and have the fewest side effects are desirable.

Menstrual suppression involves the use of hormonal regimens to decrease blood loss and number of menstrual cycles per year or to eliminate menses all together. The goals may also include management of associated bloating, nausea and vomiting, headaches, mood and behavioral changes, and cyclic exacerbation of seizures or migraines. The ultimate goal of menstrual suppression is to improve quality of life for the young woman and/or her caregivers.

Treatment options are addressed in Chapter 29.3 and considerations for individuals with DD in Table 28.1.

✋ Caution

It is essential to ascertain the goals of menstrual suppressive therapy, discuss the risks and benefits of all available treatment modalities, and provide the least invasive choice tailored to the individual's unique needs.

Sexuality, sexual education, and contraception

Young women with DD develop sexual interests that vary with their level of functioning. Adolescents with DD may participate in consensual sexual experiences, the appropriateness of which should be assessed individually. Women with mild intellectual disability are as likely to be sexually active as the general population. With more severe DD, the likelihood of sexual activity decreases. Families should be counseled that consensual relationships can be healthy experiences when young women are provided with developmentally appropriate sexual education to reduce the risk of consequences of sexual activity. Education should include discussions of their body and genital anatomy. Sexual behavior and its expression should be explained, e.g. discussing masturbation as a private sexual activity, and explaining appropriate and inappropriate sexual touching. Adolescents with DD

Table 28.1 Contraception and menstrual suppression considerations for individuals with developmental delay

Method	Contraception	Menstrual suppression	Considerations for the DD population
Barrier methods	+	−	Latex sensitivity Requires manual dexterity
Oral contraceptive pill	+	+(with extended or continuous use)	Venous thromboembolism (VTE) risk for immobile patients: consider low-dose or second-generation progestin Metabolism: antiepileptics may increase cytochrome P450 hepatic microsomal oxidative enzymes and decrease efficacy Feeding/swallowing problems
Transdermal patch	+	+(with extended or continuous use)	VTE risk for immobile patients Metabolism: antiepileptics may increase cytochrome P450 hepatic microsomal oxidative enzymes and decrease efficacy Best location may be lower back if tendency to removal
Vaginal ring	+	+(with extended or continuous use)	Requires manual dexterity for self-insertion Not usually prescribed for caregiver to insert
Depot medroxyprogesterone acetate (DMPA)	+	+	Weight gain association may affect transfer Risk of osteopenia
Copper intrauterine device (IUD)	+	−	May require anesthesia for insertion
Levonorgestrel (LNG)-intrauterine system (IUS)	+	+	May require anesthesia for insertion Requires uterus of adequate size 5–6 cm
Etonogestrol implant	+	+	May require anesthesia for insertion More unscheduled bleeding

should be provided with developmentally appropriate information on STIs, the human papillomavirus (HPV) vaccine, contraception, sexual orientation, and health implications of pregnancy.

> ### ★ Tips and tricks
>
> • Comprehensive, accurate sexual health education should be provided at an appropriate level to all young women with simple language, repetition, anatomically correct dolls, and role-playing.
> • Caregivers should be encouraged to take an active part in the education.

While sexuality is a normal part of development, adolescents with disabilities are at increased risk of abuse. Dependence on others for self-care, exposure to multiple caregivers and environments, lack of capacity to communicate abuse, underdeveloped social skills, passive or obedient behavior, and a lack of mobility to physically remove themselves from an abusive situation contribute to risk. Encouraging adolescents with DD to develop skills such as learning about personal space, body language, self-advocacy, and communication, including electronic-based communication, could assist them if placed in a vulnerable position. A request from caregivers for contraception should prompt an assessment of safety with a discussion of the living, working, and social environments of the young woman.

> ✋ **Caution**
>
> • Adolescents with DD are more than twice as likely to experience abuse compared to their peers.
> • Healthcare providers should monitor for early indicators of abuse.

Protection against pregnancy can be provided with reversible contraceptive methods. The appropriate method should consider medical comorbidities, desire for menstrual suppression, and method compliance (Table 28.1).

Families may request permanent tubal occlusion procedures or hysterectomy. These requests are wrought with ethical and legal restrictions which limit their application for women who do not have the capacity to consent themselves. It is imperative that less invasive methods of contraception (or menstrual suppression) are employed before consideration of a permanent procedure. Counseling should include a discussion of the limitations of surgical procedures, including lack of benefit for cyclic behavior, catamenial exacerbations of problems such as seizures, and protection against STIs and abuse. In the rare situations where, after exhausting less invasive options, surgery may be considered to be in the best interests of the DD individual, it is advisable to seek counsel of an ethicist or ethics committee. The healthcare provider must be aware of local laws governing the performance of these procedures.

Further reading

Burke L, Kalpakjian C, Smith Y, Quint H. Gynecologic issues of adolescents with down syndrome, autism, and cerebral palsy. *J Pediatr Adolesc Gynecol* 2010;23: 11–15.

Murphy N, Elias ER. Sexuality of children and adolescents with developmental disabilities. *Pediatrics* 2006;118(1): 398–403,

Savasi I, Spitzer RF, Allen LM, Ornstein MP. Menstrual suppression for adolescents with developmental disabilities. *J Pediatr Adolesc Gynecol* 2009;22:143–149.

29.1 Tampons and menstrual hygiene products

Stephanie Stockburger and Hatim A. Omar

Division of Adolescent Medicine, Department of Pediatrics, University of Kentucky, Kentucky Children's Hospital, Lexington, KY, USA

Menstruation is a major event in the progression of puberty for young women and usually occurs between ages 8 and 13 years. The average duration of menses is 4 days with median blood loss of about 30 mL per month. There are a number of catamenial (menstrual hygiene) products available.

★ Tips and tricks

- Physicians historically avoid discussion of menstrual hygiene products during female adolescent visits. However, the topic is important to discuss so that the teen is fully informed of the risks, benefits, and proper uses of different products.
- Although tampon use requires a "learning curve," even young teens and virgins can, if motivated, typically learn to insert them, even at the time of first menses.
- Inability to insert a tampon may signal hymenal anomalies, such as a hymenal band (see Chapter 9).

Menstrual pads

Menstrual pads are disposable and have an adhesive backing that sticks to the crotch of the woman's underwear (outside of the vagina). They are typically made of absorbent wood cellulose fibers (like paper) with a layer of perforated plastic on top to wick moisture away from the skin. Absorbency varies: super maxi pads (most absorbent), maxi pads, thin maxi pads, mini pads and panty liners (least absorbent). Menstrual pads are available with wings that wrap around the sides of the panty crotch which help keep them in place but may also abrade the inner thigh. Pads with deodorant are also available which may have a pleasant odor but can cause local irritation and mask a vaginal infection.

Tampons

Tampons are disposable cotton cylinders and are worn inside the vagina to absorb menstrual flow. They are inserted with plastic or cardboard applicators (or by hand) and have a cotton string on the end which aides in tampon removal. Tampons are considered to be medical devices by the FDA and require a label with absorbency standards. Tampons tend to be more comfortable than menstrual pads, more cosmetically appealing, and may be worn during activities such as gymnastics and swimming. The disadvantages of tampon use include risk of toxic shock syndrome (TSS), albeit rare, irritation, dryness, initial difficulty with insertion and removal, and users may have higher incidence of urinary tract infections.

Practical Pediatric and Adolescent Gynecology, First Edition. Edited by Paula J. Adams Hillard.
© 2013 John Wiley & Sons, Ltd. Published 2013 by John Wiley & Sons, Ltd.

🔬 Science revisited

- TSS is caused by an exotoxin produced by *Staphylococcus aureus* called toxic shock syndrome toxin-1 (TSST-1).
- A half of reported TSS cases are menstrual and associated with highly absorbent tampons.
- The exotoxins cause disease because they are superantigens which activate large numbers of T cells and result in massive cytokine production.
- **DIAGNOSTIC CRITERIA:**
  - Fever greater than 102°F
  - Hypotension, orthostatic syncope or dizziness
  - Diffuse macular erythroderma
  - Desquamation of skin 1–2 weeks after onset of illness, particularly involving palms and soles
  - Multisystem involvement of three or more of the following organ systems: gastrointestinal, muscular, mucous membranes, renal, hepatic, hematologic, or central nervous system
  - Negative cultures for another pathogen as well as negative tests for Rocky Mountain spotted fever, leptospirosis, or measles are also part of the criteria, if tests were obtained
- TSS may result in multiorgan failure and may be fatal.

✋ Caution

FDA guidelines for decreasing the risk of contracting TSS
- Select appropriate tampon absorbency for menstrual flow.
- Follow package directions for proper tampon insertion.
- Limit wear-time per tampon to no more than 8 hours.
- Avoid using tampons overnight.
- Consider alternating tampons with pads.

Menstrual cup

A menstrual cup is shaped like an inverted bell with a stem and is inserted into the vagina to collect (rather

✋ Patient/parent advice

Helpful tips for tampon insertion
- Tampon insertion may be easiest when flow is heaviest.
- Sit on the toilet or stand with one foot propped up such as on the toilet bowl.
- For the first few tries, place a water-based lubricant on the cotton tip.
- If the tampon is felt within the vagina or is painful after insertion, it is likely not inserted far enough.
- Aim towards the small of back when inserting.

than absorb) menstrual fluid. Most menstrual cups are reusable and are made out of silicone or natural rubber. The benefits to using menstrual cups are that they are environmentally and economically friendly and may be worn for up to 12 hours. Their disadvantages are the learning curve with insertion and removal, the need to empty and rinse the cup every 12 hours and boil it between periods. The menstrual cup is not widely used in the US.

Padded panties and reusable menstrual pads

Padded panties and reusable menstrual pads are made from soft washable fabric. The benefits are that they are environmentally and economically friendly, as well as soft and chemical free. The disadvantage is that the fabric pads must be rinsed and washed. Washable pads are not widely used in the US.

Sea sponges

Sea sponges are used similarly to a tampon (inserted into the vagina) and absorb menstrual flow. They may be washed, dried, and reused for up to 6 months. They are cost-effective, absorbent, and environmentally friendly. The disadvantages include that they need to be boiled prior to use and may leak and be messy (especially during removal). The risk of TSS is not well established.

Miniform

The miniform is a small and discrete pad that fits between the labia minora. The miniform falls out when the woman urinates. The disadvantages include that it absorbs only a small amount of fluid, may be displaced during movement, must be changed with each urination, is costly, and is not widely available.

Further reading

Kanugo S, Omar HA. Tampons and menstrual hygiene products. In: Hillard PJ (ed). *The 5 Minute Obstetrics and Gynecology Consult*. Philadelphia, PA: Wolters Kluwer, Lippincott Williams & Wilkins, 2008, p. 322.

Omar HA, Aggarwal S, Perkins KC. Tampon use in young women. *J Pediatr Adolesc Gynecol* 1998;11(3):143–146.

Omar HA, Greydanus DE, Tsitsika AK, *et al. Pediatric and Adolescent Sexuality and Gynecology*. New York, NY: Nova Science Publishers, Inc, 2010, p. 319.

29.2 Normal menses

Paula J. Adams Hillard

Department of Obstetrics and Gynecology, Stanford University School of Medicine, Stanford, CA, USA

The onset of the first menstrual period is an event that occurs in the context of maturation of the hypothalamic–pituitary–ovarian axis and pubertal growth (see Chapter 14). Breast growth signals increasing estrogen production; the first menstrual period typically occurs at approximately Tanner stage 4 breast growth. No evidence of breast development by age 13 represents two standard deviations from the mean age of 10 years and should be evaluated. Typically the first menstrual period begins approximately 2–2½ years after the onset of breast growth (thelarche). Failure to achieve menarche by age 15 years or more than 3 years after the onset of breast development should be evaluated.

length, becoming more regular with time. However, most cycles range from 21–45 days, even in the first gynecologic year (Table 29.2.1). Although this range is wider than typically seen in adult women, cycles that are consistently outside of this range are statistically uncommon, and deserve evaluation. By the third year after menarche, 60–80% of cycles are 21–34 days in length, as is typical in adults. An individual girl's normative cycle length is established around the sixth gynecologic year, around age 18 years. Early menarche is associated with an earlier onset of ovulatory cycles. In girls with menarche younger than age 12 years, virtually all cycles are ovulatory by the first year after menarche. In contrast, if menarche occurs after age 12 years, it can take as long as 8–12 years for all cycles to be ovulatory.

⬡ Science at a glance

- **Primary amenorrhea:** defined as no periods by age 15 years (or more than 3 years after the onset of breast development, based on evidence from multiple US studies.
- **Secondary amenorrhea:** a menstrual interval of greater than 90 days is abnormal, even in the first gynecologic year.

☆ Tips and tricks

There is an international movement to use clear and precise "menstrual dimensions" to describe menstrual periods, rather than imprecisely defined medical terms such as menorrhagia or menometrorrhagia.

- **Regularity:** irregular, regular, or absent
- **Frequency:** frequent, normal, or infrequent
- **Duration:** prolonged, normal, or shortened
- **Volume:** heavy, normal, or light

Menstrual cycles in the initial several years after menarche are frequently anovulatory, and variable in

---

Practical Pediatric and Adolescent Gynecology, First Edition. Edited by Paula J. Adams Hillard.
© 2013 John Wiley & Sons, Ltd. Published 2013 by John Wiley & Sons, Ltd.

Table 29.2.1 Menstrual parameters in adolescents

Clinical description		Normal limits
Frequency (days)	Frequent	<21
	Normal	**21–45**
	Infrequent	>45
Regularity	Absent	
	Regular	**Approximately monthly**
	Irregular	Cycles <21 or >45 days
Duration of flow (days)	Prolonged	>8
	Normal	**3–7**
	Shortened	<3
Volume (mL)	Heavy	>80
	Normal	**5–80 (3–6 pads/day)**
	Light	<5

Menstrual bleeding lasts 2–7 days in 80–90% of adolescents. Bleeding that is prolonged beyond 7 days, particularly after an interval of longer than 4–6 weeks, has been associated with anovulation, and deserves an evaluation for causes of anovulation, such as polycystic ovary syndrome (PCOS). PCOS occurs in 5–10% of adults, and the signs and symptoms typically begin during adolescence (see Chapter 50). As many as one-third of girls with irregular menses have been found to have elevated androgens. A careful examination for signs of androgen excess (hirsutism and acne) is warranted (see Chapter 50). While PCOS is the most common cause of infrequent menses in adolescents, many other less common conditions can also cause infrequent periods, and the cause of irregularity should be determined prior to therapy with hormonal medications (birth control pills).

Menstrual bleeding is associated with a mean blood loss of 30 mL/cycle. Chronic blood loss of greater than 80 mL/cycle is associated with anemia, although practically this parameter is of little clinical utility. On average, girls use three to six tampons or pads per day with normal menses, and bleeding that results in use of more than a pad every 1–2 hours would be considered heavy. Heavy, but regular (monthly), bleeding is frequently an early or the only sign of bleeding disorders, such as von Willebrand (VW) disease. VW disease is found in approximately 1% of the general population and up to 24% of women with heavy menstrual bleeding.

Parents, patients, health educators, and coaches should be provided with information about normal menstrual cycles in adolescents, and encouraged to seek an evaluation for cycles that are outside of normal parameters (Table 29.2.1). It is incorrect to assume that because menstrual cycles are somewhat more irregular in adolescents than in adults, that "anything goes" with regard to menstrual cyclicity and regularity. Medical conditions that can significantly impact current and future health and well-being may not be detected and appropriately managed if irregular, heavy, or prolonged bleeding is written off as part of normal adolescence.

✋ Caution

It is important to ascertain if menstrual periods fall within normal limits, as menstrual abnormalities in teens can be associated with medical conditions that have implications for future bone health (e.g. eating disorders) or future cardiovascular health (PCOS).

✋ Patient/parent advice

- The first menstrual period should begin by age 15 years.
- Normal menstrual cycles are between approximately 21 days and 45 days. Cycles longer than 90 days are distinctly uncommon. Bleeding that occurs more frequently than every 21 days or less frequently than every 45 days should be investigated to determine a cause prior to initiating therapy.
- Bleeding should typically last between 3 and 7 days.
- Bleeding heavier than one pad every 1–2 hours is abnormal and deserves investigation.

Further reading

Hillard, PJA. Menstruation. Adolescents: What's normal, what's not. In: Gordon CM, Welt C, Rebar RW *et al.* (eds). The Menstrual Cycle and Adolescent Health. *NY Acad Sci* 2008;1135:29–35.

James AH, Kouides PA, Abdul-Kadir R, *et al.* Von Willebrand disease and other bleeding disorders in women: consensus on diagnosis and management from an international expert panel. *Am J Obstet Gynecol* 2009;201:12 e1–8.

Practice Committee of American Society for Reproductive Medicine. Current evaluation of amenorrhea. *Fertil Steril* 2008;90:S219–225.

29.3

Menstrual suppression

Kelly Kantartzis and Gina Sucato
University of Pittsburgh School of Medicine, Pittsburgh, PA, USA

Menstrual suppression, the use of hormones to delay or eliminate menses, has become increasingly popular among young women. These regimens provide effective treatment for a wide range of menstrual problems experienced by adolescents. In addition, as a result of better patient understanding, provider acceptance, and increased marketing, menstrual suppression is becoming more common among contracepting adolescents.

Regimens

The traditional combined oral contraceptive (COC) pill regimen is 21 days of hormonally active pills, followed by 7 days of placebo. This regimen is an arbitrary one, and pills can be prescribed in a variety of regimens, ideally resulting in menses at periodicities ranging from every other month to never. Common regimens include 42, 63, or 84 days of continuous hormones followed by a 7-day hormone-free interval. Pills can also be taken continuously until bleeding occurs spontaneously at which time a hormone-free interval is initiated or continuously even if bleeding persists. Irregular or breakthrough bleeding is the most common side effect and typically decreases in frequency with length of use. The number of unexpected bleeding days also decreases with more frequently scheduled hormone-free intervals. Irregular bleeding is often the reason for regimen discontinua-

tion, but amenorrhea rates can approach up to 72% with continuous use for 1 year. Continuous pills more effectively suppress ovarian follicular development than do pills with a 7-day hormone-free interval, as do pills with a 4-day hormone-free interval.

Extended use of the vaginal ring (etonogestrel 120 µg/ethinyl estradiol 15 µg) and the transdermal patch (norelgestromin 6 mg/ethinyl estradiol 0.75 mg) demonstrate similar bleeding patterns compared to COCs and may be an alternative for patients with poor pill adherence. Although the vaginal ring package insert recommends that one ring only be used for up to 28 days, the rings contain sufficient medication for use for up to 35 days, and thus can be replaced once every calendar month. This eliminates the need for additional refills potentially not covered by insurers, which sometimes poses barriers to continuous pill and patch regimens. Extended cycling with the transdermal patch must be used with caution; systemic estrogen levels are estimated to be 1.6 times higher with the patch than with a standard low-dose COC pill and 3.4 times higher than with the vaginal ring. Given the greater theoretical risk of venous thromboembolism conferred by these higher estrogen levels, the transdermal patch is rarely a first-line choice for extended cycling.

Long-acting progestin-only contraception, including depot medroxyprogesterone acetate (DMPA) and the levonorgestrel intrauterine device (LNG-IUD), is associated with initial irregular bleeding. Similar to

Practical Pediatric and Adolescent Gynecology, First Edition. Edited by Paula J. Adams Hillard.
© 2013 John Wiley & Sons, Ltd. Published 2013 by John Wiley & Sons, Ltd.

combined hormonal contraception, irregular bleeding decreases with time and amenorrhea rates with DMPA and the LNG-IUD range between 45% and 71% at 1 year. Despite earlier warnings cautioning against the placement of the LNG-IUD in nulligravid women, recent studies have shown that an IUD can be safely placed in teenagers with a very low risk of expulsion (<10%) and almost no risk of uterine perforation. The etonogestrel subdermal implant is rarely used for menstrual suppression given its unpredictable bleeding patterns and low likelihood of amenorrhea (reported in some series as <20%). Similarly, the progestin-only pill infrequently results in amenorrhea.

Gonadotropin-releasing hormone (GnRH) agonists (e.g. Lupron®) can induce a hypoestrogenic environment in approximately 4 weeks, resulting in amenorrhea rates of over 75%. However, given the potential impact on bone mineral density in an adolescent, GnRH agonists are usually reserved for short-term use in oncology patients or as a final option after adolescents have failed all other treatments for serious conditions such as menorrhagia resulting in anemia or severe endometriosis.

Indications

Adolescents and their families may request less frequent menstruation for a variety of indications. (Table 29.3.1). Surveys of high-school age adolescents in the US and Europe have found that almost three-quarters of those surveyed preferred to menstruate less frequently than monthly or never. Other adolescents may seek amenorrhea only for a specific event or time interval, such as during a sports season or a class trip. In addition, patients with physical disabilities and the parents of patients with severe mental disabilities may request less frequent and more predictable menstruation to assist with menstrual hygiene (see Chapter 28).

Menstrual-related conditions, such as premenstrual syndrome, menorrhagia, and dysmenorrhea, may improve with traditional cyclic contraceptive use. However, many women whose symptoms persist during the hormone-free interval report better symptom resolution with elimination of the hormone-free interval. Improvements in pain scores among women with cyclic pelvic pain can be quite dramatic.

Table 29.3.1 Indications

- Patient preference
- Menstrual-related problems:
  - Dysmenorrhea
  - Pelvic pain
  - Menorrhagia
  - Premenstrual syndrome
  - Endometriosis
  - Recurrent ovarian cysts
- Chronic conditions with cyclic exacerbations:
  - Epilepsy
  - Migraines or other headaches
  - Asthma
  - Cystic fibrosis
  - Porphyria
- Hematologic abnormalities:
  - Anemia
  - Thrombocytopenia
  - von Willebrand disease
- Malignancy
- Menstrual hygiene:
  - Developmental delay
  - Physical disabilities

Many medical conditions and diseases demonstrate symptom variability throughout the menstrual cycle. For example, migraines and other types of headaches often worsen in the premenstrual or menstrual phase of the cycle. Headaches may improve with cyclic oral contraceptive use, but again patients whose headaches persist during the hormone-free interval have fewer and less severe headaches with extended regimens. Of note, the use of combined hormonal contraceptives in women who have migraine with aura is judged by the World Health Organization to represent an unacceptable health risk.

The heavy menstrual bleeding resulting from hematologic conditions, such as von Willebrand disease or platelet function disorders, often responds well to management with contraceptive hormones. Unfortunately, these methods may be contraindicated or inadequately effective in oncology patients, especially those undergoing blood and marrow transplant in whom heavy bleeding can be significant and difficult to manage. As a result, many experts recommend the use of GnRH agonists as the safest and most

Science revisited

Drug–drug interactions

• Combined hormonal contraceptives can interact with other medications also metabolized by the cytochrome P450 3A4 system.

• In patients whose medications require a steady state, e.g. lamictal and immunosuppressants, minimizing the number of hormone-free intervals can minimize serum drug-level fluctuations.

• It is critical that all healthcare providers are aware of the patient's medications in case further dosing adjustments are warranted.

effective method to induce short-term amenorrhea in these patients. In our clinical experience, leuprolide acetate (depot suspension 11.25 mg IM) every 3 months is an effective regimen, with infrequent reports of side effects such as hot flashes, mucous membrane dryness, or mood changes.

Menstruation in adolescents with physical or cognitive disabilities can be difficult for the patient, her caregivers, or both (see Chapter 28). Many gynecology visits for developmentally delayed adolescents, particularly those with additional diagnoses such as autism spectrum disorders, are for menstrual-related complaints and involve caregiver requests for menstrual suppression, often specifically with DMPA. DMPA has many benefits including a high likelihood of achieving amenorrhea, elimination of pill taking, and no estrogen, which may be beneficial in immobile women as these girls have a higher risk of venous thromboembolism due to their immobility. However, the hypoestrogenic environment that can occur may limit its long-term use in adolescents, especially those already at risk for poor bone health because of decreased mobility or chronic steroid use. Other methods may be difficult for patients to use. Patches may be inadvertently removed; girls may not be able to place their own vaginal rings. The LNG-IUD may be an ideal treatment given its overall high rate of amenorrhea, low risk of serious side effects, and minimal maintenance. Placement in women with special needs may require conscious sedation or general anesthesia, which may bring additional risks.

Side effects and concerns

Irregular bleeding

Irregular or unexpected bleeding is the main side effect of attempting menstrual suppression and the main reason for method or regimen discontinuation. The highest rates of irregular bleeding usually occur when a regimen is started; breakthrough bleeding is almost universal in the first 3 months of use. The frequency of unexpected bleeding declines significantly with time.

Evidence at a glance

Bleeding patterns after 1 year of continuous hormone use

• Combined oral contraceptives: amenorrhea rate – 50–70%
• DMPA: amenorrhea rate – 45–70%
• Levenorgestrel IUD: amenorrhea rate – 50%
• Transdermal patch*: amenorrhea rate at 3 months – 10%
• Vaginal ring: median number or bleeding or spotting days – 14 days in months 9 through 12 of use
• Subdermal etonorgestrel implant: mean number of bleeding or spotting days – 19 days in months 9 through 12 of use

*Information only available for 3 months of continuous patch use.

Among combined hormonal contraceptives, no formulation or regimen has emerged as the most likely to minimize breakthrough bleeding. Limited data suggest that the use of pills containing an estrane progestin (e.g. norethindrone) may result in less breakthrough bleeding regardless of estrogen dose. However, given the paucity of data, finding the right regimen for a particular patient needs to be individualized and often relies on trial and error.

Management of irregular bleeding includes reassurance, changing pill formulations, shortening the interval between scheduled withdrawal bleeds (e.g. from 84 to 63 days), switching to a different method of suppression, combining various methods, or instituting an unscheduled hormone-free interval. There is evidence to support the use of a 3- or 4-day hormone-free interval as an effective strategy for resolving persistent irregular bleeding in women using combined hormonal methods continuously. Patients should be instructed that hormone-free intervals should not occur more frequently than every 3 weeks to ensure contraceptive efficacy.

✳ Tips and tricks

Strategies for management of irregular bleeding that occurs with extended cycling

• Reassurance
• Prescribe short-term high-dose nonsteroidal anti-inflammatory drugs (e.g. ibuprofen 800 mg PO TID for 5 days)
• Shorten the interval between scheduled withdrawal bleeds
• Institute a 4-day hormone-free interval after 5 days of unexpected bleeding
• Combine two methods, such as an estrogen containing method with an LNG-IUD, or during early DMPA use

---

Bone health

Given the majority of a woman's peak bone mass is attained by the age of 18 years, the effect of long-term use of hormonal contraception on adolescent bone health is an important clinical question. Studies on oral contraceptives and bone health have yielded inconsistent results, with no consensus on the ideal ethinyl estradiol dose to optimize bone health. Likewise there are limited data available that address bone health in adolescents with use of the transdermal patch, vaginal ring, or extended cycles of COC pills.

Multiple studies have shown that while using DMPA, adolescents have decreased bone mineral density compared to adolescents using no contraception or oral contraceptive pills. Because of these findings, the FDA issued a black box warning advising caution when prescribing DMPA for more than 2 years; statements from a number of professional organizations including the American College of Obstetrics and Gynecology and the Society for Adolescent Health and Medicine have concluded that

the benefits should be weighed against potential risks. Recent studies have shown recovery of bone mineral density after discontinuation. Bone loss may be mitigated by consuming more than 1200 mg of calcium daily. In contrast, the LNG-IUD and the subdermal implant have no known effects on bone health in women.

Patient concerns

Patients and their families often ask if suppressing menses could have negative health consequences, such as infertility or cancer. Extended regimens have no known impact on return to fertility. Similarly, endometrial biopsies obtained in women using continuous hormones have shown no evidence of hyperplasia or malignancy. Overall, most experts believe menstrual suppression is safe for both short- and long-term use.

✋ Patient/parent advice

• Menstrual suppression can have a number of benefits to health, and can help manage medical problems such as heavy bleeding, pain, and other medical conditions.
• Menstrual suppression has *not* been associated with future health problems; there is no increased risk of infertility.
• Almost everyone has unscheduled (unpredictable) bleeding in the first few months of use.
• The longer a method is used, the greater the likelihood of no bleeding.

Conclusion

Many adolescents experience significant health benefits from menstrual suppression and many prefer fewer menses. Patient counseling about potential side effects is crucial given that management of these side effects, especially irregular bleeding, can be an ongoing and individualized process. Patients and their families can be reassured that menstrual suppression has not been associated with any long-term negative health consequences and may improve contraceptive effectiveness.

Pearls

• Menstrual suppression can result in many health benefits, but achieving complete amenorrhea can be difficult.
• Important steps in initiating menstrual suppression:
  ○ Understanding patient preferences
  ○ Careful management of patient expectations:
    – Provision of preventive guidance about breakthrough bleeding
    – Development of an individualized plan to manage unexpected or irregular bleeding.

Further reading

ACOG Committee Opinion No. 392, December 2007. Intrauterine Device and Adolescents. *Obstet Gynecol* 2007;110(6):1493–1495.

Gerschultz KL, Sucato GS. Eliminating monthly periods with combined hormonal contraception. *Womens Health (Lond Engl)* 2007;3(5):541–545.

Tolaymat LL, Kaunitz AM. Long-acting contraceptives in adolescents. *Curr Opin Obstet Gynecol* 2007;19(5):453–460.

30.1 When and how to perform a gynecologic exam

Paula J. Adams Hillard

Department of Obstetrics and Gynecology, Stanford University School of Medicine, Stanford, CA, USA

Indications

The gynecologic exam allows an assessment of common medical concerns that present to a primary clinician. These concerns include questions about pubertal growth, menstrual disorders (periods that are too frequent, too infrequent, too heavy, or painful), pelvic and abdominal pain, vulvar rashes and itching, vaginal discharge, contraception, and sexually-transmitted infections (STIs). The extent of the exam required for each of these concerns varies: from a simple inspection of the external genitalia, to an internal speculum and/or bimanual exam; and should be individualized on the basis of the specific symptom as well as historical information, including history of voluntary sexual activity or involuntary sexual abuse or rape. While primary pediatricians or other clinicians may or may not feel comfortable providing pelvic examinations, depending on the clinician's age, gender, experiences during residency training, and duration of the relationship that they have with a young girl or adolescent, the American Academy of Pediatrics (AAP) argues that the primary care office with the primary clinician who has established rapport and trust with the patient is often the best setting in which to perform this examination. If a clinician does not feel comfortable providing this service, or there are specific symptoms or findings, referral to a gynecologist may be warranted (Table 30.1.1). However, as many general gynecologists have not had experience with young girls or young adolescents, and there may be specific problems, referral to a specialist in adolescent gynecology or reproductive endocrinology who has experience in addressing these uncommon problems may be appropriate (Table 30.1.2).

The AAP indicates that examination of the external genitalia should be included as part of the annual comprehensive physical exam of children and adolescents of all ages. Inspection should be performed to confirm normal anatomy, assess pubertal development, and look for any unusual vulvar rashes, lesions, infection, or trauma. Making genital inspection a part of a complete examination has the effect of normalizing the experience, rather than setting it apart as exceptional. It should be explained to parents and girls that this is part of a thorough exam. Because a young girl typically trusts her primary clinician, this setting can be less uncomfortable to her.

Because the American College of Obstetricians and Gynecologists (ACOG) now recommends that cervical cancer screening should begin at age 21 years (with very few exceptions, including primarily HIV infection or immune suppression; see Chapter 30.2), and because screening for STIs can be performed on urine specimens or vaginal swabs, fewer adolescents now require a speculum examination.

Practical Pediatric and Adolescent Gynecology, First Edition. Edited by Paula J. Adams Hillard.
© 2013 John Wiley & Sons, Ltd. Published 2013 by John Wiley & Sons, Ltd.

Table 30.1.1 Reasons for a primary clinician to refer an adolescent to a gynecologist

- Vulvar, vaginal, or cervical lesion of unclear etiology or unresponsive to previous management
- Abnormal bleeding (heavy menstrual bleeding, amenorrhea, frequent bleeding) of unclear etiology or bleeding unresponsive to medical therapy or with anemia
- Dysmenorrhea unresponsive to NSAIDs and/or hormonal therapy
- Acute pelvic pain (concern about adnexal mass, ectopic pregnancy, pelvic infection)
- Chronic pelvic pain
- Adnexal mass
- Genital anomaly (duplication, imperforate hymen, vaginal septum, vaginal agenesis)
- Pregnancy
- Pelvic infection (if suspicion of tubo-ovarian complex or abscess or if clinician is not comfortable with management)
- Contraception in young women with chronic medical conditions
- Desire for contraceptive implant or IUD
- Genital trauma
- History of past gynecologic surgery with concerns about anatomy, risk of recurrence, genital anomalies, fertility

Table 30.1.2 Reasons to refer an adolescent to a gynecologist or specialist with greater experience in uncommon genital problems

- Genital anomaly:
  - Uterine duplication
  - Vaginal septum (transverse or longitudinal)
  - Vaginal agenesis
  - Obstructing anomaly:
    - Imperforate hymen,
    - Obstructing longitudinal or transverse vaginal septum with hematocolpos and/or hematometra
    - Cervical agenesis
    - Obstructed uterine horn
- History of specific gynecologic diagnoses:
  - Endometriosis
  - Germ cell tumor
  - Ovarian torsion
  - Lichen sclerosus
  - Vulvar aphthosis
  - Accidental vulvar trauma
  - Primary ovarian insufficiency
- Disorders of sex development (DSD): best managed with a team approach with genetics, endocrinology, urology, gynecology, social services, advocates for individuals with DSD (see Chapter 2):
  - History of unknown diagnosis with genital surgery in infancy or childhood
  - History of virilization and subsequent surgery:
    - Congenital adrenal hyperplasia
    - Partial androgen insensitivity syndrome
  - Complete androgen insensitivity syndrome
  - Sex chromosome anomalies:
    - Turner syndrome/gonadal dysgenesis
  - Disorders of gonadal development
- Menstrual suppression for medical indications:
  - Developmental delay or autism
  - Bleeding disorders such as von Willebrand disease
  - Menstrual molimina
- Contraception for adolescents with complex medical problems
- Vulvar masses or lesions

Indications for a pelvic exam have been described by the AAP (Table 30.1.3) and can be interpreted as recommendations for an exam that consists of more than a visual inspection.

Performance of the pelvic exam

The pelvic exam is performed in the context of a relationship in which trust has been established. As noted, this may be with the primary clinician, or it may be in the context of an initial adolescent gynecology visit (see Chapter 17). Issues of confidentiality will have been addressed (see Chapter 18), and the structure of the visit may have followed that outlined in Chapter 17. The need for an examination will have been explained, and the adolescent asked whether she wants her mother (or another individual – girlfriend or boyfriend or a trusted adult) to be with her for the exam. The adolescent will have been asked if she has any additional questions, and all questions will have been answered. Many, if not most, adolescents have some degree of anxiety about their first internal or complete pelvic exam, and this can be acknowledged, along with assurances of confidentiality, gentleness,

Table 30.1.3 Indications for a pelvic exam

- Persistent vaginal discharge
- Dysuria or urinary tract symptoms in a sexually-active female
- Dysmenorrhea unresponsive to nonsteroidal anti-inflammatory drugs
- Amenorrhea
- Abnormal vaginal bleeding
- Lower abdominal pain
- Contraceptive counseling for an intrauterine device or diaphragm
- Perform Pap test
- Suspected/reported rape or sexual abuse
- Pregnancy

Evidence at a glance

- Initiating cervical cytology screening before the age of 21 years does not change the rate of cervical cancer.
- Cervical cancer is extremely rare in individuals younger than age 21 years.
- Cervical cytology testing should begin at the age of 21 years in almost all young women.
- If cervical cytology testing is performed prior to age 21 years, management typically involves observation with minimal to no intervention.
- Human papillomavirus (HPV) infection is extremely common among adolescents, and thus HPV vaccination should be offered to all adolescents as scheduled at age 11–12 or as a catch-up vaccination (see Chapter 24).

✋ Patient/parent advice

- Your first complete gynecologic exam is a good first step to knowing about your health.
- Most people describe the exam as uncomfortable; it generally does not hurt.
- Be prepared:
  ○ Learn about your anatomy
  ○ Ask questions
  ○ Ask to look in a mirror if you're curious
  ○ Ask about what the clinician found.

and explanations. The exam should not be rushed, as adequate time is particularly important for the performance of a first gynecologic exam; if a previous examination had been difficult, painful, or traumatic; or if there is a past history of assault or abuse.

Before performing a complete pelvic examination you should:
- Be sure that you have already screened for any history of physical or sexual abuse.
- *Ask* if this is the first exam, and if not, what was her experience of the previous exam.
- Be sure that *she* chooses whom to have with her at the time of the exam: her mother, another relative, a friend (male or female).
- Ask, "Who have you talked with about the exam – your mother, a girlfriend?" ; "What did they say?"
- Dispel myths and address fears:
  ○ "Most people describe their first exam as uncomfortable and not painful."
  ○ "I know it may feel a little embarrassing and you've not had this complete exam done before, but I've done lots of first exams for girls your age."
- "I'll tell you what to expect for each step of the exam *before* I touch or do anything."
- "If at any time the exam is too painful, you need to tell me. I have lots of tricks that I can tell you to make it easier."
- Describe the pelvic exam to the extent that the patient wants to hear about it, prior to asking her to undress:
  ○ A plastic model can be used to demonstrate pelvic anatomy.
  ○ If your patient wants to see the speculum, you can demonstrate this before the exam.
- Allow privacy for her to change, but be explicit about what clothing to remove:
  ○ "You'll need to take *everything* off, except your socks; that means your panties and your bra, because we're going to do a breast exam and a complete pelvic exam."
  ○ Provide an appropriately sized gown and sheet.
  ○ Describe how you want her to put on the gown, e.g. "so that it opens in the back."
  ○ Indicate: "I'll be back in a few minutes to give you time to change, and I'll knock on the door before I enter."
- A breast exam may be performed as indicated. Breast self-exam may be discussed in older teens.
- Perform any other indicated examinations:

○ Thyroid
○ Abdomen:
– If abdomino-pelvic pain, assess all quadrants, liver, spleen, and assess for myofascial trigger points or localized tenderness, abdominal masses, excessive stool in left lower quadrant
○ If polycystic ovary syndrome (PCOS) is suspected, inspect for the presence of:
– Hirsutism. "When I'm suspicious about hormones being out of balance I look for any signs of more than average hair growth. I don't see much, but I need to ask, do you do anything to remove hair on your face, like bleaching, shaving, waxing, or threading?" Observe upper lip, sideburns, chin, upper and lower back, periareolar area, midline chest, upper and lower abdomen, inner thighs.
– Acanthosis nigricans of the neck, beneath breasts, axillae.

The steps in performing the first pelvic exam are:
• Drape the patient with a large sheet over the abdomen and legs (preferably cloth, rather than paper).
• Show the patient how to slide to the end of the table.
• If the table will allow, raise the head so that the patient is not lying flat.
• Assist the patient with placement of feet in the stirrups.
• Tell the patient you need to check to see if she has scooted to the right place at the end of the table.
• While still draped, ask the patient to let her knees fall apart, with inner thighs relaxed.
• Tuck the sheet around the patient's legs, keeping knees draped but being sure the drape is lowered in the middle, "So I can see you, and you can see me."
• Ask if the patient would like a mirror to see what you are seeing.
• "First of all, you'll feel me touch on your thighs."
○ If she is really anxious, "Does that hurt?". The answer is invariably , "No".
• "Next you'll feel me touch the area around the outside of your vagina."
○ "Does that hurt?" Again, if there are no lesions, the answer is typically "No".

• Gently inspect the pubic hair, noting Tanner staging, any lesions, inguinal adenopathy, the skin of the labia minora and majora, any inflammation or lesions such as ulcers, fissures, warts, vesicles.
• Visualize the hymen and note configuration and any partially obstructing hymenal bands, microperforation, vaginal septae, enlargement of Bartholin's or Skene's glands.
• "Next you'll feel me touch with one finger at the outside of your vagina. Most people describe that as pressure." (Use the lubricated index finger of the non-dominant hand.)
• Place gentle pressure posteriorly, while saying, "You have some strong muscles at the opening of your vagina.""
○ Assess whether muscles are tightly contracted; if so, "I want you to see if you can tighten those muscles even more."
○ Most girls are able to do this, but if unaware of the pelvic floor muscles, they may not be able to tighten further. "Try to tighten the same muscles that you would use if you were sitting on the toilet peeing; if you were expecting a really important phone call, you'd use those muscles to stop peeing."
○ "Those muscles are the key to the entire exam, and until you let them relax, we won't be able to do the exam."
• If unable to relax the pelvic floor muscles, do *not* attempt to insert a speculum.
○ Tell the patient that relaxing the muscles is necessary for the exam. Let her try again, and if she is still unable to relax the muscles, reschedule the exam if it is not urgent, and encourage her to practice relaxing the muscles.
• If patient is able to relax the pelvic floor muscles:
○ "Next I'm going to gently look inside your vagina with the speculum, which is about the width of my finger."
○ "Do you want to see the speculum?" If yes, demonstrate it and state that it has been warmed (with water or on a heating pad).
• Gently insert the warmed and sparingly lubricated speculum over the top of your index finger while withdrawing this finger. Keep gentle pressure posteriorly (anterior pressure causes urethral discomfort).
• Insert the speculum to its length before opening it, telling patient she will feel more pressure. The diameter of the speculum is smallest at the hinge/fulcrum,

177

the area which should be at the hymenal ring when the speculum is completely inserted.

• Note any vaginal discharge, taking specimens for KOH/saline microscopic prep or trichomonas culture.

• Visualize the cervix, take specimens (Pap or endocervical swab for gonorrhea and chlamydia) with warning, "I'm going to use a Q-tip to take a sample, and this will feel crampy" (if placed in the endocervix) or "scratchy" (if using a pap spatula).

• Note any mucopurulent discharge or friability of the cervix suggesting cervicitis.

• If the patient had expressed interest in using a mirror, ask if she wants to see her cervix.

• Tell the patient you are going to remove the speculum, and remind her to let her muscles relax.

• After the speculum exam, "We're done with the hardest part of the exam. You did really well. Next I'm going to place one finger in your vagina to be sure that things feel normal."

• Lubricate *only* the index finger of the dominant hand for single-finger bimanual exam; lubricating the thumb only leads to smearing lubricant over the perineum and clitoris.

• Place the *single* finger (index finger of dominant hand) *pronated* at introitus and remind the patient to "relax those same muscles again."

• Insert the index finger to the second knuckle before telling patient "You'll feel my finger moving inside;" then rotate the hand to supination.

• Throughout the exam, but particularly during the bimanual exam, observe the patient's nonverbal communication, body language, and facial expressions. Gentle humor may help.

• Palpate the cervix, assessing uterine position by palpating the anterior and posterior fornix, telling patient, "You'll feel me moving your uterus, and that may feel a bit different from what you've felt before."

• Assess uterine characteristics:
  ○ Size (normal size compared to pregnancy gestational age, e.g. "8-week size")
  ○ Shape (regular contour vs bumpy, as with uterine fibroids)
  ○ Position (anteverted, anteflexed, axial, retroverted, retroflexed)
  ○ Consistency (firm = normal vs softened as in pregnancy)

  ○ Mobility (mobile or fixed)
  ○ Tenderness (normal = nontender)
• Similarly, assess adnexae:
  ○ Palpable normal ovaries
  ○ Describe any discrete mass (vs fullness in adnexae):
    – Size (preferably in cm vs fruit—grapefruit, orange, lemon),
    – Consistency (cystic vs firm),
    – Tenderness (normal = nontender)
  ○ If unable to palpate ovaries, state in the chart :
    – "No adnexal masses appreciated" or
    – "Unable to assess adnexae due to body habitus" if overweight or obese.

• If deemed necessary, a rectovaginal exam can assess for posterior uterine tenderness or nodularity, as might be seen with endometriosis. Describe each step of the exam to the patient.

• If unable to do a vaginal bimanual exam (because the patient is a young adolescent or she is unable to tolerate) and this is felt to be essential, the clinician can assess the pelvis using rectal examination alone.

• At the end of exam, provide a summary:
  ○ "Your exam looks completely normal" or
  ○ If there are any abnormal findings, describe briefly, stating, "You can get dressed and we'll talk more about it."

• Remind the patient to slide back from the edge of the table before sitting up.

• Provide a wipe/tissue to clean up/remove lubricant from the perineum, "to wipe the goopy stuff off".

• Warn her that there may be some spotting, and offer a pad or tampon.

• Provide feedback, "You did a great job" if true. If she tolerated the exam poorly, "You did the best that you could. It's clear that the exam was hard for you. Next time you'll know better what to expect."

An adolescent's successful completion of her first gynecologic exam can be empowering, and can allow her to feel some mastery and ownership of her ability to take charge of her own health. The hope is that with this examination in which she is able to learn about her own body, her interest in keeping it healthy will increase. The first pelvic exam, performed in a gentle, collaborative, respectful manner, can set the stage for a lifetime of gynecologic health and good preventive health screening health habits.

✋ Caution

- Before performing the first gynecologic exam, always screen for a history of physical or sexual abuse.
- Decide what is the most important part of the exam, and start with that part. For example, if there is concern regarding uterine tenderness, start with a gentle bimanual exam; the speculum exam can be omitted if necessary.
- If the patient is unable to tolerate the exam, *stop* immediately if she indicates that she is unable to proceed:
  - You will not be able to get adequate information if she is in significant pain, and the exam has the potential to further traumatize her.
  - Alternatives for information gathering, such as a transabdominal pelvic ultrasound, clinician or self-collected vaginal swabs for STI testing, or repeating an exam at a later date may be necessary.

Further reading

American College of Obstetricians and Gynecologists. *Toolkit for Teen Care*, 2nd edn. Washington DC: ACOG, 2010.

Braverman PK, Breech L. American Academy of Pediatrics. Clinical report–gynecologic examination for adolescents in the pediatric office setting. *Pediatrics* 2010;126:583–590.

Emans SJ. Office evaluation of the child and adolescent. In: Emans SJ, Laufer M (eds). *Goldstein's Pediatric and Adolescent Gynecology*, 6th edn. Philadelphia: Lippincott Williams & Wilkins, 2012, pp. 1–20.

30.2 Cervical cytology screening

Paula J. Adams Hillard

Department of Obstetrics and Gynecology, Stanford University School of Medicine, Stanford, CA, USA

Guidelines for cervical cytology screening (traditionally termed the Pap test or Pap smear, short for Papanicolau smear) in adolescents have changed a great deal in the last 30 years. In the past, guidelines from the American Cancer Society (ACS), the American College of Obstetricians and Gynecologists (ACOG), and the American Society of Colposcopy and Cervical Pathology (ASCCP) recommended the initiation of screening based on the age of initiation of vaginal intercourse. Cervical intraepithelial neoplasia (CIN), the potentially premalignant cervical changes that can progress to an invasive cervical cancer, is caused by infection with certain high-risk types of the sexually-transmitted human papillomavirus (HPV). As additional knowledge has been gained about the epidemiology and natural history of infection with HPV, as well as the natural history of CIN, it has become apparent that, while many adolescents acquire an infection with HPV after the onset of sexual activity, 90% of these infections resolve within 24 months in otherwise healthy teens with an intact immune system (see Chapter 44.2). HPV vaccination of girls and boys at the recommended age of 11–12 years or as a "catch-up" vaccine has the potential to minimize the risk of acquisition and transmission of HPV, and to ultimately lower the risks of cervical, vaginal, vulvar, and anal cancers.

Cervical cancer is truly rare in adolescents, and cervical cytology screening does not appear to change the rate of cervical cancer in this age group. Thus,

> ### ✋ Caution
>
> - Cervical cancer is rare in adolescents.
> - HPV acquisition is common in adolescents.
> - Cervical cytology screening does not change the rate of cervical cancer in adolescents.
> - Cervical cytology screening should begin at age 21 years in most adolescents.
> - *Exceptions*:
>   - Adolescents with HIV:
>   - Screen twice in first year after HIV diagnosis
>   - Annual screening after first year.
>   - Adolescents with immunocompromise (organ transplant recipients, long-term steroid use):
>   - Initial screen after the onset of sexual activity
>   - Screen twice in first year after sexual debut
>   - Annual screening after first year.
> - HPV testing is *not* recommended at any time, including prior to HPV vaccination (see Chapter 24) in adolescents. If obtained, a positive result should not influence management.
> - The diagnosis of a non-HIV STI is not an indication for earlier cervical cytology screening.
> - Pregnancy does not alter screening guidelines.

Table 30.2.1 Management of adolescents with abnormal cervical cytology

Cytologic/histologic finding	Management
ASC-US, LSIL, CIN 1	Repeat cytology in 1 year Colposcopy indicated if HSIL or if persistence x 2 years Persistence of CIN 1 >24 months, strongly consider ongoing monitoring
ASC-H	Colposcopy If *no* CIN 2 or 3, repeat cytology every 6 months with repeat colposcopy if *any* cytologic abnormality If two consecutive normal cytology, repeat at age 21 years
HSIL	Colposcopy with endocervical sampling: "see and treat" with LEEP is unacceptable If *no* CIN 2 or 3, repeat colposcopy/ endocervical sampling and cytology at 6-month intervals If HSIL persistent at 1 year, repeat biopsy and thorough vaginal exam If HSIL persists at 24 months and no vaginal lesions, perform diagnostic excision
AGC	Colposcopy with endocervical sampling by clinician with expertise in dysplasia Endometrial sampling not required unless morbidly obese, or with abnormal bleeding, oligomenorrhea, or suspicion of endometrial cancer
CIN 2, 3	Observation with colposcopy and cytology every 6 months up to 24 months *or* Ablation or excision provided there is satisfactory colposcopy If colposcopy unsatisfactory, treatment is recommended If CIN 2 on biopsy, observation is preferred, but treatment is acceptable During observation, if colposcopic appearance of lesions worsens or HSIL cytology or colposcopy persists x 1 year, repeat biopsy is indicated Persistent CIN 2- or 3-confirmed histology for 24 months, treatment is recommended CIN 3: therapy is recommended

ASC-US, atypical squamous cells of undetermined significance; ASC-H, atypical squamous cells, cannot rule out high-grade squamous intraepithelial lesion; LSIL, low-grade intraepithelial lesion; HSIL, high-grade squamous intraepithelial lesion; CIN, cervical intraepithelial neoplasia; AGC, atypical glandular cells.

ACOG now recommends that cervical cytology screening begin at age 21 years in most healthy adolescents, regardless of the age of onset of sexual activity.

Healthy adolescents who have previously had cervical cytology testing performed prior to age 21 years should not be rescreened until age 21 years. Table 30.2.1 describes the management of adolescents in whom an abnormal cervical test has been obtained. In general, observation and conservative management is emphasized, as the vast majority of lesions, including CIN 2, will regress in this population.

Cervical loop electrosurgical excision procedures (LEEP) are associated with an increased risk of preterm labor and premature rupture of membranes in a subsequent pregnancy. Consent for colposcopy, biopsy, and treatment of cervical dysplasia is generally considered analogous to consent for diagnosis and treatment of STIs, for which minors are typically allowed to consent. Individual state laws should be consulted. Parental involvement should be encouraged, as parental guidance and support can be helpful. In addition, the procedure will be billed, and an explanation of benefits for insurance purposes can compromise confidentiality.

Because adolescents have high rates of STIs, screening and treatment for *Chlamydia trachomatis* and *Neisseria gonorrhoeae* should be performed before cervical treatment procedures.

✋ Patient/parent advice

- For almost all adolescents, the first Pap test should be done at age 21 years.
- The Pap test is not the same as a pelvic exam:
  ○ A pelvic exam (using a speculum – a metal instrument that spreads the walls of the vagina) may be needed to check for infection or to look for causes of vaginal discharge or bleeding.
  ○ A Pap test *may* be done at the same time, but this is not always the case.
- An abnormal Pap test does *not* mean you have cancer; most abnormal pap tests in teens show mild changes.
- Mild changes on a Pap test usually go away on their own. Mild changes include:
  ○ ASC-US: atypical squamous cells of undetermined significance
  ○ LSIL: low-grade squamous intraepithelial lesions.
- If a cervical procedure is recommended to treat an abnormal Pap test, a second opinion from another clinician is not unreasonable, as there are risks associated with cervical treatments.
- The use of condoms will help minimize the risks of some STIs, but does not eliminate the risks of getting HPV, which requires only skin-to-skin contact, not necessarily vaginal intercourse.
- HPV vaccination is safe and effective at lowering the risks of getting HPV, genital warts, and cervical cancer.

Summary

Cervical cancer screening before the age of 21 years does not change the rate of cervical cancer. Current guidelines recommend that cervical cancer screening should begin in almost all adolescents at age 21 years; adolescents with chronic immunosuppression (HIV, organ transplant, or chronic steroid use) should have earlier screening. Current guidelines for treatment of CIN in adolescents emphasize observation for management of CIN 1, and indicate that observation is the preferred treatment for CIN 2. The guidelines consider the adverse impact of screening in adolescents – unnecessary colposcopic procedures and the potential risks of cervical excision procedures on future pregnancy outcomes.

Further reading

ACOG Committee on Adolescent Health Care. Cervical Center in Adolescents: Screening, Evaluation, and Management. Committee Opinion #463. American College of Obstetricians and Gynecologists. *Obstet Gynecol* 2010; 116:469–472.

Kahn JA, Slap GB, Bernstein DI, *et al.* Personal meaning of human papillomavirus and pap test results in adolescent and young adult women. *Health Psychol* 2007;26(2): 192–200.

Wright TC Jr, Massad LS, Dunton CJ, Spitzer M, Wilkinson EJ, Solomon D. 2006 Consensus guidelines for the management of women with abnormal cervical screening tests. 2006 ASCCP-Sponsored Consensus Conference. *J Low Genit Tract Dis* 2007;11:201–222.

31 Sexually-transmitted disease screening

Michael G. Spigarelli

Division of Adolescent Medicine, University of Utah, Salt Lake City, UT, USA

If screening is to be effective, it must be understood that all potential sexually-transmitted disease (STD) infections must be screened for, and not just suspected or known infections tested for in symptomatic individuals. With all STD infections, asymptomatic carriage is the expected norm as this is typical for the vast majority of the time, making screening followed by appropriate treatment the most effective way to prevent disease-related sequelae, as well as to decrease the impact and burden of disease within the population. Properly accomplished screening will by definition produce many appropriately negative tests. Current estimates indicate that the rate of STD screening is exceedingly low, with only 2% of adolescent females screened when asymptomatic and only 14% tested when actually symptomatic.

This chapter will discuss the basic approach to screening in female adolescents, and will encompass who to screen, when to screen, and how to accomplish that screening.

Who should be screened?

All sexually-active adolescent and young adult females up through age 25 years should be screened for the appropriate sexually-transmitted infections (STIs). This age cut point was chosen because women who are sexually active and younger than this age have the highest incidence of infection and the highest number of recent partners; the vast majority of those infections are asymptomatic.

In order to accomplish this screening, it is important for healthcare providers to be comfortable discussing sexual activity with adolescents. This requires time to provide an explanation of confidentiality and to discuss the topic in private, away from parents or guardians (see Chapters 17 and 18). All states recognize the right to screen, diagnose, and treat STIs confidentially, so long as the adolescent is above the age of consent (see Chapter 19); this should be discussed with all adolescents, and appropriate time dedicated to this important aspect of healthcare. It is typically easiest to introduce a specific provider-patient time for confidential discussions during each visit with an adolescent, in order to allow personal issues to be routinely discussed. It is important not to ask sensitive questions in front of the parent or guardian, as this places the adolescent in a "no-win" situation where she may feel the need to lie to protect her privacy or feel compelled to reveal information, both of which have the potential to damage her future healthcare (see Chapter 17).

What screening should be done and when?

Current evidence supports testing for *Chlamydia trachomatis*, *Neisseria gonorrhoeae*, and human immunodeficiency virus (HIV) infection at least annually

Practical Pediatric and Adolescent Gynecology, First Edition. Edited by Paula J. Adams Hillard.
© 2013 John Wiley & Sons, Ltd. Published 2013 by John Wiley & Sons, Ltd.

> ### ★ Tips and tricks
>
> • It is important to insist that a portion of each adolescent healthcare visit be a confidential time with the adolescent and the provider, as this allows the discussion of sensitive or embarrassing topics without fear of disclosure.
> • This helps to establish health literacy and trust, while providing effective and needed care.

> ### ✋ Patient/parent advice
>
> • Establishing a relationship based on trust between an adolescent and her care provider is critically important.
> • This will allow sensitive issues to be discussed and improve future healthcare decisions and delivery.

for women that are sexually active. Some providers recommend testing more frequently in high-prevalence groups, including adolescents, those with a new sexual partner, homeless youths, inconsistent condom users, injection drug users, sex workers, and those with previous pregnancies or STIs.

Cervical cancer (Papanicolaou or Pap testing) screening should be initiated at age 21 years, based upon both a low incidence of clinically significant disease and limited screening utility for precancerous lesions in younger women (see Chapter 30.2).

Routinely screening those who are asymptomatic for other infections, including syphilis, trichomoniasis, bacterial vaginosis, herpes simplex virus, human papillomavirus, hepatitis A virus, and hepatitis B virus is not recommended. Anyone diagnosed with either chlamydia or gonorrhea should be screened for other STDs, including chlamydia, gonorrhea, syphilis, and HIV if not previously done at the same visit.

Pregnancy

There are additional screening recommendations for pregnant patients as a result of the potential complications for both the mother and soon to be born infant.

C. trachomatis and *N. gonorrhoeae* screening is recommended at the first prenatal visit; women aged 25 years or younger and those at increased risk for chlamydia (previous treatment for chlamydia during the pregnancy; new or more than one sex partner) should also be retested every 3–6 months (and preferably during the third trimester) to prevent maternal postnatal complications and chlamydia infection in the infant.

HIV screening is recommended as early in pregnancy as possible, with a retest in the third trimester (preferably before 36 weeks' gestation) for those at high risk (illicit drug user, diagnosis of other STDs, having multiple sex partners during pregnancy, living in a high HIV prevalence areas, or with an HIV-infected partner). Rapid HIV screening is recommended for any woman in labor if HIV status is not documented, in order to determine the duration of antiretroviral prophylaxis if required.

A serologic test for syphilis should be performed in all pregnant women at the first prenatal visit. This screening should be repeated later in pregnancy (around 28 weeks' gestation) and at delivery for those who are at high risk for syphilis or who live in areas of high syphilis morbidity.

In addition, all pregnant women should receive hepatitis B surface antigen (HBsAg) screening during a prenatal visit (preferably during the first trimester), even if they have been previously vaccinated or tested. Unscreened women and those at high risk of hepatitis infection (having more than one sex partner in the previous 6 months, those treated for an STD, recent or current injection-drug users, or those with an HBsAg-positive sex partner) or with clinical hepatitis should be retested at the time of admission to the hospital for delivery.

How to screen

Chlamydia and gonorrhea urogenital screening can be accomplished using urine, endocervical swabs, or vaginal swab specimens. Rectal and oral screening (for those engaging in receptive oral or anal intercourse) can be achieved for both organisms utilizing a swab specimen.

Provider-obtained samples for chlamydia and gonorrhea, including endocervical, vaginal, oral or anal swabs, have the advantage that the provider's knowledge and experience can detect symptoms of other infections or conditions that would not be tested for without direct observation. The two drawbacks are -based limitations (as it necessitates a clinic visit for the examination) and the invasiveness of the procedure, which may limit the number of adolescents who are willing to be screened.

Patient-obtained sampling is a convenient alternative, allowing an individual to provide a urine specimen or vaginal swab without having to undergo a formal pelvic exam. This has the advantage of reducing the time required and increasing the number of screenings through increased patient comfort, but with the drawback that an experienced provider is not able to obtain other testing or initiate treatment if something had been observed during the exam.

With adolescent patients, these two approaches can and are used within the same practice. Typically it is recommended that at least one provider-based screening visit occurs each year, while an additional visit approximately 6 months later has the potential for patient-obtained sampling if the patient is more comfortable with that approach.

> ### ✋ Caution
>
> Exclusive reliance upon self-administered STD screening swabs can miss other important disease-related and anatomic issues in adolescent females.

Endocervical specimens have been the historical method used for screening, and as such, numerous tests, including nucleic acid amplification tests (NAATs) which detect the presence of bacterial DNA, cell culture, direct immunofluorescence, enzyme immunoassay (EIA), and nucleic acid hybridization tests are all readily available for such samples. NAATs are the most sensitive tests for these specimens and are approved for use with urine. These are available for both chlamydia and gonorrhea screening.

Some NAATs are approved for use with vaginal swab specimens, including either a provider- or self-collected sample. However, most NAAT and nucleic acid hybridization tests are not yet FDA approved for use with rectal or oropharyngeal swab specimens.

Laboratories may offer screening tests on liquid-based cytology specimens collected for Pap smears, utilizing NAAT testing, although these may be less sensitive than cervical swab specimens. It is important to discuss what specimens and samples can be appropriately tested utilizing local laboratories, based upon FDA approval of the tests.

It is important to note that Gram staining, traditionally used for identifying gonorrhea in males, is not sufficient with endocervical, pharyngeal, or rectal specimens to detect gonorrheal infection, and therefore is not recommended. Specific testing, utilizing NAATs for example, for *N. gonorrhoeae*, is recommended, because of the easy availability of highly sensitive and specific testing methods, and because a specific diagnosis can enhance partner notification and treatment.

Nonculture chlamydia or gonorrhea tests do not have the ability to provide antibiotic susceptibility or viability results as the methods only detect the presence of DNA, not living bacteria; nucleic acid from dead bacteria can still be detected in the 6-week window following treatment. Therefore, in cases of suspected or documented treatment failure, as well as of abuse or rape, clinicians should perform both culture and antimicrobial susceptibility testing.

> ### ⚛ Science revisited
>
> • Nucleic acid amplification tests (NAATs) are exceedingly sensitive and specific tests for detecting STDs.
> • They detect DNA from the organism tested for, and as such can provide evidence that the bacteria was present, but cannot provide antibiotic sensitivity or proof of a living organism; thus, caution should be applied when performing a test within 4–6 weeks after STD treatment, as the test may be falsely positive.

HIV screening can be accomplished by standard serologic approaches or using oral swabs to detect antibodies to the HIV virus. Typical serologic tests involve a two-step process, beginning with an enzyme-linked immunosorbent assay (ELISA) followed by a confirmatory Western blot test. ELISA testing is not used alone to diagnose HIV because of a high false-positive rate, and thus before a positive result is reported, it is confirmed by the Western blot, which allows for a remarkably accurate test with very low false-positive and false-negative rates. Rapid testing methods based upon oral plasma or serum samples are available that allow the preliminary results to be obtained in minutes; as with the ELISA testing, positive results require confirmatory Western blot testing before final diagnosis can be made. These tests detect antibodies and if the patient is tested early after infection, it may be that the level of antibodies produced is not sufficient to be detected. This issue forms the basis for recommending annual HIV screening in sexually-active populations.

Conclusion

Screening for STDs in adolescents is an important step to diagnosing and treating these conditions. The

exceedingly low rates of screening leave many adolescents and young adults with undiagnosed, untreated STDs, which are then spread to others, continuing the cycle of infection and transmission. Routine screening has the ability to decrease the numbers of those infected and iteratively reduce the individual and societal costs associated with infection.

Further reading

American Medical Association Department of Adolescent Health. Guidelines for Adolescent Preventative Services (GAPS). 2008 Centers for Disease Control and Prevention. Sexually transmitted diseases treatment guidelines, 2010. *MMWR* 2010;59(No. RR-12):1–110.

Tebb KP, Wibbelsman C, Neuhause JM, Shafer MA. Screening for asymptomatic chlamydia infections among sexually active adolescent girls during pediatric urgent care. *Arch Pediatr Adolesc Med* 2009;163(6):559–564.

32 Unintended pregnancy: options and counseling

Kaiyti Duffy[1] and Rachael Phelps[2]
[1]University of Illinois at Chicago College of Medicine, Chicago, IL, USA
[2]Planned Parenthood of the Rochester/Syracuse Region, University of Rochester, Rochester, NY, USA

Unplanned pregnancy in adolescents is a serious public health concern. Approximately 750 000 teen-agers each year become pregnant. Of those, 59% result in live births, 27% in terminations, and 14% in fetal loss. In some instances, these pregnancies are wanted and/or planned but the vast majorities are not. Because many teen pregnancies are diagnosed in primary care offices, providers delivering care to adolescents need to be able to provide comprehensive, nonbiased pregnancy options counseling to ensure that young women make the best decisions for their unique situations.

☆ Tips and tricks

When providing pregnancy options counseling, providers should:
- Ask open-ended questions.
- Reflect: "I am hearing you say that you…"
- Validate: "Many young women feel…"
- Give the patient control: "Which would you prefer?"
- Pay attention to nonverbal cues.
- Communicate acceptance: tone, eye contact.
- Use silence: let her finish.

Providers should avoid:
- False reassurances: "You'll be fine."
- Over-identification: "I know how you feel."
- Medical jargon: "Have you had previous terminations?"
- Loaded and/or judgmental statements: "Do you want to keep the baby?"
- Giving advice: "I think you should…"

Reproduced from Goodman S, Wolfe M, TEACH Trainers Collaborative Working Group. *Early Abortion Training Workbook,* 3rd Edition. San Francisco: UCSF Bixby Center for Reproductive Health Research & Policy, 2007, with permission.

The DECISION model

The DECISION model was created by a committee of experts as part of the Adolescent Reproductive and Sexual Health Education Project (ARSHEP), a project of the nonprofit organization Physicians for Reproductive Choice and Health. It is intended as a guide for providers in diagnosing a pregnancy in teen patients and providing unbiased pregnancy options counseling.

D: Determine the reason for the visit

Some young women seek medical attention because they have a suspicion they are pregnant. However, they may present with unrelated symptoms. A complete history should establish the concerns. Other young women have no idea that they are pregnant and are completely taken off guard by the possibility. If any part of the clinical history suggests the possibility of pregnancy, a urine pregnancy test should be performed in the office to confirm or rule out the diagnosis. Urine pregnancy tests become positive 2 weeks after unprotected intercourse, about the time of a missed menses. Prompt diagnosis of pregnancy in teens is key to ensuring early access to prenatal care or pregnancy termination services.

✋ Caution

At this point in the interview, if the provider does not feel that they can provide unbiased counseling, including all pregnancy options, they must refer the patient to someone who can.

E: Evaluate feelings

After the sample is collected and before the results are available, providers can explore the possible results. Some useful questions for the provider to ask include:
- "What are you feelings about the result?"
- "Have you ever wanted to get pregnant?"
- "How do you feel about the sexual encounter that brought you here today?"
- "Do you have any friends who are pregnant or who have had a baby? How do you feel about that?"

C: Confirm pregnancy results

Negative test

If the test is negative, it is essential to determine the date of the last act of unprotected sex. If the event occurred within the last 14 days, a pregnancy cannot yet be ruled out and the patient should be informed that she needs to return for a repeat test. If unprotected sex occurred within the past 5 days, the patient is a candidate for emergency contraception (see Chapter 34.6).

Additionally, the provider should determine how the patient feels about the result. If she is disappointed, it is important to explore why the young woman was seeking pregnancy. In counseling a young woman who is seeking pregnancy, it is beneficial to work through with her the realities of parenthood and to explore the possible benefits of waiting. The provider can explore the patient's family support, relationship with her partner, and how pregnancy and child bearing fits in with long-term goals. If the patient is convinced that this is the life choice for her, preconception counseling can be provided, including a recommendation for folic acid supplementation.

If the patient is relieved, the provider can work with the adolescent to prevent a future pregnancy, including abstinence and contraceptive counseling. Patients who choose contraception should be provided with the method the same day and encouraged to "quick start" rather than waiting for their menses. For depot medroxyprogesterone acetate, the implant, the patch, the ring, and oral contraceptive pills, this provides earlier protection from pregnancy without posing any risk to an early undetected pregnancy.

✋ Caution

For all sexually-active adolescents, it is important to inquire about potential reproductive coercion and contraception sabotage by partners.
- "Has your partner ever tried to mess up your birth control?"
- "Will your partner use a condom if you ask him to?"
- "Has your partner ever pressured you to become pregnant when you did not want to be?"

Positive result

After disclosing the news of the positive result, the provider must again assess how the patient feels. Some patients know right away what they want to do. Others need more counseling. Providers can begin by saying: "When faced with an unplanned pregnancy, young women generally have three options:

parenthood, adoption, and pregnancy termination. Would you like any more information about these options?"

If the patient already knows what she wants to do, providers can ensure that she has all the information she needs and that her decision is being made without coercion, and then refer her to the appropriate professionals to enable her choice.

In the event the patient needs additional counseling, move onto the next step.

I: Identify personal circumstances

Every young woman's situation is different. You should start by placing the pregnancy within the context of her life:
• "How do you picture the next year of your life? The next 5 years?"
• "How does this pregnancy affect where you want to be?"

Additionally, it is worth exploring how her personal/spiritual/religious beliefs will affect her decision process:
• "Do your parents/friends/partner have particularly strong opinions about any of these options?"
• "When you think about going through with any of the options, what do you feel? What are your fears?"

S: Assess support

In choosing to parent, place a child for adoption, or terminate a pregnancy, a young woman needs to count on the support of her partner, friends, parents or other trusted adults. First, discuss who the patient identifies as her support network:
• What role would these people play in her decision process?
• What role would they play if each of the three choices were carried out?

Second, explore the young woman's relationship with the man by whom she is pregnant:
• Are they in a relationship?
• Have they ever discussed parenthood?
• Would he be willing and/or able to help support a baby?
• What are his opinions about adoption? Abortion?

Finally, you should discuss whether there is an adult in whom she can confide to discuss her options. If so, when will she contact him/her? If not, help her

identify someone. A patient at potential risk of poor coping with her pregnancy decision is likely to experience stigma, secrecy, internal conflict, or lack a support system.

I: Address immediate concerns

In choosing how to proceed, the patient must consider the immediate concerns regarding each of the available choices. If she is going to continue her pregnancy, she needs to be started on prenatal vitamins and referred for prenatal care. If applicable, she needs to be referred to a Medicaid enrollment liaison. If she chooses to parent, she must also start thinking about where and with whom she will live, and how she will support herself and a baby. Will her coparent be involved? If she chooses adoption, she will need to work with a social worker and an adoption agency. It is possible to choose either an open or closed adoptions depending upon the agency and the wishes of the birth and adoptive parents.

If the patient decides to terminate, she must act on her decision within a finite timeframe. Abortion is legal in 50 states but restrictions vary. As of December 2012, 37 states required some parental involvement in a young woman's decision to have an abortion. Twenty-five states require a mandatory waiting period (usually 24 hours) between the counseling and the procedure. More information can be found at http://www.guttmacher.org/sections/abortion.php?pub=spib.

In addition to legal restrictions, a young woman must be able to locate an abortion provider (over 90% of counties lack an abortion provider), secure transportation to and from the provider, and be able to fund the procedure. In the first trimester, women can obtain a medication abortion (up to 9 weeks) or an aspiration abortion, which cost between $350 and $500. Only 17 states provide funding for Medicaid enrollees to obtain an abortion. Young women in the remaining states must pay for the procedure out of pocket. While abortion is legal up to 24 weeks in most states, abortions in the second trimester are more difficult to obtain due to expense and availability.

After considering the immediate concerns connected with each decision, the patient may be ready to make a decision on the spot, in which case appropriate local referrals should be provided. However, she may need more time to consider all of the information discussed.

Evidence at a glance

- Abortion is an extremely safe medical procedure. In fact, abortion is more than 10 times safer than childbirth.
- The vast majority (88%) of pregnancy terminations occur in the first trimester. Serious complications relating to aspiration abortions in this time frame are extremely rare. Approximately 2.5% of women experience minor complications and less than 0.5% have more serious complications that require some additional medical intervention.
- Medication abortion is also extremely safe. Serious complications are rare, occur in less than 0.5% of cases, and are comparable to those associated with miscarriage.

O: Offer a timeline

If the young woman leaves the office without having made a decision, it is important to establish a timeline as her next steps are time sensitive. Helpful questions include:

- How much time do you need to make your decision?
- When do you plan to involve a parent/another adult in your decision?
- If you choose to continue the pregnancy, by what date will you make an appointment for prenatal care?
- If you decide to terminate the pregnancy, by what date will you schedule an appointment?

N: Next steps

At the end of the visit, provide the patient with written resources and necessary referrals. Ask if she has any more questions and whether you can follow-up with her by phone in a couple days. Remind her of the timeline and the timeliness of her decision. Finally, schedule a future visit.

Patient/parent advice

There are many additional resources available to young women experiencing an unintended pregnancy. They include:

- **Pregnancy Options Workbook**
www.pregnancyoptions.info
This workbook, which can be downloaded from the site, includes factual information about each option as well as exercises to help your patient come to a decision.

- **Backline**
www.yourbackline.org
Backline is a website that supports women and their loved ones who are facing difficult decisions around pregnancy. It is dedicated to addressing the broad range of experiences and emotions surrounding pregnancy, parenting, adoption, and abortion. Visit their website for more information or call their talk-line on 1-888-493-0092.

- **Mom, Dad I'm Pregnant**
www.abortioncarenetwork.org/mom-dad
This website has resources for teens, both boys and girls, facing pregnancies. It offers advice on how to inform parents as well as how to work through the pregnancy options. It also has great resources for parents to help them best cope with the situation and provide teens with needed support.

- **Faith Aloud**
www.faithaloud.org/faith/faith-counseling.php
This website connects teens with specially trained religious counselors and clergy (Roman Catholic, Jewish, Unitarian-Universalist, Protestant, Christian, and Buddhist) who provide religious support and guidance throughout the pregnancy decision-making process. People of no particular religious faith are equally welcome to receive services. All counselors have the minimum of a Master's degree and have also completed specialized training in pregnancy options counseling.

Further reading

Committee on Adolescence. American Academy of Pediatrics. Counseling the adolescent about pregnancy options. *Pediatrics* 1998;101(5):938–940.

Gamble S, Strauss L, Parker W, Cook D, Zane S, Hamdan S. Abortion Surveillance – United States, 2005. *MMWR* 2008;57:1–32.

Paul M, Lichtenberg E, Borgatta L, Grimes D, Stubblefield P, Creinin M (eds). *Management of Unintended and Abnormal Pregnancy: Comprehensive Abortion Care.* Oxford: Wiley-Blackwell, 2009.

33.1 Contraceptive counseling for healthy teens

Stephanie B. Teal

University of Colorado, Denver School of Medicine, Aurora, CO, USA

Adolescence is, by its very nature, a time of change, and as clinicians we must be prepared to adapt our counseling styles to meet the changing psychological and cognitive development of our adolescent patients (see Chapter 20). Different techniques are required to guide the early adolescent on healthy reproductive behaviors than for a late adolescent. In counseling, it is important to remember that sexual activity in adolescents arises from more than physical imperatives; aspects of development expressed through sexuality include testing models of intimacy, practicing adult relationship patterns, and negotiating their own desires in the face of another's. Keeping the patient's developmental needs in mind during counseling allows the clinician to help the young woman meet her needs with maximum safety, resulting in better health outcomes. Further, knowledge-based or education-based counseling may be less effective in adolescents.

Two normal cognitive aspects of adolescence are idealized expectations and the minimization of personal susceptibility to negative consequences that befall others. Thus, discussions of risks of pregnancy, early motherhood, and sexually-transmitted infections (STIs) are less likely to translate into behavior change, as it is difficult for the adolescent to integrate her knowledge of these issues into an accurate perception of personal risk. The ultimate goal of adolescent contraceptive counseling is to help the young woman find a contraceptive method that is acceptable to her, and that is easily within her ability to use safely and consistently.

Most parents and providers are aware of the process of physical growth and development that youngsters go through as they become adults. However, they may be less familiar with the uniquely human experience of adolescence – the process of cognitive, psychosocial, and moral growth and development that transforms dependent children into independent, self-sufficient members of society (see Appendix 1.9.2). Adolescents of different ages are at different points on this spectrum of growth, and consideration of the hallmarks of each stage guides contraceptive counseling.

Early adolescence (11–14 years of age)

Approximately 5% of girls are sexually active when they enter early adolescence. By the time they leave this stage of development, 20% of them will have engaged in some form of exploratory sexual activity. It is helpful to provide this type of information to young adolescents and their parents by explaining that early adolescence is to sexuality what toddlerhood is to stair and street safety – it is the ideal time for anticipatory guidance that protects children from harm without provoking harmful experimentation.

Practical Pediatric and Adolescent Gynecology, First Edition. Edited by Paula J. Adams Hillard.
© 2013 John Wiley & Sons, Ltd. Published 2013 by John Wiley & Sons, Ltd.

The physical changes of puberty make early adolescents extremely self-conscious. They tend to be modest, but behave as if they are on stage, performing in front of an imaginary audience. Accordingly, if a young adolescent appears to have already lost her modesty, e.g. presents in the office in a tight tank top and shows more interest in heterosexual activity than comparing herself to other girls, the clinician should be aware that her physical and social development may be ahead of her cognitive development. Potential causes ranging from normal but precocious physical maturation to chronic sexual abuse should be considered, and the young adolescent's awareness of, and comfort with, her development investigated.

★ Tips and tricks

Talking with teens and parents
- Statements like, "I bet that everyone tells you that you look older than you are. That can be flattering when you are young, but it is also hard because sometimes people expect you to act older than you are. Have you had that problem? Do people expect you to do things you don't feel ready to do?" can help introduce the topic.
- Framing the discussion as the next installment in an ongoing preventative health and safety dialogue with the parents and/or patient can break the ice.
- A statement like, "Years ago, before you could sit-up, your doctor's discussion about stair safety probably seemed as unnecessary as the discussion I would like to have about intimacy and interpersonal relationships" can get a two- or three-way conversation started.

At this stage of development it is sufficient for patients and their parents to become conscious of the intimacy-related dangers that lie ahead and acknowledge the need to develop guidelines like "look both ways before you cross the street" that will be protective for a lifetime. The topics that should be covered in broad anticipatory terms include:
- **Criteria and guidelines for moving from one level of intimacy to the next and back again.** To develop into an autonomous sexual being, the patient must understand that there are numerous ways to experience intimacy and express sexual attractions.
- **Criteria and guidelines for intimate partner selection.** The patient should be encouraged to apply the criteria she uses for choosing girlfriends to selecting intimate partners; that is, how she recognizes the people who seem fun to hang around with, but do not actually treat her well.
- **Misperceptions and misunderstanding that can become entrenched concerns.** To avoid risky sexual behavior, the patient must have enough factual information to ignore myths about the causes of infertility and about contraceptive safety and side effects. For example, girls who have been told that they will get pregnant if they do not use birth control may believe they are sterile if they do not conceive after several episodes of unprotected sex.

Middle adolescence (15–17 years of age)

By the beginning of middle adolescence, approximately 20% of girls will have engaged in sexual activity. By the time they leave this developmental stage, 70% will have had sexual intercourse. Since sexual experimentation is normative at this stage of development, the focus of counseling should be on helping patients and their parents understand that protection against the potential morbidities of recklessness, depression, pregnancy, infection, and cervical cancer must be normative, too. The quest for an identity makes middle adolescents narcissistic and self-absorbed; they develop a sense of personal invulnerability to risk that allows them to experiment with different roles and lifestyles.

The first goal of counseling middle adolescents is to help them and their parents expand and formalize the guidelines they considered during early adolescence into a rubric that will be protective for a lifetime. Talking to family members, adult friends, trusted teachers, and counselors about the particulars of moving from one level of intimacy to the next should be encouraged because each culture has its own normative values and behavioral expectations.

Adolescents at this stage should understand that even if they use dual protection – a contraceptive and a prophylactic – no method of contraception is perfect. The risk of becoming pregnant or acquiring a STI increases with the number of sexual encounters and the number of sexual partners. Taking a thorough partner history, routine periodic STI testing, and frequent discussions about fidelity can be as good or better protection against STIs than using a condom.

The second goal of counseling is to promote normal cognitive development by encouraging adolescents to engage in theoretical role experimentation. Asking questions such as "How old do you want to be when you have your first baby?" "Why do you want to be that age?" "What about your boyfriend, your best friend, your older sister, or your mom?" "What would be the worst part of getting pregnant, a sexually-transmitted infection, or telling a boy you liked a lot you did not want to have sex with him, or that he had to use a condom? Why?" gets the process started and provides a segue to discussing how to keep intimate relationships safe.

As adolescents mature they begin to rely more on those in their peer group for information and decision-making. Teens are more likely to smoke, use alcohol, become sexually active and participate in other risky behaviors if these behaviors are common among their social network. The same is true of contraceptive behavior. It is therefore important to counsel teens on how common contraception use is.

★ Tips and tricks

• Building safety and rapport with the middle adolescent can be facilitated by letting her know you are aware of her need to deal with conflicting emotions and are willing to help her reason them into a cognitive perspective that minimizes her risk-taking behavior.

• For example, "What do you think is the best way to get out of a tight, sexually-risky situation:
  ◦ Avoiding being alone with guys
  ◦ Creating a distraction that changes the mood
  ◦ Just getting up and leaving
  ◦ Speaking up and expressing your concerns or
  ◦ Living with it and the consequences?
  ◦ Why?
  ◦ What do you usually do in these situations?
  ◦ Why?"

Late adolescence (18–21 years of age)

By the time youth reach late adolescence, 70% will have had sexual intercourse. By the time they leave this developmental stage, too many will have been pregnant (3 in 10 US girls will get pregnant at least once by age 20) and had a STI. The focus of counseling at this stage of development should be on helping patients make both safe sex and the avoidance of sexual morbidity a means of attaining the intimacy they want and deserve.

Young women at this stage of development tend to be less concerned about their bodies and identities. As they begin to develop a sense of their futures, they learn to think causally and become capable of anticipating events and reasoning through problems. The acquisition of these skills diminishes but does not eliminate the need for risky, provocative experimentation and the propensity for magical thinking, and late adolescents still benefit from adult oversight. A clinician's verbal reminder about the necessity of taking a thorough sexual history from her partner, routine periodic testing for STIs, and frequent discussions about fidelity and using condoms can be a badly needed reality check for a late adolescent who believes she has found the love of her life. While the ensuing discussion should also include a reminder of the physical and emotional harms that STIs can cause, scare tactics and threats about future sterility should be avoided. Fears about infertility are a deterrent for effective contraceptive use and a motivator for seeking pregnancy prematurely.

Directive and nondirective counseling

Several schema exist that describe and categorize counseling approaches to promote health behavior changes. For this chapter, a variety of more subtly described methods have been grouped into "directive" versus "nondirective" counseling.

Counseling adolescents is different from counseling adults or children because adolescents need both the information and education typically provided to adult patients as well as the guidance that is typically provided to children. Accordingly, both professionals and parents find that a directive approach works best with this age group, in contrast to a permissive–indulgent method such as motivational interviewing or narrative therapy.

A directive counseling approach directs the adolescent's contraceptive behavior (initiation and continuation) in a rational, issue-oriented manner by setting high standards and expectations for mature behavior, firmly enforcing rules, and encouraging independence and individuality by recognizing rights and offering choices. A directive method is not the same as a dictatorial approach, in which the patient is told what option is best for her.

Adolescents usually define the opportunity costs and benefits of childbearing in terms of the circumstances of their romantic relationships rather than a long-term life course plan. Their intent to avoid conception tends to be as fickle as their intimate affairs because most do not know how many children they want or when they want to have them. Focusing on contraceptive behavior rather than childbearing intentions precludes the need to know.

Evidence at a glance

Directive counseling

• What adolescents want and benefit from most is evidence-based discussions that simultaneously direct and guide the choices they make and teach them the skills they need to make healthy decisions. There is good evidence that this approach works; it minimizes risk-taking behaviors, maximizes contraceptive use, and improves patient satisfaction.

• Providers who primarily care for adults can be uncomfortable with such directive counseling, as consumer choice, patient autonomy, and personal decision-making have such high value in our society.

• Studies demonstrate that when it comes to making decisions about behaviors that can have long-term effects on their lives, adolescents dislike and suffer as much from no guidance and unlimited options as they do from lectures and rigid, externally imposed rules.

• Asking a sexually-active teen, especially in early or mid-adolescence, "what do you want to use for birth control?" implies that her preference will be equivalently valid without the input of the provider's knowledge, experience, and expertise.

✋ Caution

• It can be easy to become frustrated with adolescents, as any parent can attest. Identifying common triggers that arise in adolescent contraceptive counseling can help providers maintain an appropriate therapeutic alliance with a trying patient.

• It is appropriate for adolescents to try out different roles, some of which are distasteful. Behaviors should not be conflated with personal identity. Remember, the purpose of these roles is to evaluate the reactions they provoke.

• In adults, ambivalence is experienced as psychologically unpleasant. In early and mid-adolescents, however, the positive and negative aspects of a subject, such as having a baby, can both be present in a person's mind at the same time without a resultant urge to resolve the conflict one way or another. Talking to a patient who does not desire a baby any time soon, but does not want to start contraception, can trigger a provider to feel they "care more than the patient does." Remember, directive counseling towards passive contraceptive methods (depo-Provera, subdermal implants, intrauterine devices) can take advantage of this unresolved ambivalence.

Some sexually active teens claim they do not need contraception. The simplest and easiest way to begin to understand the reproductive behavior of such young women is to ask them why not. This question is preferable to the alternative – asking about childbearing intentions – particularly during adolescence.

However, the responses adolescents give to open-ended questions like, "Why aren't you using birth control?", e.g., "I don't know" or "I just didn't think about it," are often not helpful in understanding the reasons for their behavior. The goal is to help the adolescent understand the difference between her desires and her intentions (i.e. the conscious commitment to try to achieve a goal), and to help her feel that she can and wants to exercise as much control over this part of her life as she does over other parts. At a minimum, she should not leave the clinic thinking that nothing will happen if she continues to have unprotected sexual intercourse. Optimally, the conversation will help her decide if she intends to have a baby now or not. Even if she remains ambivalent, however, she may agree that "whatever happens, happens" is not an acceptable way to become pregnant and for this reason may accept a trial period of contraception while she decides when she really wants to start a family, with whom, and what she plans to do to ensure it happens as she desires.

Counseling adolescents about contraception can be highly rewarding. Engaging a sexually active youngster to accept a long-acting contraceptive method, or adhere to a short-acting method, is a health intervention that may impact her life far beyond any other medical services we provide. The author recently cared for a married 29-year-old woman with a Master's degree and two young children, who told me about receiving a contraceptive implant at age 13 after a miscarriage. She told me, "the doctor said, 'I have just the right thing for you,' and she explained all the side effects that were normal. That doctor saved my life."

Further reading

Bruckner H, Martin A, Bearman PS. Ambivalence and pregnancy: adolescents' attitudes, contraceptive use and pregnancy. *Perspect Sex Reprod Health* 2004;36(6):248–257.

Nathanson CA, Becker MH. The influence of client-provider relationships on teenage women's subsequent use of contraception. *Am J Public Health* 1985;75:33–38.

Resnick MD, Bearman PS, Blum RW, *et al*. Protecting adolescents from harm. *JAMA* 1997;278:823–832.

Acknowledgements

The author wishes to acknowledge the contributions of Catherine Stevens-Simon MD (deceased) and Jeanelle Sheeder PhD to this chapter.

33.2 Contraceptive counseling for teens with medical illness

Melissa Gilliam and Amy K. Whitaker
The University of Chicago, Chicago, IL, USA

Unplanned and adolescent pregnancies are particularly deleterious in women with medical illness. Many disease states, such as uncontrolled diabetes and seizure disorder, pose serious risk to a developing fetus; others, such as systemic lupus erythematosus (SLE) and cardiac disease, may worsen in pregnancy and increase risk from the disease. Thus, the selection of an effective contraceptive method for a sexually-active adolescent patient with a medical illness is crucial.

> ### ✶ Tips and tricks
>
> It is important to note that no method of contraception is contraindicated in an adolescent based on her age or parity alone.

Condoms and long-acting reversible contraceptives: the two ends of the contraceptive efficacy spectrum

The primary role for the male condom in adolescents with medical illness is to decrease the transmission of sexually-transmitted infections (STIs) (see Chapter 34.1). Clinicians should counsel all adolescents who are at risk for STIs and unintended pregnancy to use both latex condoms and a more effective method of contraception.

Long-acting reversible contraceptive (LARC) methods, intrauterine devices (IUDs), and contraceptive implants, are highly effective in preventing pregnancy. LARC methods have few contraindications and typical-use failure rates are less than 1% (Table 33.2.1), making them appealing for this population. Evidence for use of IUDs and implants among adolescents supports their safety and efficacy, and adolescent users have high reported rates of satisfaction and continuation (see Chapters 34.4 and 34.5).

Systemic lupus erythematosus

The health risks of pregnancy in adolescents with SLE are considerable, including worsening of disease, fetal loss, pre-eclampsia, growth restriction, and maternal morbidity and mortality. It is therefore of critical important that adolescents with SLE have a highly effective method of contraception.

Contraceptive management for adolescents with SLE depends on the severity of the disease, as SLE can be complicated by involvement of many organ systems, including ophthalmic, cardiovascular, and renal. Some patients with SLE are at increased risk of thromboembolic disease, particularly those with antiphospholipid antibodies or severe nephrotic syndrome. Thus, organ involvement, presence of antiphospholipid antibodies (or unknown status),

Practical Pediatric and Adolescent Gynecology, First Edition. Edited by Paula J. Adams Hillard.
© 2013 John Wiley & Sons, Ltd. Published 2013 by John Wiley & Sons, Ltd.

⚠ Caution

- While there are no medical contraindications to behavioral and barrier birth control methods, these methods are associated with high typical-use failure rates (Table 33.2.1).
- The 2010 Center for Disease Control (CDC) U.S. Medical Eligibility Criteria (USMEC) for Contraceptive Use states that "women with medical conditions associated with a high risk of adverse consequences from unintended pregnancy should be advised that use of barrier or behavioral methods may not be an appropriate choice due to high typical-use failure rates."
- Conditions that may occur in adolescents and that are associated with increased risk for adverse health events as a result of unintended pregnancy are listed in the USMEC (http://www.cdc.gov/reproductivehealth/unintendedpregnancy/USMEC.htm).

Table 33.2.1 Percentage of women experiencing an unintended pregnancy during the first year of typical use and the first year of perfect use of contraception and the percentage continuing use at the end of the first year: United States of America

Method (1)	% of Women Experiencing an Unintended Pregnancy within the First Year of Use		% of Women Continuing Use at One Year[3] (4)
	Typical Use[1] (2)	Perfect Use[2] (3)	
No method[4]	85	85	
Spermicides[5]	28	18	42
Fertility awareness-based methods	24		47
Standard Days method[6]		5	
TwoDay method[6]		4	
Ovulation method[6]		3	
Symptothermal method[6]		0.4	
Withdrawal	22	4	46
Sponge			36
Parous women	24	20	
Nulliparous women	12	9	
Condom[7]			
Female (fc)	21	5	41
Male	18	2	43
Diaphragm[8]	12	6	57
Combined pill and progestin-only pill	9	0.3	67
Evra patch	9	0.3	67
NuvaRing	9	0.3	67
Depo-Provera	6	0.2	56
Intrauterine contraceptives			
ParaGard (copper T)	0.8	0.6	78
Mirena (LNg)	0.2	0.2	80
Implanon	0.05	0.05	84
Female sterilization	0.5	0.5	100
Male sterilization	0.15	0.10	100

Emergency Contraception: Emergency contraceptive pills or insertion of a copper intrauterine contraceptive after unprotected intercourse substantially reduces the risk of pregnancy.[9] (See Chapter 6.).

Table 33.2.1 (*Continued*)

Method (1)	% of Women Experiencing an Unintended Pregnancy within the First Year of Use		% of Women Continuing Use at One Year[3]
	Typical Use[1] (2)	Perfect Use[2] (3)	(4)
Lactational Amenorrhea Method: LAM is a highly effective, *temporary* method of contraception.[10] (See Chapter 18.)			

Reproduced with permission from Trussell J. Contraceptive Efficacy. In Hatcher RA, Trussell J, Nelson AL, Cates W, Stewart FH, Kowal D, (eds). *Contraceptive Techology: 19th Revised Edition*. New York, NY: Ardent Media, 2007.

Notes:

[1]Among *typical* couples who initiate use of a method (not necessarily for the first time), the percentage who experience an accidental pregnancy during the first year if they do not stop use for any other reason. Estimates of the probability of pregnancy during the first year of typical use for spermicides, withdrawal, fertility awareness-based methods, the diaphragm, the male condom, the oral contraceptive pill, and Depo-Provera are taken from the 1995 National Survey of Family Growth corrected for underreporting of abortion; see the text for the derivation of estimates for the other methods.

[2]Among couples who initiate use of a method (not necessarily for the first time) and who use it *perfectly* (both consistently and correctly), the percentage who experience an accidental pregnancy during the first year if they do not stop use for any other reason. See the text for the derivation of the estimate for each method.

[3]Among couples attempting to avoid pregnancy, the percentage who continue to use a method for 1 year.

[4]The percentages becoming pregnant in columns (2) and (3) are based on data from populations where contraception is not used and from women who cease using contraception in order to become pregnant. Among such populations, about 89% become pregnant within 1 year. This estimate was lowered slightly (to 85%) to represent the percentage who would become pregnant within 1 year among women now relying on reversible methods of contraception if they abandoned contraception altogether.

[5]Foams, creams, gels, vaginal suppositories, and vaginal film.

[6]The Ovulation and TwoDay methods are based on evaluation of cervical mucus. The Standard Days method avoids intercourse on cycle days 8 through 19. The Symptothermal method is a double-check method based on evaluation of cervical mucus to determine the first fertile day and evaluation of cervical mucus and temperature to determine the last fertile day.

[7]Without spermicides.

[8]With spermicidal cream or jelly.

[9]ella, Plan B One-Step and Next Choice are the only dedicated products specifically marketed for emergency contraception. The label for Plan B One-Step (one dose is 1 white pill) says to take the pill within 72 hours after unprotected intercourse. Research has shown that all of the brands listed here are effective when used within 120 hours after unprotected sex. The label for Next Choice (one dose is 1 peach pill) says to take 1 pill within 72 hours after unprotected intercourse and another pill 12 hours later. Research has shown that both pills can be taken at the same time with no decrease in efficacy or increase in side effects and that they are effective when used within 120 hours after unprotected sex. The Food and Drug Administration has in addition declared the following 19 brands of oral contraceptives to be safe and effective for emergency contraception: Ogestrel (1 dose is 2 white pills), Nordette (1 dose is 4 light-orange pills), Cryselle, Levora, Low-Ogestrel, Lo/Ovral, or Quasence (1 dose is 4 white pills), Jolessa, Portia, Seasonale or Trivora (1 dose is 4 pink pills), Seasonique (1 dose is 4 light-blue-green pills), Enpresse (one dose is 4 orange pills), Lessina (1 dose is 5 pink pills), Aviane or LoSeasonique (one dose is 5 orange pills), Lutera or Sronyx (one dose is 5 white pills), and Lybrel (one dose is 6 yellow pills).

[10]However, to maintain effective protection against pregnancy, another method of contraception must be used as soon as menstruation resumes, the frequency or duration of breastfeeds is reduced, bottle feeds are introduced, or the baby reaches 6 months of age.

Science revisited

• When prescribing contraception for adolescent women with medical illness, an invaluable resource is the Centers for Disease Control and Prevention Medical Eligibility Criteria for Contraceptive Use (USMEC, http://www.cdc.gov/reproductivehealth/unintendedpregnancy/USMEC.htm).

• Based on the model of the World Health Organization's (WHO's) MEC, the USMEC provides evidence-based guidance on the safety of contraceptive method use for women with specific characteristics and medical conditions.

Categories of medical eligibility criteria for contraceptive use from the USMEC:

1: A condition for which there is no restriction for the use of the contraceptive method.

2: A condition for which the advantages of using the method generally outweigh the theoretical or proven risks.

3: A condition for which the theoretical or proven risks usually outweigh the advantages of using the method.

4: A condition that represents an unacceptable health risk if the contraceptive method is used.

Evidence at a glance

• The SELENA (Safety of Estrogen in Lupus: National Assessment) trial was a randomized, double-blind, placebo-controlled trial of oral contraceptives in women with a diagnosis of SLE but stable or inactive disease.

• The number of lupus flares among oral contraceptive users was equal to those among women in the placebo group.

and disease severity will determine contraceptive choice for these adolescents. Specifically, providers should refer to the USMEC guidance regarding the end organ that is affected. Thromboembolic risk factors are contraindications for combined hormonal contraceptives (CHCs), while immunosuppres-

sion and thrombocytopenia are not. In fact, most adolescents with SLE can use the full array of contraceptives.

Antiphospholipid antibodies significantly limit contraceptive selection for adolescents and young women with SLE. For example, the USMEC rates the levonorgestrel-releasing IUD (LNG-IUS), progestin-only methods, and CHCs as category 3 (the risk of use usually outweighs the advantages). Thus, the copper IUD is the method most suitable for women with positive antibodies.

Anemias

Contraception in young women with sickle cell disease (SCD) or thalassemia prevents unintended pregnancies and has medical benefits since it regulates and even eliminates menses. Some women with SCD will experience crises with their menstrual cycles (catemenial crises). Heavy menses can worsen the anemia associated with SCD, and dysmenorrhea can exacerbate the pain of SCD crises.

CHCs can be used safely in these women. Depot medroxyprogesterone acetate (DMPA) and older progestin-only contraceptives are associated with decreased rates of sickling. In the case of iron-deficiency anemia, CHCs decrease menstrual blood flow. All progestin-only methods of contraception are safe to use in women with SCD, thalassemia, or iron-deficiency anemia without limitations.

Both the copper IUD and the LNG-IUS can be used by adolescents with SCD, thalassemia, or iron-deficiency anemia. If an adolescent opts to use the copper IUD, providers should counsel her about the possible risks of increased blood loss. The LNG-IUS can improve iron-deficiency anemia.

HIV/AIDS

Condoms, in conjunction with a highly effective method of contraception, are critical for youth with a known transmissible infection such as human immunodeficiency virus (HIV). For adolescents and young adults with HIV, the effect of hormonal contraceptives on disease progression or acquisition and interaction with antiretroviral therapies should be considered.

Evidence at a glance

- Overall, data indicate that CHCs do not increase the risk of HIV acquisition.
- There are currently no data that suggest that CHCs should not be prescribed to women at risk for HIV acquisition.
- CHCs do not increase HIV disease progression.
  - Studies have considered viral load, survival, and CD4 count.
- While studies show no increased transmission to uninfected partners, a few studies suggest that CHCs increase the amount of virus in the genital tract or the amount of viral shedding.
- The strongest evidence supports no increased risks associated with acquisition, disease progression or disease transmission with CHC use among women with HIV.

While adolescents with HIV or acquired immune deficiency syndrome (AIDS) can use all CHCs, consideration must be given to interactions with antiretroviral (ARV) therapy. The USMEC recommends using oral contraceptives with at least 30 µg of ethinyl estradiol to optimize effectiveness.

There are minimal data on the interaction of the single-rod implant and ARVs. Yet, it would be prudent to enforce that condom use is essential for both disease and pregnancy prevention. The higher serum levels of DMPA and the frequency of dosing suggest that the contraceptive efficacy of DMPA would be preserved in adolescents using ARVs.

Adolescents with HIV can safely use progestin-only contraception (POC) methods. Yet, controversy does exist. Studies of DMPA use among some high-risk populations have shown increased transmission and acquisition. However, it must be recognized that these conclusions are based on a small number of subjects and a small effect size. Thus, providers can be very comfortable prescribing POC methods to adolescents and young adults with HIV.

The IUD raises slightly different considerations for adolescents and young adults with HIV/AIDs. While the supporting data are sparse, questions have been raised about the potential for infectious complications. Thus, while still safe to use, all IUDs are rated a category 2 for initiation and continuation among young women at risk for or infected with HIV. However, there is additional guidance for young women with AIDs. Specifically, for women with AIDS, providers should consider whether the benefits outweigh the risks of infection when initiating IUD use and should monitor users for pelvic infection. Finally, if the patient is clinically well and on ARV therapy, then the benefits of IUD use outweigh the risk for a young woman with AIDs.

Seizures and migraines

Preventing pregnancy in young women with seizure disorders is an important consideration due to the teratogenicity of some seizure medications. Similarly, young women with catamenial epilepsy can benefit from hormonal contraception. Yet, providers of contraception to young women with seizures must be careful to consider potential drug interactions. Anticonvulsants that induce the P450 enzymes can increase the metabolism of both the estrogen and progestin components of CHCs, perhaps making these methods less effective. These medications include: phenytoin, carbamazepine, barbiturates, primidone, topiramate, and oxcarbazepine. Women using these medications should use an oral contraceptive containing a minimum of 30 µg of ethinyl estradiol, and their use is considered category 3 by the USMEC; other contraceptive methods should be considered. Similar considerations apply for progestin-only pills; again another method should be considered. Conversely, some anticonvulsants such as lamotrigine are less effective with CHCs, as anticonvulsant drug levels are decreased during oral contraceptive use; this finding is not evident with POP use.

DMPA is not associated with a decrease in contraceptive efficacy for women with seizures. DMPA may be particularly appropriate, as small studies have shown fewer seizures in young women using DMPA. DMPA may require more frequent dosing in young women using anticonvulsants. There are few data regarding the LNG-IUS and interaction with anticonvulsants, although interactions are not thought to occur.

Many young women experience headaches and some of these may not have previously been diagnosed as migraines. Clinicians should take a careful headache history to be able to make a diagnosis of migraines or migraines with aura in order to determine safe contraceptive use. Overall, all methods of contraception are safe to use by women with a history of headaches. However, if a patient experiences worsening headaches with the contraceptive method, then the method should be discontinued. Nonmigrainous headaches are category 1 for initiation and category 2 for continuation. Women with migraines who use CHCs are at increased risk of ischemic stroke (two to four fold). When women have other risk factors for stroke (such as hypertension or smoking), the use of CHCs should be reconsidered.

Women with migraine with aura are considered to be at unacceptably high risk of stroke and CHCs are contraindicated at all ages (category 4). Consultation with a neurologist may be necessary, as aura may be hard to distinguish.

Progestin-only methods of contraception are safe to use (category 1) in young women who have a history of headaches. Women with migraine with aura should be monitored for worsening of headache symptoms.

All intrauterine methods can be used in women with headaches. However, the LNG-IUS is rated category 2 for initiation of use, but category 3 for women who develop migraines with aura during use.

Hypertension and cardiovascular disease

With the decreasing estrogen content of COCs, their cardiovascular safety has improved dramatically, with a decrease in severe adverse effects, such as stroke, myocardial infarction, and deep vein thrombosis.

Although risk for cardiac disease increases in cigarette smokers, in the healthy adolescent population, the advantages of using CHCs outweigh the risks in cigarette smokers because adolescents are at low risk of cardiovascular disease. There are no restrictions for use of any of the progestin-only methods or IUDs in smokers at any age.

For women with hypertension, even young women with well-controlled disease, the USMEC warns that risks outweigh advantages of CHC use, and that in severe hypertension ($\geq$160/$\geq$100 mmHg) or if vascular disease is present, CHCs represent an unac-

ceptable health risk. However, the American College of Obstetricians and Gynecologists (ACOG) allows for a trial of CHC use in otherwise healthy women under 35 years old with well-controlled, monitored disease who do not smoke or have vascular disease. Studies have not demonstrated significant changes in blood pressure with progestin-only methods, so these methods may be used without restriction in mild hypertension (up to 159/99 mmHg), and advantages outweigh risks in severe hypertension or when vascular disease is present. Although the advantages of DMPA use with mild hypertension outweigh the risks, DMPA's risks outweigh its advantages if there is more severe disease or vascular involvement, an uncommon condition in adolescents.

Hormonal contraceptive agents have been shown to induce both favorable and unfavorable changes in the serum lipid profile. It is not clear, however, whether any of these changes in serum lipids increase the risk for cardiovascular disease, particularly in the adolescent. Adolescent patients with known hyperlipidemias are not limited in their choice of contraceptive method, but should be assessed for other cardiovascular risk factors. Use of a CHC method should be based on the type and severity of the disease. ACOG recommends frequent monitoring after starting a CHC in patients with hyperlipidemia until stabilization is observed.

There are no contraindications to the use of the copper IUD in any form of cardiovascular disease.

Diabetes and insulin resistance

Hormonal contraception has been associated with adverse changes in carbohydrate metabolism and insulin resistance. While CHCs and DMPA may impair glucose tolerance and elevate insulin levels, clinically significant effects have not been reported. The etonorgestrel implant induces mild insulin resistance without a significant change in serum glucose levels. POPs and the LNG-IUS do not significantly impair carbohydrate metabolism.

For women without diabetes, alterations in carbohydrate metabolism are not clinically significant. A Cochrane review shows that for women without diabetes, CHCs have minimal effect on carbohydrate metabolism. For women with a history of gestational diabetes, the use of a low-dose COC has a minimal risk of impaired glucose tolerance and does not influence the risk of developing diabetes.

Although there are theoretical concerns about prescribing hormonal contraception for women with insulin-requiring diabetes, the studies examining its use by women with well-controlled, uncomplicated diabetes are reassuring. Current data suggest that modern CHCs have little effect on glycemic control or the insulin requirements of diabetic women. Current or past COC use and duration of use are not associated with glycosylated hemoglobin elevations, or the development of complicated disease. Similarly, the LNG-IUS has no clinical effect on glycosylated hemoglobin, fasting serum glucose, or daily insulin requirements in women with diabetes. In contrast to COCs and the LNG-IUS, diabetic users of DMPA have a nonclinically significant increase in fasting blood glucose.

The USMEC indicates that the advantages of hormonal contraception generally outweigh the risks for both noninsulin- and insulin-dependent diabetic women. However, for women with nephropathy, retinopathy, neuropathy, or other vascular disease, CHC and DMPA should not be used, whereas use of POPs, the contraceptive implant, and the LNG-IUS are acceptable. ACOG recommends that use of CHCs by diabetic women should be limited to otherwise healthy women under 35 years who do not smoke.

Risk of venous thromboembolism

All users of CHCs, including adolescents, have an increased risk of venous thromboembolism (VTE), including pulmonary embolism (PE) and deep vein thrombosis (DVT), due to the estrogen component of CHCs. Although the risk of VTE is reduced with the lower doses of estrogen in modern COCs, users still have a three to four fold elevated risk of VTE compared with nonpregnant nonusers.

☆ Tips and tricks

It is important to remember that VTE occurs substantially more frequently in pregnant women than in users of CHCs.

Use of CHCs particularly increases the risk of VTE in women with thrombophilic disorders, such as the factor V Leiden mutation. Laboratory screening may be indicated to identify thrombophilic disorders in women with a family history of VTE or thrombophilic disorder, but *routine screening is not currently recommended*, and a family history of VTE is not a contraindication to use of CHC.

Due to the increased risk of thromboembolism, USMEC recommends that individuals who are less than 3 weeks postpartum, have a personal history of VTE, or have a known thrombogenic mutation do not use CHCs. Additionally, updated CDC criteria for contraception in the postpartum period discourage use of CHCs for up to *6 weeks postpartum* for women with risk factors for VTE, including obesity and smoking. Because prolonged immobilization is also a risk factor for VTE, USMEC recommends that CHCs should be discontinued when major surgery with prolonged immobilization is anticipated.

For the copper IUD and for progestin-only methods of contraception, the USMEC gives no restrictions or states that the advantages generally outweigh the risks of methods used for all conditions related to VTE, including a personal history of, or an acute DVT or PE.

Depressive disorders

Mood changes are commonly cited as one of the side effects of hormonal contraception and as a reason for discontinuation. Despite these reported potential effects on mood, there does not appear to be a significant risk of worsening depressive symptoms among women with depressive disorders who use hormonal contraception. The USMEC gives a category 1 to all methods of contraception for women with depressive disorders.

Conclusion

Contraceptive management of young women with medical disease merits careful consideration of the risk of pregnancy, the risk of contraception, and potential drug interactions with current medications. There are many highly effective methods of contraception that these young women can use safely.

Evidence at a glance

Moods and contraception

• Several large studies have found no increase in depressive symptoms among adolescent users of COCs or DMPA.

• Two small prospective studies of adolescents using DMPA showed no worsening of depressive symptoms, and one showed a decrease in depressive symptoms after 1 year of DMPA use.

• The *ACOG Practice Bulletin* on hormonal contraception in women with coexisting medical conditions states "in women with depressive disorders, symptoms do not appear to worsen with use of hormonal methods of contraception."

Further reading

American College of Obstetricians and Gynecologists. The use of hormonal contraception in women with coexisting medical conditions. ACOG Practice Bulletin No. 73. *Obstet Gynecol* 2006:107:1453–1472.

Centers for Disease Control and Prevention. U.S. Medical Eligibility Criteria for Contraceptive Use, 2010. *MMWR Early Release* 2010;59. Available at http://www.cdc.gov/reproductivehealth/unintendedpregnancy/usmec.htm

World Health Organization. *Medical Eligibility Criteria for Contraceptive Use*, 4th edn. Geneva: WHO, 2009. Available to purchase at http://www.who.int/reproductive health/publications/family_planning/9789241563888/en/index.html

34.1

Barrier methods

Uri Belkind and Susan M. Coupey

Division of Adolescent Medicine, Children's Hospital at Montefiore/Albert Einstein College of Medicine, Bronx, NY, USA

Barrier methods of contraception work by preventing spermatozoa from reaching the upper female genital tract. These methods may be used alone or, to improve efficacy, in combination with a spermicide.

These methods (Table 34.1.1) can be broadly divided into male-controlled options, the male condom, and female-controlled methods such as the female condom, diaphragm, contraceptive sponge, Lea's shield, or cervical cap (FemCap).

Barrier contraceptive methods are safe options for adolescents; however, with the availability of a wider array of highly effective hormonal methods, their use has decreased in the last few decades, with the exception of the male condom. Because of the need for consistent use with every act of intercourse, something difficult to achieve for most adolescents, barrier methods do not protect against pregnancy as effectively as hormonal contraceptive methods. Available data, which are not adolescent-specific, show that efficacy varies by method, with failure rates ranging from as low as 2% per year for perfect use of the male condom, to as high as 32% per year for typical use of the contraceptive sponge or cervical cap (Table 34.1.1; see also Appendix 1.12.2 for comparison with other methods). Adequate counseling is fundamental in attaining the highest levels of efficacy through consistent use.

Male condom

Use of the male condom is very common in adolescent sexual relationships and is often recommended as a back-up or second method to prevent sexually-transmitted infection (STI), especially human immunodeficiency virus (HIV).

> ### ☆ Tips and tricks
>
> • All sexually active adolescents are at high risk of contracting STIs and they should use male condoms with every act of intercourse.
> • Male condoms are compatible with all other contraceptive methods, except female condoms.
> • When adolescents are using male condoms alone for contraception, always counsel or prescribe (for those younger than 17) emergency contraception as a back-up plan in case the condom breaks, slips off, or they forget to use one.

The condom acts as a physical barrier by covering the penile glans and shaft. It is available in a wide array of shapes, sizes, colors, and thicknesses (0.03–0.1 mm), as well as with or without a reservoir tip. Condoms

Practical Pediatric and Adolescent Gynecology, First Edition. Edited by Paula J. Adams Hillard.
© 2013 John Wiley & Sons, Ltd. Published 2013 by John Wiley & Sons, Ltd.

Table 34.1.1 Barrier methods of contraception

	Male condom	Female condom	Diaphragm	Contraceptive sponge	Lea's shield	FemCap
Failure rate: Perfect use (%)*‡	2	5	6	9–20†	9–15^Δ	9–26†
Typical use (%)*‡	15–71	21	16	16–32†	N/A	16–32†
Frequency of dosing	Single use	Single use	With each intercourse Lasts up to 2 years	Single use Effective for up to 24 hours	With each intercourse Multiple uses	With each intercourse Multiple uses
Continuation rates (%)ᵚ	53	49	57	N/A	N/A	N/A
Side effects	Latex sensitivity§		Poor fitting may result in pelvic discomfort or dyspareunia May predispose to UTIs Risk of TSS	May predispose to UTIs Risk of TSS	May predispose to UTIs Risk of TSS	May predispose to UTIs Risk of TSS
Advantages for teens	Protection against STIs Inexpensive Easily accessible	May be inserted up to 8 hours before intercourse Easily accessible Female-driven Protection against STIs	Effective for up to 6 hours, longer reapplying spermicide May decrease the risk of cervical neoplasia	Over-the-counter Effective for up to 24 hours	Effective for up to 8 hours, longer reapplying spermicide No fitting necessary	May be left in place for up to 48 hours
Disadvantages for teens	Reduced sensation Lack of spontaneity Problems with erection Lack of cooperation	Expensive Visible outer ring may be unattractive	Available by prescription only Requires a pelvic exam for fitting Must be left in place for 6 hours after intercourse	Must be left in place for 6 hours after intercourse Some women may experience problems with removal	Available by prescription only Must be left in place for 8 hours after intercourse May be felt by partner	Available by prescription only Must be left in place for 8 hours after intercourse

N/A, data not available; UTI, urinary tract infection; TSS, toxic shock syndrome.

*During the first 12 months.

‡Adolescent-specific data only for male condom: failure rate for <20-year olds 13.9–71.7% depending on poverty and relationship status.

†Affected by parity. Failure rate higher in parous women.

^ΔData from a single study.

ᵚFirst year continuation rates.

§Latex-free condoms are widely available.

are most commonly made from latex rubber, but are also made of polyurethane, synthetic elastomers (Tactylon), or natural membrane (lambskin), and are available with or without lubricant or spermicide.

> ✋ **Caution**
>
> Adolescents with latex allergy should be counseled regarding latex-free condom options.

The pregnancy rate with typical use of male condoms is approximately 15% per year, but can be as high as 70% in female adolescents of lower socioeconomic status cohabiting with their sexual partner, mainly due to improper/inconsistent use, most notably the failure to use a condom during every act of sexual intercourse. Efficacy is not increased with spermicide-lubricated condoms, and the spermicide may irritate the vaginal walls of the female partner. Efficacy is theoretically increased with the concomitant use of vaginal spermicide.

Advantages of male condoms include their wide accessibility for adolescents. Condom purchase does not require a prescription and condoms are inexpensive. In addition, condoms are often available free of charge in schools, health centers, and health fairs.

Male condoms offer several noncontraceptive benefits, the most notable of which is protection against STIs. Another potential benefit for adolescent males is prolonged intercourse and prevention of premature ejaculation.

There are few side effects of condom use except for latex sensitivity causing allergic reactions for which synthetic alternatives are available. Factors that may lead to nonuse of male condoms include reduced sensation, reduced spontaneity, difficulty maintaining an erection, lack of partner co-operation, and genital irritation.

> ✋ **Patient advice**
>
> **Recommendations for correct male condom use**
> - Condoms can be easily and discreetly carried by both male and female adolescents.
> - Use a new condom for each act of intercourse.

> - Store condoms in a cool, dry place and out of direct sunlight.
> - Do not use condoms that show evidence of damage or obvious signs of age.
> - Condoms should be handled with care to prevent tearing or puncture.
> - Put the condom on before genital contact.
> - Hold the tip of the condom, unroll it onto the erect penis, and leave space at the tip to collect semen – ensure that no air is trapped in the tip of the condom.
> - Ensure adequate lubrication – use only water-based lubricants with latex condoms.
> - If a condom breaks, it should be replaced immediately. If ejaculation occurs after breakage, the immediate use of spermicide may prevent pregnancy.
> - Following ejaculation, the base of the condom should be held and withdrawal should occur while the penis is still erect.
> - Never re-use a condom.

Female-controlled barrier contraception methods

These methods include the female condom, the diaphragm, contraceptive sponges, Lea's shield, and the cervical cap or FemCap. Some of these methods are used in conjunction with spermicides. Although their use has declined, and fewer than 1% of all women aged 15–19 years use these methods, the absence of systemic effects makes them an option for adolescents who have contraindications to hormonal methods.

> ✋ **Caution**
>
> - Rarely, abnormalities in vaginal anatomy may interfere with a satisfactory fit, decreasing the effectiveness of some female-controlled barrier methods.
> - Some female barrier contraceptive methods and spermicide use increase vaginal colonization with *Escherichia coli* and thus increase the risk of vaginal and urinary tract infections.

Female condom

This is a soft, loose-fitting, single-use polyurethane, lubricated sheath that is 7.8 cm in diameter and 17 cm in length between two flexible support rings. The internal ring, at the closed end of the sheath, is inserted into the vagina. The external ring remains outside the vagina after insertion and confers some protection to the labia and the base of the penis during intercourse.

In the first year of use, the pregnancy rate for the female condom ranges from 5% with perfect use to 21% with typical use (Table 43.1.1), presumably due to inconsistent use or "misrouting" of the penis between the sheath and the vaginal wall.

Advantages, as with the male condom, include protection against STIs with minimal, if any side effects.

Diaphragm

This dome-shaped silicone cup with a flexible rim is used with spermicide and inserted into the vagina before intercourse. The dome covers the cervix while the posterior rim rests against the posterior vaginal fornix and the anterior rim fits snuggly behind the pubic bone. The diaphragm ranges in sizes from 50 to 95 mm and must be fitted properly, by an experienced provider, to ensure efficacy and avoid pelvic discomfort or dyspareunia.

The pregnancy rate in the first year perfect and typical use is 6%, and 16%, respectively (see Appendix 1.12.2 for comparison with other methods). There are no specific data on failure rates in adolescents, and adolescents infrequently choose to use the diaphragm.

Contraceptive sponge

The sponge is a single-use, one-sized, pillow-shaped polyurethane sponge containing 1 g of nonoxynol-9 (N9) spermicide. It has a concave dimple on one side that is placed against the cervix and a woven polyester loop on the other that facilitates removal. It is moistened with tap water prior to use and inserted deep into the vagina. It should not be used in the presence of vaginal bleeding, including, menses.

Efficacy of the sponge varies with parity. For nulliparous women the pregnancy rate is 9% and 16% per year and for multiparous women 20% and 32%

per year with perfect and typical use, respectively (see Appendix 1.12.2 for comparison with other methods).

> ✋ **Caution**
>
> Frequent use of N9 may cause irritation with vulvovaginal mucosal disruption, which may increase susceptibility to HIV infection.

Lea's shield

This is a single-sized, oval device made of medical-grade silicone that fits over the cervix and serves as a barrier to the passage of sperm as well as a vehicle to hold spermicide against the cervical os. Since it is available only in one size, it does not need to be fitted, but is available by prescription only and it is recommended that the provider allow the woman to practice comfortable insertion and removal in the office. After the patient inserts the shield, the provider should check that the device covers the cervix and the loop used for removal fits behind the symphisis. Once inserted, it can stay in place for up to 48 hours.

Data on its effectiveness are lacking, and there are no data specific for adolescents, but initial studies showed 1-year failure rates of 9–15% with perfect use.

> **Evidence at a glance**
>
> - There are no systemic effects of spermicides on early pregnancy.
> - There is no association between the use of spermicides and birth defects.

FemCap

This is a hat-shaped silicone cap placed over the cervix with a brim that is applied to the vaginal fornices. The broader part of the rim should be placed against the posterior vaginal wall for stabilization and the device is pushed deeply into the vagina, creating a vacuum between the cervix and the rim of the cap. It is used in combination with spermicides. It is available in three sizes from 22 to 30 mm; choice of size is based on parity.

Efficacy has not been studied as extensively as with other methods but seems to be related to parity with failure rates of 9% and 16% in nulliparous women and 26% and 32% in parous women with perfect and typical use, respectively.

Further reading

Hatcher RA, Trussell J, Nelson AL, *et al. Contraceptive Technology*, 20th revised edn. New York: Ardent Media, 2011.

Greydanus DE, Patel DR, Rimsza ME. Contraception in the adolescent: An update. *Pediatrics* 2001;107:562–573.

Rieder J, Coupey SM. The use of nonhormonal methods of contraception in adolescents. *Pediatr Clin North Am* 1999;46:671–694.

34.2 Oral contraception

Emily M. Godfrey[1] and Melissa Kottke[2]

[1]Department of Family Medicine, University of Washington, Seattle, WA, USA
[2]Department of Gynecology and Obstetrics, Emory University School of Medicine, and Jane Fonda Center for Adolescent Reproductive Health, Atlanta, GA, USA

Combined hormonal oral contraception (COC) is one of the most popular birth control methods used by teenagers in the US. Because the COC is often considered synonymous with "birth control," its familiarity may be appealing to adolescents. In that the majority of teens are healthy and eligible for COC use, clinicians who see adolescent females should become comfortable providing this service.

⚛ Science revisited

Mechanism of action
- COC pills contain both estrogen and progestin and work by suppressing ovulation.
- COCs act on the reproductive tract by suppressing the release of gonadotropin-releasing hormone (GnRH) from the hypothalamus, and by suppressing follicle-stimulating hormone (FSH) and luteinizing hormone (LH) from the pituitary. COCs can also help thicken cervical mucus, which can act as a barrier to sperm penetration.

Modern COCs contain low-dose estrogen, with most having a dose from 20 to 35 µg to minimize estrogen-related adverse effects. The progestin in COCs varies according to different properties and levels of androgenic activity.

COCs are a highly effective form of contraception, although they are not considered the most effective. In a perfect world, when an adolescent takes a pill every single day at the same time every day, the failure rate is less than 1%. In a more typical world, however, in which many teens may miss a pill, either because they forget or are delayed in filling their prescription, or take the pills incorrectly, the failure is greater – about 9% (see Appendix 1.12.2 for comparison with other methods).

Good and poor candidates

Most adolescents can use COCs. It is rare that adolescents will have a medical condition making the use of COCs inappropriate. Should an adolescent have a health condition or characteristic that may be of concern, healthcare providers should check the United States Medical Eligibility Criteria (USMEC) prior to prescribing COCs (http://www.cdc.gov; see Chapter 33.2). The USMEC provides evidence-based guidance about the safety and efficacy of COCs for an adolescent with a particular condition or characteristic. The USMEC can assist with restricting use when there is evidence of risk, but also facilitating use where there is evidence of safety. Some common medical conditions for which teens *can* use COCs include:

Practical Pediatric and Adolescent Gynecology, First Edition. Edited by Paula J. Adams Hillard.
© 2013 John Wiley & Sons, Ltd. Published 2013 by John Wiley & Sons, Ltd.

- Family history of breast cancer
- Concomitant use of medications, such as antibiotics, antifungals, antiparasitics, and nucleoside reverse transcriptase inhibitors
- Benign ovarian tumors
- Sickle cell disease
- Insulin- or noninsulin-dependent diabetes mellitus (without evidence of vascular disease)
- Obesity
- Inflammatory bowel disease (mild)
- Migraine without aura
- Smoking.

> ### ☝ Caution
>
> - Most adolescents can use COCs.
> - Adolescents with certain characteristics or medical conditions may have contraindications to COC use.
> - Candidates should meet the USMEC guidelines (http://www.cdc.gov/reproductivehealth/unintendedpregnancy/USMEC.htm) prior to initiating the method.
> - Healthcare providers should use good clinical judgment when counseling about COC use.
> - Adolescents who have a history of prior COC failure or have difficulty remembering to take a pill daily might be considered as poor candidates for COC use.

Noncontraceptive benefits

COCs can be considered as a treatment for any of the conditions listed in Table 34.2.1., even when the adolescent is not sexually active. Prescribing COCs for the treatment of certain disorders in the nonsexually active adolescent has not been shown to encourage sexual activity.

Initial visit

Each adolescent visit should include a conversation about sexuality (see Chapter 20). Discussion of contraception should not be limited to those adolescents who endorse previous or current intercourse. Each visit with a young person is an opportunity for educa-

Table 34.2.1 Conditions that occur frequently in adolescents for which COCs can have a beneficial effect

- Dysmenorrhea
- Premenstrual syndrome
- Benign breast disease
- Iron-deficiency anemia
- Acne
- Menstrual irregularities

Adapted with permission from Hatcher RA, Zieman M, Cwiak C, *et al*. A Pocket Guide to Managing Contraception. Tiger, GA.: Bridging the Gap Foundation, 2009, p. 128. Bridging the Gap Communications.

tion not only about current behaviors, but also as preparation for future behaviors, establishing an environment where sexuality and issues surrounding sexual health can be safely discussed, as well as imparting knowledge that the young person can share with her friends (see Chapter 33.1).

According to the World Health Organization Selected Practice Recommendations, the only component of an exam that is necessary prior to initiating COCs is blood pressure. For an asymptomatic teen, there is no need for a pelvic exam. Pap smears should begin at age 21 years. The Center for Disease Control and Prevention recommends screening for gonorrhea and chlamydia for sexually-active females under the age of 25 years; this can be done with a self-collected vaginal swab or urine specimen. In teens who have been sexually active, an office-based urine pregnancy test is appropriate.

> ### ☝ Patient/parent advice
>
> - Reinforce clinic policies on confidentiality regarding reproductive health and contraception with both the teen and parent.
> - Be specific about what you can and cannot keep confidential and why.
> - Reassure the parent regarding the safety of COCs and the potential to protect future fertility. Parents have a wide range of concerns from cancer to infertility.

Which pill?

Most teens can succeed with most pills. In COC use, the most important consideration is that the selected pill is actually taken. Thus, if there is something that will increase her consistent and correct use of a certain pill, then that factor can dictate the pill choice. For example, if her trust level of a pill is high because her sister or mother is using it, then that might be the best pill for her. If she has financial concerns, a generic brand or one that allows the lowest co-pay is appropriate. Important in this selection is reassurance from the provider that if this pill does not work for her, there are many others from which to choose.

Extended or continuous use of COC may be of interest to teens, particularly those who are trying to minimize or avoid menstrual symptoms and those who are active and find unpredictable menses disruptive. This can be accomplished by prescription of a product dedicated to extended cycles which are now available in generic forms or with any monophasic combined pill. Some teens will need reassurance that menstrual blood will not "build up" inside of them.

> ### ☆ Tips and tricks
>
> • Using a "demo" pill pack during initial conversations may provide an opportunity to ask questions and may encourage correct use.
> • Using this pack may facilitate discussion of when to expect menses with the hormone-free placebo pills (also known as the "different color pills").
> • The "demo" can facilitate discussions of how to extend the cycle or skip periods if the patient chooses.

When to start

Starting the pill on the day of her visit, also called Quick Start, is a concrete and convenient way to initiate COCs (Figure 34.2.1). This is easier to understand

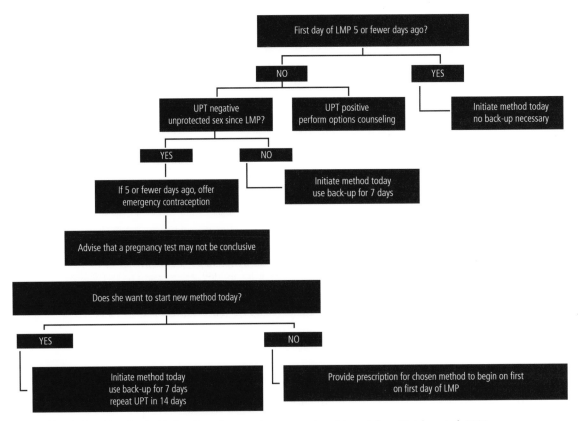

Figure 34.2.1 Algorithm for Quick Starting a hormonal contraceptive. Adapted from Hatcher *et al.* 2009. LMP, last menstrual period; UPT, urine pregnancy test.

and remember than the traditional recommendation of waiting to start the pills when the next cycle begins. It allows the clinician to immediately engage the motivated patient and potentially prevent pregnancies that could occur while waiting for the next cycle to begin.

Length of prescription

Clinicians can help improve COC use by giving a prescription for an entire year, remembering that this will require 13 packs for those who are using COC cyclically, and more for those who are using them continuously. If your clinic has the capacity, providing the actual pill packs may improve continuation.

Follow-up visits

A follow-up visit to reinforce consistent use, recheck blood pressure, and trouble-shoot side effects that may interfere with continuation may be a good idea. During the follow-up visit, things to discuss include:
• Is she remembering to take a pill every day? Reinforce that the pill needs to be taken every day to be effective. Endorse that it is difficult to remember to take a pill every day, especially when you feel well.
• Is she experiencing any side effects that concern her? The most common side effects are nausea, breast tenderness, and breakthrough bleeding. Management clues for addressing these side effects are mentioned below.
• What is she doing to avoid sexually-transmitted diseases (STDs)? Remind her that COCs do not

protect from STDs, so encourage prevention activities like consistent condom use, screening for STDs, partner testing, and monogamy.

Management of problems

Missing pills
Most of the evidence regarding missing pills relates to COCs with 30–35 μg of estrogen. Some limited evidence suggests that there may be a higher risk of pregnancy when 20 μg estrogen pills are missed than the 30–35 μg pills. Thus, a more cautious approach is suggested for adolescents taking 20 μg estrogen pills.
• **Missed one or two active pills (or starts new pack 1–2 days late)**: an active pill should be taken as soon as possible and then pills taken daily, one each day. Back-up contraception is not needed.
• **Missed three or more active pills (or starts new pack three or more days late)**: in general, an active pill should be taken as soon as possible as well as the pill scheduled for that day (or two pills at the same time), then pills taken daily, one each day. Back-up contraception, such as condoms or abstinence, is recommended for 7 consecutive days. To maximize protection against unwanted pregnancy, consider prescribing emergency contraception. If missed pills are in the third pill week, the active hormone pills should be completed and a new pill pack started without taking the inactive pills.
• Adolescents who are taking COCs containing 20–25 mcg and who miss two or more pills should follow the instructions for "missed three or more active pills."

Nausea
• Nausea can be improved by taking the pill with food or at night time before bed.
• Pills with lower estrogen doses may also help.

Vomiting/diarrhea
• Vomiting within 2 hours after taking an active pill: another active pill should be taken.
• Severe vomiting or diarrhea for 24 hours or more: pills should continue to be taken (if she can). Pre-treatment with an antiemetic can be considered. If the vomiting or diarrhea persists for 2 days or more, she should be instructed about missed pills as outlined earlier.

✋ Patient advice

• Try to fit taking your pill into a routine you do every day. Try taping your pill pack to your toothpaste or setting it on your alarm clock.
• Get others involved. Ask a friend, family member, or partner to remind you, "Have you taken your pill today?"
• Arrange reminders. Set your cell phone alarm to go off every day at a time when you will be able to take your pill, or sign up for reminders through services like www.bedsider.org

Breast tenderness
• Breast tenderness often improves with time.
• A more supportive bra and/or analgesics such as ibuprofen or acetaminophen may be suggested.

Menstrual abnormalities
Menstrual abnormalities, such as breakthrough spotting or bleeding, are common among COCs users (see Appendix 1.12.4 for comparison with other hormonal methods). Menstrual abnormalities may be slightly higher with the lowest dose COCs (20 μg estrogen) than with pills containing 30–35 μg estrogen. These abnormalities are even more common among adolescents who are using extended or continuous COCs, especially during the first 6 months of use.

🖐 Patient advice

• Irregular bleeding is common in the first 3–6 months of use and usually improves with time.
• Irregular bleeding does *not* imply that the risk of pregnancy is increased, as long as the regimen is being used consistently.
• Consistent daily pill use (taking a pill daily) is important.
• Breakthrough bleeding is more common in teens who miss pills.

If bleeding persists or is bothersome, you should evaluate for common causes such as pregnancy, inconsistent pill use, interactions with other medications, cervicitis, and cigarette smoking.

There is no evidence that COCs with different formulations of estrogen or progestin result in better bleeding patterns than others. However, if an adolescent requests another type of COC, allowing her to switch may consequently impact her bleeding patterns and can improve her overall satisfaction with COC use. If bleeding is occurring more in the second half of her cycle, some may benefit from a pill with a higher dose of estrogen or a tricyclic pill.

Birth control method switching

Some teens already using another birth control method may wish to switch to COCs; other teens who are on the birth control pill may wish to switch to an alternative birth control method. To lower the chance of getting pregnant, there should be no gap when switching between different types of contraceptive methods. Patients should be discouraged from waiting for their next period before switching to a new method (Table 34.2.2).

COC failure and potential exposure in early pregnancy

COC exposure around the time of conception has not shown to be associated with congenital malformations. Should an adolescent report or suspect an unplanned pregnancy during COC use, COCs should be stopped immediately and the adolescent should receive comprehensive options counseling and be referred appropriately (see Chapter 32). An adolescent who becomes pregnant while using COCs should be counseled about using a more effective birth control method post pregnancy.

⚗ Science revisited

• A meta-analysis of 12 prospective cohort studies reported a nonsignificant relative risk for major congenital malformations, heart defects, and limb reduction defects among women exposed to COCs either early in pregnancy, after the last menstrual period, or within 1 month of conception
• One additional prospective study found a slight increase in risk of low birth weight, but no increase in risk of neonatal or infant death among women who were exposed to COCs in early pregnancy.

Table 34.2.2 Contraception method switching: how to switch to or from COCs

Switching from	Switching *to*						
	COCs	Patch	Ring	Progestin shot ("Depo")	Progestin implant	Hormone IUD	Copper IUD (nonhormone)
COCs	*No gap:* take first pill of new pack the day after taking any pill in the old pack	Start patch *one day before* stopping pill	*No gap:* insert ring the day after taking any pill in the pack	First shot *7 days before* stopping pill	Insert implant *4 days before* stopping pill	Insert hormone IUD *7 days before* stopping pill	Can insert copper IUD *up to 5 days after* stopping pill
Patch	Start pill *1 day before* stopping patch						
Ring	Start pill *1 day before* stopping ring						
Progestin shot ("Depo")	Can take first pill up to *15 weeks after* the last shot						
Progestin implant	Start pill *7 days before* implant is removed						
Hormone IUD	Start pill *1 day before* IUD is removed						
Copper IUD	Start pill *7 days before* IUD is removed						

Adapted with permission from Reproductive Health Access Project: http://www.reproductiveaccess.org/fact_sheets/switching_bc.htm

---

♀ Pearls

- COCs can be used by most teens, even those who have specific medical conditions.
- COCs can help alleviate many common medical problems during adolescence.
- COC counseling should focus on the importance of compliance and avoidance of missed pills.
- Providers can assist patient success in using COCs by:
  - Initiating pills using "quick start," rather than waiting until the next menstrual period
  - Prescribing a 1-year prescription, and
  - Avoiding unnecessary screening exams and tests.
- A continuous or extended use regimen may also be prescribed.
- Some teens may experience side effects, most of which can be managed with counseling and reassurance.

Further reading

Centers for Disease Control and Prevention (CDC). U.S. Medical Eligibility Criteria for Contraceptive Use, 2010: adapted from the World Health Organization Medical Eligibility Criteria for Contraceptive Use, 4th edition. *MMWR Recomm Rep* 2010;59:1–86.

World Health Organization. *Selected Practice Recommendations for Contraception Use*, 2nd edn. Geneva: WHO, 2004.

Zieman M, Hatcher RA, Cwiak C, *et al. A Pocket Guide to Managing Contraception*. Tiger, GA: Bridging the Gap Foundation, 2010, p. 128

34.3

Transdermal and vaginal combination methods

Sherine Patterson-Rose and Paula Braverman

Division of Adolescent Medicine, Cincinnati Children's Hospital Medical Center, Cincinnati, OH, USA

While similar to combined oral contraceptive pills (COCs) in mechanism of action and hormonal composition, the transdermal patch (OrthoEvra[R]) and the transvaginal ring (NuvaRing[R]) simplify compliance by eliminating the need for daily use. The patch contains 0.75 mg of ethinyl estradiol (EE) and 6 mg of norelgestromin, while the ring contains 0.015 mg of EE and 0.120 mg of etonogestrel. Both methods of delivery avoid gastrointestinal absorption and first-pass metabolism through the liver, resulting in steady blood levels of hormones, unlike the daily peaks with COCs. Both have similar side effects and contraindications to COCs and are as effective in primarily preventing ovulation (Table 34.3.1).

Evidence at a glance

- The patch is associated with circulating estrogen levels that are 60% higher than the pill.
- Studies have shown that both the patch and the ring can be used in extended cycle regimens.
- Studies have shown that effectiveness of the patch decreases in women over 90 kg (>198 lbs). However, these findings may be similar among all COCs and further trials are needed.

- Studies of acceptability of the patch and ring in adolescents demonstrate that attitudes toward the methods were related to:
  - Distrust in the contraceptive effectiveness of a new method
  - Media coverage of the method and its side effects
  - Influence of partner and peers
  - Specific method concerns.
- Adolescents' concerns about the patch have included visibility and possible health risks.
- Concerns about the ring have included:
  - Vaginal insertion
  - Anticipated reaction of their sexual partner.

Prescribing

A routine history and physical exam should be conducted, including blood pressure and weight, to determine any medical contraindications to use. Specifically, for those patients requesting the patch, a history of skin sensitivity or exfoliative dermatologic disorders should be elicited. For the ring, the patient needs a level of comfort with inserting and removing a device intravaginally. A pelvic exam is not required prior to prescribing either method. While routine tests are not

Practical Pediatric and Adolescent Gynecology, First Edition. Edited by Paula J. Adams Hillard.
© 2013 John Wiley & Sons, Ltd. Published 2013 by John Wiley & Sons, Ltd.

Table 34.3.1 Summary of features of transdermal patch and intravaginal ring method of contraception

	Transdermal patch (ORTHOEVRA[R])	Intravaginal ring (NUVARING[R])
Failure rate*		
Perfect use	0.3%	0.3%
Typical use	9%	9%
Frequency of dosing	Weekly × 3 weeks; then 1-week break	Inserted × 3 weeks; then 1-week break
Continuation rate at 1 year**	10.9 per 100 person years	29.4 per 100 person years
Discontinuation	Rapid return to fertility upon discontinuation	Rapid return to fertility upon discontinuation
Side effects	Skin reaction: dermatitis, hyperpigmentation	Vaginal symptoms: vaginitis, leukorrhea
	Nausea	Nausea
	Headache	Headache
	Breast discomfort, engorgement or pain	Breast discomfort, engorgement or pain
	Increased risk of venous thromboembolism	Increased risk of venous thromboembolism
Advantages for teens	Easier compliance	Easier compliance
	Ease of concealment	Ease of concealment
	Steadier hormonal levels than COCs	Steadier hormonal levels than COCs
Disadvantages for teens	Visibility concerns	Intravaginal application
	Possibility of a patch detachment	Possible interference with sex

*See Appendix 1.12.2 for comparison with other methods.
**Reproduced with permission from Raine TR, Foster-Rosales A, Upadhyay U, Boyer CB, Brown BA, Sokolof A, Harper CC. One-year contraceptive continuation and pregnancy in adolescent girls and women initiating hormonal contraceptives. *Obstet Gynecol* 2011;117(2):363–371. Lippincott Williams & Wilkins.

necessary, a pregnancy test is advised when planning to initiate the method prior to the next normal menses. For those patients with a family history of venous thromboembolism in a first-degree relative, a thrombophilia work-up may be indicated prior to use.

Method initiation

1. If having menses and not using hormonal contraception or the intrauterine device (IUD), there are three options:
• Start on the first day of menses; no additional contraception is needed.
• Start on the first Sunday after menses (patch) or days 2–5 of menses (ring); back-up contraception is required for the first week.
• Immediate start on any cycle day (Quick Start; see Figure 34.2.1). Studies have shown this is acceptable if a pregnancy test is negative; back-up contraception is required for the first week. A repeat pregnancy test

should be considered 2 weeks later in case of recent unprotected sexual activity.
2. For switching from another combined hormonal contraceptive, see Appendix 1.12.5.
3. Following abortion or miscarriage:
• **First trimester:** the patch or ring may be started within the first 5 days following an abortion without need for additional contraception.
• **Second trimester/postpartum:** the patch can be started 3–4 weeks and the ring 4 weeks after delivery for non-breastfeeding postpartum teenagers and those with a second trimester pregnancy loss. An additional method of contraception should be used for the first week.

Management

Patch

The patch should be changed on the same day of each week, alternating the site of attachment. Patches can be applied to the upper arms, upper and lower back, or lower abdomen.

✋ Patient advice

Patch

• If a patch is partially or completely detached for less than 24 hours, try to reapply it. If it does not adhere, remove the patch and apply a replacement. If more than 24 hours have elapsed or the time period is unknown, start a new patch cycle immediately, using back-up contraception for the first 7 days.

• If there is a delay in changing the patch at the start of a cycle in week 1, apply a new patch and use back-up contraception during the first week. Emergency contraception should be offered if the teenager has had unprotected sex.

• For a delay during week 2 or 3 of the cycle:
  ○ If less than 48 hours, apply the new patch immediately, keeping the same patch change day. No back-up contraception is needed.
  ○ If more than 48 hours, start a new 4-week cycle immediately, using back-up contraception for the first week. Emergency contraception should be offered if the teenager has had unprotected sex.

• If there is a delay in the fourth week of the patch cycle, remove the patch as soon as possible. The next patch will start on the usual patch change day. No back-up or emergency contraception is needed.

Ring

The ring is left in place for 3 weeks and then removed for 7 days. After the ring-free interval, a new ring is placed on the same day of the week that the first ring was inserted.

✋ Patient advice

Ring

• If the ring has been left in place for up to 4 weeks, the woman remains protected. The ring should be removed and a new ring placed after a 1–week-free interval. If the ring has been left in place for more than 4 weeks, pregnancy should be ruled out. Back-up contraception is needed until the new ring has been in place for 7 days.

• If the ring becomes disconnected, it should be discarded and replaced. A disconnected ring does not alter contraceptive efficacy.

• If the ring has been expelled for less than 3 hours, rinse with cool to lukewarm water and re-insert.

• If the ring has been expelled for more than 3 hours:
  ○ During week 1 or 2, it should be re-inserted as soon as possible and a back-up method should be used for 7 days.
  ○ During week 3, the ring should be discarded. Either insert a new ring 7 days later after a withdrawal bleed or insert a new ring immediately, restarting the 3-week cycle. With the latter method, spotting may occur.

★ Tips and tricks

Plan a follow-up visit 6–8 weeks after method initiation to review the side effects and compliance.

Patch

• The patch continues to maintain contraceptive efficacy in weeks 2 and 3 of the cycle even with a 48-hour delay in changing the patch.

• Mild contact dermatitis may be treated with a topical steroid cream; if symptoms persist or are severe, discontinue the patch.

• Prescribe an extra patch in case of detachment

Ring

• Contraceptive efficacy is maintained up to 3 hours per 24-hour period if the ring is removed.

• Have the patient practice insertion and removal of the ring in the office to ensure comfort with use.

✋ Caution

Refer to the USMEC categories and prescribing criteria for medical conditions that represent an unacceptable health risk with use of the method (category 4; http://www.cdc.gov/reproductivehealth/unintendedpregnancy/USMEC.htm).

Drug–drug interactions

• Antiretroviral (ARV) therapy: may decrease or increase the bioavailability of hormones from the patch and the ring.
• Anticonvulsant therapy: some anticonvulsants may reduce the efficacy of the patch and the ring.
• Antibiotic therapy:
  ○ Rifampicin and rifabutin may reduce the effectiveness of the patch and the ring.
  ○ Most antibiotics, antifungal agents, and antiparasitic agents do not have significant interactions

⚗ Science revisited

• **Venous thromboembolism (VTE) risk:**
  ○ Studies have shown conflicting evidence regarding the frequency of venous thrombotic events among women using the transdermal patch as compared to COCs containing norgestimate. A recent well-controlled study found no increased VTE risk in women under age 40 years when comparing the patch to an COC with a second-generation progestin.
  ○ One recent study has shown an increased risk of VTE with the ring compared to standard COCs (including a third-generation progestin). This study included an adolescent population but since this is the first report of this type, further studies are needed.
• **Bone mineral density (BMD).** Studies with young adult women have shown that both the vaginal ring and the patch produce no change in BMD and demonstrate a positive influence on bone turnover over 1–2 years. Similar studies are needed in postmenarchal adolescents.

✋ Patient/parent advice

• Neither the patch nor the ring prevents transmission of sexually transmitted infections (STIs) or HIV infection.
• Keeping track of the patch or ring change days on a calendar may aid in adherence.

Patch

• Do not use lotions or creams in the area of patch application.
• Do not tape, paste or cut the patch.
• Activities such as exercise, showers or swimming can be done without concern for detachment.

Ring

• The ring should be kept refrigerated prior to use.
• Ring placement in the vagina can be facilitated by loading the ring into an empty tampon inserter.
• Squatting may aid with removal of the ring.
• If the ring is removed, it should be rinsed with cool to lukewarm water prior to reinsertion.

♀ Pearls

• The patch and the ring are excellent forms of contraception for adolescents.
• While specific tests are not required prior to prescribing, a detailed history and physical exam will help exclude contraindications.
• When prescribing these methods, it is useful to review brief management scenarios.
• Follow-up in 6–8 weeks to review side effects and compliance.

Further reading

Jick SS, Hagberg KW, Hernandez RK, Kaye JA. Post-marketing study of ORTHO EVRA and levonorgestrel oral contraceptives containing hormonal contraceptives with 30 mcg of ethinyl estradiol in relation to non-fatal venous thromboembolism. *Contraception* 2010;81:16–21.

Massaro M, Di Carlo C, Gargano V, Formisano C, Bifulco G, Nappi C. Effects of the contraceptive patch and the vaginal ring on bone metabolism and bone mineral density: A prospective, controlled, randomized study. *Contraception* 2010;81:209–214.

Raine TR, Epstein LB, Harper CC, Brown B, Boyer CB. Attitudes toward the vaginal ring and transdermal patch among adolescent and young women. *J Adolesc Health* 2009;45:262–267.

Raine TR, Foster-Rosales A, Upadhyay U, Boyer CB, Brown BA, Sokolof A, Harper CC. One-year contraceptive continuation and pregnancy in adolescent girls and women initiating hormonal contraceptives. *Obstet Gynecol* 2011; 117(2):363–371.

34.4 Intrauterine devices

Sophia Yen

Department of Pediatrics, Division of Adolescent Medicine, Stanford University School of Medicine, Stanford, CA, USA

For physicians who wish to help their adolescent patients prevent unplanned pregnancies, knowledge about intrauterine devices (IUDs) is crucial. Two types of IUDs are currently available in the US: the levonorgestrel intrauterine system (LNG-IUS) and the copper T380A (Table 34.4.1).

Per 2007 American College of Obstetricians and Gynecologists (ACOG) guidelines, IUDs may be considered first-line contraception in both parous and nulliparous adolescents. The 2006–2008 National Survey of Family Growth found that only 3.6% of US sexually-active adolescents use the IUD. However, this is a significant increase from 2002 when only 0.2% of adolescents reported using the IUD.

Because they require little to no patient effort for use, IUDs have a very low failure rate. The first year typical failure rate for the copper T380A IUD is 0.8% and for the LNG-IUS it is 0.2%. This puts the IUD in the same range as tubal ligation for efficacy. The discontinuation rate at 1 year for adults is 22% for the copper T380A IUD and 20% for the LNG-IUS. A major reason for discontinuation of the IUD is its side effects (Table 34.4.1).

Barriers to use of IUDs by adolescents include cost, confidentiality, fear of side effects, and lack of knowledge of the IUD as an option. Cost depends on insurance coverage. Some countries or states cover birth control because they have found it to be cost-effective. In the US, for every $1 spent on family planning,

> ## ✋ Patient advice
>
> ### Benefits of the IUD
> - Lowest failure rate of most contraceptives
> - Long-term efficacy (5 or 10 years)
> - Patient does not have to think about the method
> - Cost-effective
> - Rapid return to fertility after removal
> - Appropriate in many cases where estrogen-containing birth control is not
> - LNG-IUS can be used to treat menorrhagia and endometriosis (off-label indication)

the government saves $4 in future expenses. Most states give adolescents the right to receive confidential contraceptive services without parental permission and/or notification (see Table 18.4 and the Guttmacher Institute's "State Policies in Brief: Minors' Access to Contraceptive Services" available at http://www.guttmacher.org/statecenter/adolescents/html).

Many myths pervade both public and medical opinions of IUD use in adolescents. These pose significant barriers to adoption of the IUD by adolescents. The truths about IUDs are rather different.

Practical Pediatric and Adolescent Gynecology, First Edition. Edited by Paula J. Adams Hillard.
© 2013 John Wiley & Sons, Ltd. Published 2013 by John Wiley & Sons, Ltd.

Table 34.4.1 Comparison of the LNG-IUS and copper IUD.

	LNG-IUS	Copper IUD
Failure rate		
Perfect use	0.1*†	0.6*†
Typical use	0.2*†	1.0*†
Discontinuation at 1 year	20%	22%
Frequency of dosing	5 years	10 years
Common side effects	Lighter menses Possible amenorrhea (20–60% of users at 1 year) Intermenstrual spotting and bleeding in first months of use	Possible menorrhagia Possible increased dysmenorrhea Unscheduled bleeding in the first month after insertion
Advantages for teens	Lighter menses Possible amenorrhea Less dysmenorrhea	Longer duration of action
Disadvantages for teens	Higher cost	Possible menorrhagia Possible increased dysmenorrhea

*% of women experiencing an unintended pregnancy in the first year of use.
†See Appendix 1.12.2 for comparison with other methods.

Evidence at a glance

The truths about IUDs

- IUDs do not increase an adolescent's risk of pelvic inflammatory disease (PID) beyond a slight increased risk in the first 20 days after insertion (a risk that is present for women of all ages).
- The risk of PID with IUD placement with no infection present at the time of insertion is 0–2% and increases to 0–5% when there is a documented infection at the time of insertion.
- The LNG-IUD may decrease the risk of PID because the progestin effect on cervical mucus may lower the risk of ascending infection.
- IUDs do not increase an adolescent's risk of acquiring sexually-transmitted infections (STIs).
- Past use of an IUD has not been found to be associated with infertility; past history of chlamydia infection *is* associated with infertility.

Which IUD is preferable?

This depends on the patient's preferences, including whether they want 5 or 10 years of protection. Cost may be a factor – the LNG-IUS is generally more expensive than the copper IUD. Some adolescents may have concerns about hormonal therapy, and prefer a nonhormonal IUD. In general, adolescents tend to select the LNG-IUS because of its better side effect profile, resulting in lighter periods and greater prospects of amenorrhea.

Insertion of the IUD

Contraindications to IUD initiation are listed in Table 34.4.2.

Postpartum IUDs should be placed either within 48 hours or later than 4 weeks postpartum. Postpartum IUDs that are placed within 48 hours after delivery of the placenta are associated with lower expulsion

Table 34.4.2 WHO category 4 contraindications to IUD initiation (conditions that represent an unacceptable health risk if the method is used)

- Pregnancy
- Current purulent cervicitis
- Current chlamydial infection
- Current gonorrhea infection
- Pelvic tuberculosis
- Current pelvic inflammatory disease (PID)
- Anatomic distorted uterine cavity
- Cervical cancer
- Endometrial cancer
- Unexplained vaginal bleeding before evaluation
- Postpartum puerperal sepsis

rates than those placed after 48 hours to 4 weeks postpartum.

An IUD can be placed without regard to timing of menses, as long as the woman is not pregnant.

✋ Caution

- All adolescents should be screened for gonorrhea and chlamydia before IUD insertion.
- Screening at time of insertion is acceptable and increases the rate of IUD insertion.
- Patients who have positive screens and are treated promptly do not suffer increased morbidity.
- Routine prophylactic antibiotics are not recommended.
- Active cervicitis is a contraindication to placement of an IUD.

Common side effects during insertion include: vasovagal syncope, variable amounts of pain, and diaphoresis. Rare side effects during insertion include vomiting, cervical laceration, and uterine perforation. For a few days after insertion, patients may have spotting or light bleeding with mild cramping. Irregular bleeding is common for the first several months after LNG-IUS insertion.

★ Tips and tricks

- An adolescent's first pelvic exam should not include an IUD insertion; she should first be "walked and talked" through her first speculum exam to assess her tolerance and to allow her to give a truly informed consent to an IUD insertion procedure.
- Many patients experience pain or discomfort with IUD insertion. In one study, 86% of adolescents reported mild to severe pain with insertion.
- Premedication with 400 μg of buccal misoprostol 2–4 hours prior to insertion may be used to soften a nulliparous cervix and make insertion easier for patient and provider.
- Nonsteroidal anti-inflammatory drugs for analgesia, such as 600–800 mg ibuprofen, 1–2 hours before the procedure and 6 hours after the insertion help decrease the pain experienced by patients.
- Practitioners may also use a paracervical or intracervical nerve block to help reduce the pain experienced during insertion.
- A Graves speculum should be used for IUD insertion instead of the usual Pederson speculum. The Graves speculum allows more space for the instrumentation used in IUD placement.

Follow-up

There are no evidence-based guidelines for follow-up after IUD insertion, although many clinicians suggest an "IUD check" at 6–8 weeks after insertion to assess tolerance by history, assure that the string is visible on examination, and assess patient satisfaction.

The complication rate for IUDs is quite low at about 1.8 per 100 cases. Severe or prolonged cramping post insertion can be related to partial expulsion, perforation or PID. If the cramping persists, is unrelated to menses, and it bothers the patient, then the IUD should be removed.

If the strings cannot be seen on examination, contraception is not assured and pregnancy should be ruled out. If the pregnancy test is negative, a practitioner can search for the strings using an endocervical brush or cotton-tipped applicator in the endocervical canal. If the strings are still not palpable or visible, an ultrasound should be done to locate the IUD and insure that it has not been expelled or perforated the uterus.

If a pregnancy occurs with the IUD in place, first the practitioner must determine if the pregnancy is ectopic or intrauterine. Use of an IUD does not increase the risk of ectopic pregnancy over that in a woman who is not contracepting, but in the rare instance that a pregnancy occurs with an IUD in place, the risk that the pregnancy is an ectopic pregnancy is increased. Pregnancies with IUDs should be managed by an obstetrician–gynecologist. If the pregnancy is ectopic, then the IUD can remain in place during treatment of the ectopic pregnancy. If the pregnancy is intrauterine, the IUD should be removed as soon as possible after a discussion of the increased risks of spontaneous abortion, preterm delivery, and septic abortion if the IUD is left in place; there is an increased risk of spontaneous abortion if the IUD is removed as well.

Removal of the IUD is not necessary for treatment of STIs and PID, although consideration should be given to removal if symptoms fail to resolve after 72 hours of treatment.

Perforations rarely occur. If a perforation occurs at the time of insertion, the IUD should be removed immediately. The patient should then receive alternative contraception, be monitored for excessive bleeding, and followed up as appropriate. After the next menstrual cycle, another IUD insertion may be attempted.

Expulsions are higher in nulliparous patients compared with primiparas (8% versus 1.5%).

Other uses

The copper IUD can be placed up to 5 days after contraceptive failure, rape, or unprotected sex as emergency contraception (EC) (see Chapter 34.6). In one study 86% of parous and 80% of nonparous women kept the copper IUD for long-term contraception after placement for EC.

The LNG-IUS can be used for the treatment of menorrhagia because it reduces the menstrual flow on average by 75% at 3 months after insertion.

Further reading

American College of Obstetricians and Gynecologists. ACOG Committee Opinion No. 392, December 2007. Intrauterine device and adolescents. *Obstet Gynecol* 2007;110(6):1493–1495.

U.S. Medical Eligibility Criteria for Contraceptive Use 2010 Appendix E http://www.cdc.gov/mmwr/preview/mmwrhtml/rr5904a6.htm

Yen S, Saah T, Hillard PJ. IUDs and adolescents – an underutilized opportunity for pregnancy prevention. *J Pediatr Adolesc Gynecol* 2010;23:e123–e128.

Acknowledgements

Most of this chapter was based on the article written with Dr Paula J.A. Hillard.

34.5 Progestin-only contraception

Michelle M. Isley[1] and Andrew M. Kaunitz[2]

[1]Department of Obstetrics and Gynecology, The Ohio State University, Columbus, OH, USA
[2]Department of Obstetrics and Gynecology, University of Florida College of Medicine-Jacksonville, Jacksonville, FL, USA

Progestin-only pills

Progestin-only pills (POPs), also known as "mini-pills," are taken daily without a placebo week. The dose of progestin in POPs is lower than in combination pills, and therefore POPs are less forgiving if taken late or missed completely. Accordingly, POPs may only be appropriate for adolescents who are highly motivated individuals and/or those who are subfecund due to lactation. In adolescents, oral contraceptive failure rates are higher than in adults; typical use failure rates are 9%, but approach 25% in some reports focused on adolescents.

> ### ⚠ Caution
>
> Successful use of oral contraceptive pills depends on consistent daily pill-taking.

POPs are safe for teens, including those who are nursing their infant immediately postpartum. Bleeding changes are common and a main reason for contraceptive discontinuation in adolescents. Appropriate counseling about irregular bleeding and the importance of consistent use is critical.

Injectable contraception

Depot medroxyprogesterone acetate (DMPA) is a 3-month progestin-only injectable contraceptive. One factor in the decreasing rate of teenage pregnancy in the US is the increased use of DMPA in this population. DMPA represents an appealing contraceptive method for adolescents because it is long-acting (with contraceptive effects lasting beyond the recommended 3-month schedule), private, not coital- or partner-dependent, and effective.

When used perfectly, DMPA has a failure rate of less than 1%; however, as many users (particularly adolescents) do not return on time for repeat injections, the typical use failure rate is 6%. A dose of 150 mg is administered intramuscularly or 104 mg administered subcutaneously every 12 weeks. Ovulation is suppressed for at least 14 weeks, allowing for a 2-week "grace period." Although ovulation *can* return as early as 14 weeks after the last injection, ovulation is suppressed for a median of 9–10 months after the last injection. The efficacy of DMPA has not been found to be reduced by high body weight or the use of concurrent medications (including hepatic enzyme inducers), likely secondary to the high circulating levels of progestin associated with DMPA use.

Counseling for DMPA should focus on potential side effects. The most common and important

Practical Pediatric and Adolescent Gynecology, First Edition. Edited by Paula J. Adams Hillard.
© 2013 John Wiley & Sons, Ltd. Published 2013 by John Wiley & Sons, Ltd.

✋ Advice for patients/parents

Bleeding changes with DMPA
- Occur in all women using DMPA
- In many users, bleeding is irregular and unpredictable, often lasting 7 days or longer during the first few months of use.
- With time, the frequency of abnormal bleeding decreases, and rates of amenorrhea are 50% at 1 year of use and 75% after 2 years of use (Figure 34.5.1).

Weight gain with DMPA
- Common, but not consistent for all users.
- Reported in up to half of all adolescent users.

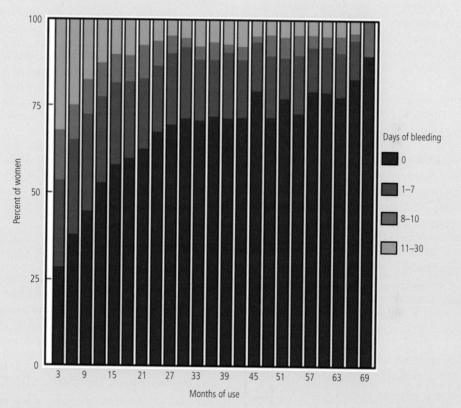

Figure 34.5.1 Percent of women and reported number of bleeding days with length of DMPA use. Based on Schwallie PC, Assenzo JR. Contraceptive use–efficacy study utilizing medroxyprogesterone acetate administered as an intramuscular injection once every 90 days. *Fertility and Sterility.* May 1973;24(5):331–339.

of these are bleeding abnormalities and weight changes. Up to one-quarter of women will discontinue DMPA within the first year of use due to bleeding irregularities; weight gain is also common reason for discontinuation.

DMPA's skeletal impact when used during adolescence, the time of accumulation of peak bone mass, has generated substantial attention and controversy.
• Due to its suppression of ovarian estrogen production, use of DMPA leads to reduction in bone mineral density (BMD) in current adolescent as well as adult users.
• Reassuringly, review of the available evidence in aggregate indicates that the decrease in BMD associated with current use of DMPA in adolescents is reversible after discontinuation of DMPA, with recovery to baseline BMD levels occurring in 1–2 years.
• Few studies have addressed fracture risk associated with use of DMPA, but none has definitely linked DMPA use with fractures either during or after use.
• Given the evidence, most authorities, including the Society for Adolescent Health and Medicine and the American College of Obstetricians and Gynecologists, agree that the advantages of using DMPA in adolescents for pregnancy prevention outweigh the risks of temporary BMD loss (Table 34.5.1).
• Both the WHO and the CDC Medical Eligibility Criteria rate DMPA in women aged 18–45 years as a category 1 method (no restriction of method use). In women aged younger than 18 or older than 45 years, DMPA is rated a category 2 (the advantages of the method generally outweigh the theoretical or proven risks).

The recommended timing of initiation for DMPA is given in Table 34.5.2.

Implantable contraception

The 3-year, single-rod contraceptive implant is widely available and provides highly effective, convenient birth control for adolescents. Multiple studies demonstrate high adolescent acceptability of the implant. Subdermal placement of the implant is readily accomplished in the office by clinicians who have completed the manufacturer-required training program. The

Table 34.5.1 Recommendations regarding DMPA use in adolescents

Society for Adolescent Health and Medicine
• "For the majority of adolescents, the benefits of DMPA outweigh potential risks. Continue prescribing DMPA to adolescent girls needing contraception with adequate explanation of benefits and potential risks".
• Recommend daily exercise and 1300 mg of and 400 IU of vitamin D to all adolescents receiving DMPA.

ACOG
• "Given the efficacy of DMPA, particularly for populations such as adolescents for whom contraceptive adherence can be challenging or for those who feel they could not comply with a daily method or a method that must be used with each act of intercourse, the possible adverse effects of DMPA must be balanced against the significant personal and public health impact of unintended pregnancy. Concerns regarding the effect of DMPA on BMD should neither prevent practitioners from prescribing DMPA nor limit its use to 2 consecutive years."
• "Practitioners should not perform BMD monitoring solely in response to DMPA use because any observed short-term loss in BMD associated with DMPA use may be recovered and is unlikely to place a woman at risk of fracture during use or in later years."

annual failure rate is less than 1%. The implant contains etonogestrel and suppresses ovulation for at least 30 months. The implant's efficacy is augmented by progestin-induced cervical mucus thickening. Return to fertility is rapid after implant removal.

Similar to other progestin-only only methods, the implant causes uterine bleeding changes. Bleeding or spotting can last for a few or many days. On average, the total number of bleeding days is less than that of women with ovulatory menses, but the schedule is irregular and unpredictable.

Progestin-only implants do not appear to adversely affect BMD. While implants cause ovulation suppression, they do not suppress ovarian estradiol production, and thus, in contrast to DMPA, do not produce a hypoestrogenic state in users.

The recommended timing of initiation for implant is given in Table 34.5.2.

Table 34.5.2 Recommended timing of injection of DMPA or insertion of progestin-only implant

Patient	Recommended timing of initiation of DMPA or implant
No hormonal contraception used in the past month	Days 1–5 of the menstrual cycle or exclude pregnancy Back-up method for 7 days after injection or insertion
Switching from a combination hormonal method	Anytime within 7 days of the last active dose (pill, patch, ring)
Switching from POP	Any day, do not skip any doses
Progestin-only implant or intrauterine device (IUD)	Same day as implant or IUD removal
Progestin-only injectable contraception	Same day as next injection would be due
First or second trimester abortion	Same day or within 5 days
Postpartum, including breastfeeding	Immediate
Any other time	Exclude pregnancy Back-up method for 7 days after injection or insertion

Use of progestin-only methods in postpartum adolescents

An especially high-risk group of adolescents are those who have given birth or experienced an induced or spontaneous abortion. Repeat pregnancy in adolescence is a serious public health problem that carries social, economic, and medical consequences. Because injectable and implantable contraception are long-acting and less likely to be used inconsistently or be discontinued as easily as daily or coital-dependent methods, promoting DMPA or implants for postpartum/postabortion contraception represents an effective approach to preventing repeat teen pregnancy.

Progestin-only methods do not impair lactation and represent appropriate choices for lactating women. While package labeling advises initiating these methods at 6 weeks postpartum, clinical experience with immediate postpartum initiation (regardless of lactation status) is reassuring and represents a sound approach to initiating injectable or implantable contraception in teens. CDC Medical Eligibility Criteria rate immediate postpartum initiation of DMPA or the implant category 1 in non-breastfeeding women and category 2 in breastfeeding women.

Evidence at a glance

- When initiated immediately or at 6 weeks postpartum, DMPA has not been shown to decrease the duration of lactation or infant weight gain.
- The use of the single-rod implant in postpartum women does not result in changes in milk volume, milk constituents, or infant growth rates.

Conclusion

Progestin-only contraceptive methods (pills, injectable, implant) are safe for most adolescents. Counseling should help candidates anticipate bleeding changes characteristically experienced by users. The efficacy and convenience of DMPA and the implant make them particularly attractive contraceptive choices for sexually-active adolescents.

Further reading

Isley MM, Kaunitz AM. Update on hormonal contraception and bone density. *Rev Endocr Metab Discord* 2011; 12:93–106.

Ornstein RM, Fisher MM. Hormonal contraception and adolescents. *Pediatr Drugs* 2006;8:25–45.

Tolaymat LL, Kaunitz AM. Long acting contraceptives in adolescents. *Curr Opin Obstet Gynecol* 2007;19:453–460.

34.6 Emergency contraception

Kaiyti Duffy[1] and Melanie A. Gold[2]

[1]University of Illinois at Chicago College of Medicine, Chicago, IL, USA
[2]Department of Pediatrics, Division of Adolescent Medicine, University of Pittsburgh School of Medicine, Pittsburgh, PA, USA

Emergency contraception (EC) offers young women a second chance to prevent pregnancy if a contraceptive was not used, or there was contraceptive failure or forced intercourse. Although a dedicated product for EC has been available commercially in the US for a decade, many adolescents still lack the knowledge and ability to access EC in a timely manner. Furthermore, few adolescent providers routinely discuss EC with their patients. By incorporating the strategies outlined in this chapter, providers can play a pivotal role in ensuring that young women obtain EC when they need it and have a chance to prevent unintended pregnancy.

When discussing sexual health with patients, providers should obtain a detailed sexual history, including number of partners, sexual behaviors, and condom and contraception use (see Appendices 1.11.1 and 1.11.2). If a young woman is interested in initiating contraception, providers provide counseling, taking into account cost, ease of use, side effects, noncontraceptive benefits, and confidentiality of the method (see Chapter 33.1). Within each conversation about contraception, providers are encouraged to introduce and discuss EC with both male and female patients. It can be beneficial to ask, "In the event that you use your method of contraception incorrectly or you forget to use it, what can you do to prevent pregnancy?" and/or "What have you heard about emergency contraception?" This allows the adolescent to demonstrate what he or she knows about emergency contraception and to discuss any myths he/she may have heard. The provider can then give more focused and tailored anticipatory guidance.

☝ Patient/parent advice

- EC is not appropriate for long-term contraception due to the fact that it is less effective, more costly, and associated with increased side effects.
- Therefore, patients are advised to use another method as everyday birth control.

Emergency contraception options

There are several pill products that can be used for EC. Providers should tell the adolescent which EC options are available to her and discuss the differences. The simplest to use are the dedicated products designed specifically as EC pills. These require administration of only one or two oral tablets. Plan B® was FDA approved for use as EC in 1999. Consisting of two doses of 0.75 mg of levonorgestrel (LNG) taken 12 hours apart, the method was replaced with generic (NextChoice®) and one-dose versions (Plan B One-Step®) in 2009. The most recently approved method

Practical Pediatric and Adolescent Gynecology, First Edition. Edited by Paula J. Adams Hillard.
© 2013 John Wiley & Sons, Ltd. Published 2013 by John Wiley & Sons, Ltd.

is a second-generation antiprogestin, ulipristal acetate (UPA). Marketed under the brand name ella™, this method was approved by the FDA in August 2010 and includes one single 30-mg oral dose of UPA.

In addition to these dedicated products, young women can use higher doses of certain regular combined estrogen–progestin or progestin-only oral contraceptive pills as EC (pills containing ethinyl estradiol and either norgestrel or LNG have been assessed for EC). This regimen is sometimes referred to as the Yuzpe regimen. The number of pills required to insure the correct dose of estrogen and/or progestin varies between brands. For more information, visit http://ec.princeton.edu. Because of their lower efficacy rates and worse side effect profile, these combination pill regimens are less commonly recommended for EC when dedicated products are available.

The copper intrauterine device can also be used for EC (see Chapter 34.4). However, young women must make an appointment for insertion within a 5-day window after unprotected intercourse and be able to pay for insertion. As such, this option is not as easily accessible as the dedicated products and will not be discussed further in this chapter.

Efficacy

All the dedicated products are safe and effective in preventing pregnancy when used correctly. Although exact efficacy rates are difficult to pinpoint, researchers estimate that the combined estrogen–progestin regimen prevents between 56% and 89% of pregnancies and the LNG-only methods prevent between 52% and 100% of pregnancies. The single-dose LNG-only regimen is as effective as the two-dose regimen. UPA has been shown to be highly efficacious with rates ranging from 62% to 85%.

The package labeling for LNG-only pills recommends initiating the regimen within 72 hours. Some studies have found LNG-only pills to be most effective the sooner they are taken after unprotected intercourse; however, research indicates reasonable effectiveness up to 120 hours after unprotected intercourse. In contrast, the efficacy of UPA remains constant up to 120 hours after unprotected intercourse and may be a better option, especially for young women seeking EC between 3 and 5 days after unprotected intercourse.

✋ Caution

- It is essential to counsel adolescent women that, in order to be effective, EC must be used with *every* act of unprotected intercourse.
- Taking EC once during a cycle does not protect a woman from pregnancy for the entire cycle.
- In fact, having additional acts of unprotected sexual intercourse a few days after EC use may increase a young woman's pregnancy risk due to the delay in ovulation.
- LNG-only EC can be used more than once during the cycle, but current UPA labeling states it should be limited to one dose per cycle.

Evidence at a glance

- Obtaining accurate efficacy rates for EC is difficult because these rates are based on an estimate of the number of pregnancies that would have occurred if no postcoital contraception was used.
- This estimate is influenced by many factors such as baseline fertility, number of acts of unprotected coitus during the cycle, and timing of intercourse relative to ovulation.
- A meta-analysis of studies comparing LNG to UPA concluded that the pregnancy rate was lower with UPA at all time points up to 120 hours.
- When taken within 24 hours, UPA users had a pregnancy rate 65% less than those using LNG up to 120 hours and 42% less than those using LNG within 72 hours after unprotected intercourse.

★ Tips and tricks

When explaining efficacy rates to adolescents, it is beneficial to be as concrete and clear as possible, e.g.: for every 100 women who have unprotected sex during the second week of the menstrual cycle, eight will get pregnant. If EC is used correctly, only one will get pregnant.

Safety

According to the U.S. Medical Eligibility Criteria for Contraceptive Use, there are no situations in which the risks of using LNG EC outweigh the benefits (UPA was not available at the time of evaluation but its safety was demonstrated in two Phase III clinical trials prior to FDA approval).

Side effects

The combined estrogen-progestin regimen is associated with significantly more side effects than the LNG-only method. UPA and LNG-only users experience similar side effects, including nausea and vomiting, abdominal pain, breast tenderness, headache, dizziness, and fatigue. Young women should be told that the discomfort usually passes within a day.

✋ Caution

If vomiting occurs within 2 hours of taking the medication, some providers recommend repeating the dose.

Women may also experience some menstrual irregularities following EC use. Research indicates that UPA appears to lengthen and the LNG-only method to shorten the cycle in which it is used. However, in both group, menses occurs within 7 days of the expected time in the majority of users.

Access

NextChoice® and Plan-B One-Step® are currently available to all women 17 years and older directly from the pharmacy without a prescription. Young women aged 16 years and under must have a prescription to obtain either drug, with the exception of nine states (Alaska, California, Hawaii, Maine, Massachusetts, New Hampshire, New Mexico, Vermont, and Washington State). A prescription is required for all women seeking ella™ regardless of age.

Facilitating correct use

During contraceptive counseling, it is beneficial to help young women to create a plan for what to do in the event of contraceptive failure. Specifically:
- Will she purchase the medication and keep it at home or wait until she needs it to get the prescription filled?

★ Tips and tricks

- Young women most often do not plan unprotected intercourse and therefore are unprepared when the need for EC arises.
- For young women under 17 years and/or those who prefer ella™, providers are advised by the major professional organizations concerned with the care of adolescents to offer and provide prescriptions in advance.
- Research indicates that young women who do receive advanced prescriptions are more likely to use EC and to use it sooner after unprotected intercourse.
- Providers can maintain a list of local pharmacies that supply EC and how much the products cost.

• Which pharmacy will she go to get her prescription filled?
• How sure is she that the pharmacy carries EC and has it in stock? This may be of particular concern with ella™.
• How will she obtain the money to purchase the prescription?

Cost

The cost of EC may pose an additional barrier to use by younger women. Though prices vary by location, Plan B One-Step and NextChoice® cost from $35 to $60 at pharmacies. ella™ may cost upwards of $55 at a pharmacy. It is possible to order ella™ from an online pharmacy, but this requires a credit card and a shipping fee. In addition to the cost of the pills, young women aged 16 years and under without advanced prescriptions may have to pay for a visit with a healthcare provider in order to obtain a prescription.

Follow-up

After using LNG-only EC or UPA, a back-up barrier method is recommended for women who then start hormonal contraception. Barriers should be used for 7 days following administration of LNG-only EC. It is unclear how long a barrier method should be used following administration of UPA. Current FDA labeling recommends that a barrier method be used with subsequent acts of intercourse that occur in that same menstrual cycle. A woman should return for a pregnancy test if her menses is 7 or more days late after using EC. For UPA users, women who "quick start" their contraceptive methods (started immediately after EC) should complete a pregnancy test at home or in the office 3 weeks after taking UPA.

Young women should also be offered testing for sexually-transmitted infections at the follow-up visit if not already done at the time of EC provision.

Conclusion

Emergency contraception is a safe and effective option for young women who have experienced a contraceptive failure. In addition to using combination oral contraceptive pills for EC, there are several designated products on the market. Young women may face issues in accessing the regimen within the recommended 120 hours. Therefore, providers should work with patients to educate them about the existence of EC and strategies for accessing the pills as quickly as possible after unprotected sexual intercourse.

Further reading

Glasier AF, Cameron ST, Fine PM, *et al.* Ulipristal acetate versus levonorgestrel for emergency contraception: a randomised noninferiority trial and metaanalysis. *Lancet* 2010;375:555–562.

Meyer JL, Gold MA, Haggerty CL. Advance provision of emergency contraception among adolescent and young adult women: a systematic review of literature. *J Pediatr Adolesc Gynecol* 2011;24:2–9.

Piaggio G, Kapp N, von Hertzen H. Effect on pregnancy rates of the delay in the administration of levonorgestrel for emergency contraception: a combined analysis of four WHO trials. *Contraception* 2011;84:35–39.

35 Hirsutism

Dianne Deplewski and Robert L. Rosenfield

The University of Chicago Pritzker School of Medicine, Section of Pediatric Endocrinology, Chicago, IL, USA

Hirsutism is defined as excessive sexual hair that appears in a male pattern in women. Approximately 5% of reproductive-age women in the general population are hirsute. Hirsutism is commonly graded according to the Ferriman–Gallwey system, which quantifies the extent of hair growth in the most androgen-sensitive areas (Figure 35.1). In adult women, a score of less than 8 is normal, 8–15 indicates mild hirsutism, and greater than 15 indicates moderate to severe hirsutism. This scoring system has limitations, mainly due to the subjective nature of the assessment, which is especially problematic when evaluating women who are blond or have had cosmetic treatment. It also does not include androgen-sensitive areas such as the sideburn, perineal, or buttock areas. Moreover, substantial hirsutism may exist in one or two areas without yielding an excessive score (focal hirsutism). In addition, the hirsutism score often does not correlate well with the androgen level. Approximately one-half of mildly hirsute women and one-sixth of moderate to severely hirsute women do not have hyperandrogenemia and thus are diagnosed with idiopathic hirsutism. Most women with a two-fold or greater elevation of androgen levels will have some degree of hirsutism. However, about one-third of women with hyperandrogenemia will have no skin manifestations, or may have seborrhea, acne, or alopecia without hirsutism. Hirsutism may be absent in young adolescents whose hyperandrogenism has not evolved fully.

Hirsutism must be distinguished from hypertrichosis, the generalized excess growth of hair distributed in a nonsexual pattern that does not result from hyperandrogenemia.

> ### ⬡ Science revisited
>
> - Sexual hair follicles and sebaceous glands both develop from the pilosebaceous unit (PSU) with growth dependent upon the presence of androgen.
> - Prior to puberty, hair is vellus (small, straight, and fair) and the sebaceous glands are small. In specific areas of the skin, terminal hairs (larger, curlier, and darker, hence more visible) develop upon exposure to increased levels of androgens at puberty.
> - In acne-prone areas of the body (e.g. the forehead and cheeks), the increased androgen levels dramatically increase the size of the sebaceous glands while the hair remains vellus.

Diagnosis

Hirsutism in over half of patients is due to hyperandrogenism (Table 35.1). Therefore, the history and examination should address risk factors for polycystic

Practical Pediatric and Adolescent Gynecology, First Edition. Edited by Paula J. Adams Hillard.
© 2013 John Wiley & Sons, Ltd. Published 2013 by John Wiley & Sons, Ltd.

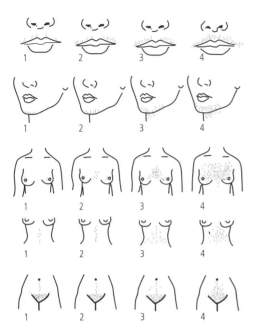

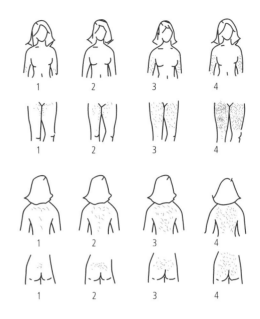

Figure 35.1 Ferriman–Gallwey hirsutism scoring system. Each of the nine body areas which is most sensitive to androgen is assigned a score from 0 (no hair) to 4 (frankly virile), and these are summed to provide a hormonal hirsutism score.

Reproduced with permission from Rosenfield RL. *Clin Endocrinol Metab.* 93:1105–1120. Copyright 2008, The Endocrine Society.

ovary syndrome (PCOS) or other endocrinopathy, virilizing disorders, and androgenic medications. Hirsutism usually develops after menarche in adolescent girls and is typically slowly progressive.

menstrual irregularity, mild hirsutism does not place patients at high risk for PCOS.

Other causes of hyperandrogenemia are infrequent. Nonclassic congenital adrenal hyperplasia is present

---

✋ **Caution**
Rapid progression of hirsutism or other signs of rapid virilization in a female of any age should raise concern for an androgen-secreting tumor.

Hyperandrogenism is most often caused by PCOS. Typical clinical features of PCOS include cutaneous signs of hyperandrogenism (hirsutism, acne, or pattern baldness), menstrual irregularity, obesity or polycystic ovaries (Chapter 50). In the presence of menstrual irregularity, even normal degrees of unwanted hair growth are usually associated with hyperandrogenemia. Conversely, in the absence of

★ **Tips and tricks**
• Hyperandrogenism should be considered in adolescent females who have inflammatory/cystic acne that appears before mid-puberty and is severe, persistent, or unresponsiveness to first-line dermatologic therapy.   • Androgenetic alopecia in girls may present as female-pattern baldness, typically affecting the crown, and manifesting early as a midline part widened in a "Christmas tree" pattern. A simple maneuver to determine scalp hair loss is the hair-pull test. Gentle traction is exerted on a group of 40–60 hairs. If more than 10 hairs are pulled out, the test is considered positive.

Table 35.1 Differential diagnosis of hirsutism in adolescents

Normal testosterone level
- Hypertrichosis:
  - Hereditary
  - Drug use:
    - Glucocorticoids
    - Phenytoins
    - Minoxidil
    - Diazoxide
    - Cyclosporine
- Idiopathic hirsutism
- Anabolic steroids

Elevated testosterone level
- Polycystic ovary syndrome
- Ovarian steroidogenic blocks
- Congenital adrenal hyperplasia:
  - Classic 21-hydroxylase deficiency
  - Nonclassic 21-hydroxylase deficiency
  - Deficiency in other adrenal enzymes necessary for cortisol biosynthesis
  - Sulfotransferase 2A deficiency
  - Cortisone reductase deficiency
- Other functional adrenal disorders:
  - Cushing syndrome
  - Cortisol resistance
- Hyperprolactinemia
- Growth hormone excess
- Insulin resistance syndromes
- Virilizing ovarian or adrenal tumor
- Thyroid dysfunction
- Drugs:
  - Testosterone
  - Valproic acid

The decision to test for hyperandrogenemia depends on how likely this abnormality is in the patient with hirsutism. Figure 35.2 illustrates a practical approach to the initial evaluation of hirsutism.

The key androgen to measure is serum (or plasma) testosterone as testosterone is the major circulating hormone that determines androgenization. However, there are many pitfalls in testosterone assays at the low levels found in women, and reliable testosterone assays are not available to many physicians.

⚛ Science revisited

Plasma free testosterone is the single most useful test to detect hyperandrogenemia when the clinical picture is discordant with the total testosterone level, since plasma free testosterone is 50% more sensitive than total testosterone in detecting hyperandrogenemia. This is because hirsute women commonly have a relatively low level of sex hormone-binding globulin (SHBG), which is the main determinant of the bioactive portion of plasma testosterone, the fraction that is free or "bioavailable" (which includes that loosely bound to albumin).

The automated testosterone assays that are used in most laboratories are generally not suitable to accurately measure female levels. Assays that yield norms substantially above 60 ng/dL are suspect.

Despite the potential advantages of assaying free testosterone, these assays are less well standardized. The most reliable free testosterone assays compute free testosterone from total testosterone and SHBG. Plasma total and free testosterone are best assessed in the early morning on days 4–10 of the menstrual cycle in regularly cycling women, the time for which norms are standardized.

The routine assay of other androgens is of little utility. Very high total testosterone (>200 ng/dL) or dehydroepiandrosterone sulfate (>700 μg/dL) heighten the risk of neoplasm, the latter indicating an adrenal source. However, women with androgenic tumors can also present with lesser elevations.

in only about 2.5% of hyperandrogenic women in the US. Androgen-secreting tumors are present in approximately 0.2% of hyperandrogenic women. Cushing syndrome, hyperprolactinemia, acromegaly, and thyroid dysfunction must be considered in the differential diagnosis of hyperandrogenism, but usually present because of their other manifestations. About 8% of women have mild, often asymptomatic, idiopathic hyperandrogenism. This may be due to abnormal peripheral metabolism of prohormones, the most common cause of which appears to be obesity. Valproic acid raises plasma testosterone.

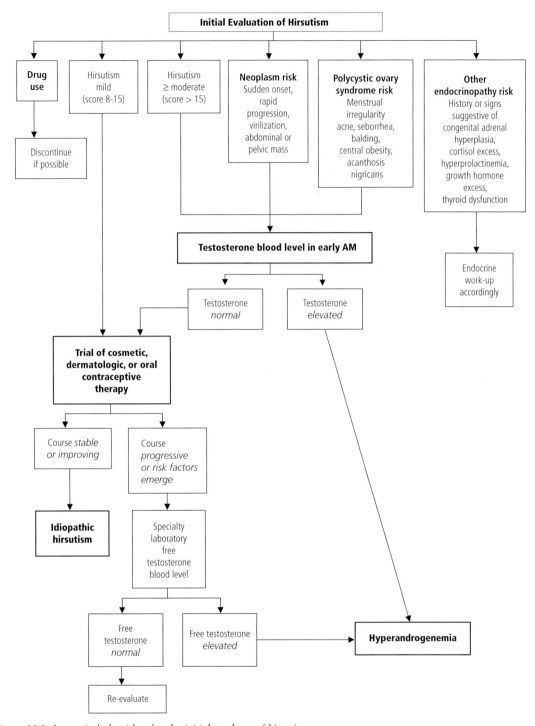

Figure 35.2 A practical algorithm for the initial work-up of hirsutism.
Reproduced with permission from Rosenfield RL. *UptoDate* 2011; as adapted, from Martin KA, Chang RJ, Ehrmann DA, Ibanez L, Lobo RA, Rosenfield RL, Shapiro J, Montori VM, Swiglo BA. Evaluation and treatment of hirsutism in premenopausal women: an endocrine society clinical practice guideline. *J Clin Endocrinol Metab.* 2008;93(4):1105–1120. The Endocrine Society.

> ### ⚛ Science revisited
>
> Testosterone arises as a by-product of ovarian and adrenal function, by either secretion or metabolism of prohormones (mainly androstenedione or dehydroepiandrosterone) in peripheral tissues, such as fat. Mid-follicular phase levels vary by about 25% around the mean, being highest in the early morning; levels are slightly lower in the perimenstrual phase of the cycle and slightly higher in mid-cycle.

> ### ✶ Tips and tricks
>
> Low SHBG levels are a clue to both testosterone excess and insulin-resistant hyperinsulinism.

> ### ✋ Caution
>
> Oral contraceptive pills normalize androgens in PCOS, and thus interfere with the assessment of androgens and diagnosis of PCOS.

Management

To many girls, unwanted hair affects quality of life. The degree of hirsutism bears no relationship to the distress it causes the patient. Some cannot tolerate a degree of superfluous hair growth that is within normal limits, while others are accepting of substantially abnormal degrees of sexual hair growth.

There are two main approaches to manage hirsutism, which may be used either individually or in combination:
• Direct methods to reduce and remove hair including cosmetic approaches, electrolysis and photoepilation (laser and intense pulse light)
• Pharmacologic therapies that target androgen production and action (Table 35.2).

Cosmetic and physical measures

Cosmetic measures are the cornerstone of care for hirsutism, but the cost of these treatments is not ordi-narily covered by health insurance programs. Simple, inexpensive cosmetic measures such as bleaching and shaving suffice for many with mild hirsutism. Depilating agents and waxing treatments are useful, but prone to cause skin irritation. Eflornithine hydro-chloride cream 13.9% (Vaniqa®) may be prescribed for the topical treatment of facial hirsutism (or off-label for focal hirsutism elsewhere), with a maximal effect by 8–24 weeks and marked improvement in 32% of patients.

For women who choose hair removal therapy, laser or photoepilation are generally preferable to electrolysis. Electrolysis involves inserting an electrode to destroy individual hair follicles, while laser devices damage hair follicles by combining relatively selective absorption of heat by dark hairs with penetration into the dermis. Light-skinned individuals are the best candidates, requiring the lower energy pulses. Those with heavily tanned or darker skin require the use of cooling procedures and adjustment of energy levels to minimize the risk of skin side effects. For women undergoing photoepilation therapy, adding eflornithine cream during treatment may yield a more rapid response. Laser treatment can cover a somewhat wider area with fewer side effects and less pain than electrolysis, temporarily reduces the need for simple cosmetic measures about four-fold for several months after a single session, and permanently reduces hair density by 30% or more with three to four treatments of a site. Both laser and electrolysis therapy require trained personnel, are repetitious, expensive, and painful, are practical only for treating limited areas, and may result in local reactions, including burns, dyspigmentation, and scarring.

Hormonal treatments

Hormonal therapies act by either suppressing androgen production or blocking the action of androgens within the skin. This causes hairs to revert toward the prepubertal vellus type. Assessments of efficacy are limited by their subjective nature, the paucity of randomized controlled trials, and the fact that treatment of hirsutism is an "off-label" use of these agents.

Pharmacotherapy is typically initiated with an estrogen- and progestin-containing oral contraceptive pill (OCP). OCPs reduce hyperandrogenism via several mechanisms including suppression of luteinizing hormone (LH) secretion (and therefore ovarian

Drug type	Active ingredient	Examples	Major mechanism	Indication	Dosage	Contraindications	Major side effects
Cell cycle inhibitor	Eflornithine HCl 13.9%	Vaniqa®	Irreversible inhibitor of ornithine decarboxylase	Focal hirsutism	Topical BID	Pregnancy, nursing	Rash, potential systemic toxicity with widespread application
Oral contraceptive pills	Ethinyl estradiol 30 µg + drospirenone; Ethinyl estradiol 35 µg + norgestimate; Ethinyl estradiol 50 µg + ethynodiol diacetate	Yasmin®; Ortho Cyclen®; Demulen® 1/50; Zovia® 1/50	Suppress ovarian function	Generalized hirsutism	1 tablet daily	Venous thrombosis, uncontrolled hypertension	Irregular menstrual bleeding, venous thrombosis
Antiandrogens	Spironolactone	Spironolactone	Competitive inhibitor of androgen-receptor binding	Severe hirsutism	50–100 mg BID PO	Lack of contraception, kidney or liver failure	Undervirilized male fetus, irregular menstrual bleeding unless oral contraceptive administered, nausea, hyperkalemia, hypotension, liver dysfunction
	Cyproterone acetate	Cyproterone acetate	Competitive inhibitor of androgen-receptor binding	Severe hirsutism	Initial: 50–100 mg daily on menstrual cycle days 5–15; Maintenance: 5 mg daily on menstrual days 5–15	Lack of contraception	Undervirilized male fetus, irregular menstrual bleeding unless oral contraceptive administered, nausea
	Ethinyl estradiol 35 µg + cyproterone acetate 2 mg	Diane®	Competitive inhibitor of androgen-receptor binding	Severe hirsutism	1 tablet daily	Venous thrombosis, uncontrolled hypertension	Irregular menstrual bleeding, venous thrombosis
	Flutamide	Flutamide	Nonsteroidal competitive inhibitor of androgen-receptor binding	Severe hirsutism	125–250 mg BID PO	Lack of contraception, liver disease	Undervirilized male fetus, liver dysfunction
	Finasteride	Finasteride	Competitive 5α-reductase inhibitor	Severe hirsutism	2.5–5 mg daily	Lack of contraception	Undervirilized male fetus
Glucocorticoids	Glucocorticoid	Prednisone	Suppresses adrenal function	Congenital adrenal hyperplasia	5–7.5 mg HS PO	Uncontrolled diabetes, obesity	Cushingoid changes, adrenal atrophy
Gonadotropin-releasing agonists	Leuprolide acetate depot	Depot Lupron®	Suppress gonadotropins	Oral contraceptive alternative	7.5 mg monthly with 25–50 µg transdermal estradiol	Osteoporosis	Osteoporosis

androgen secretion), stimulation of hepatic production of SHBG (thereby increasing the fraction of androgen bound in serum and rendering it biologically unavailable), a slight reduction in adrenal androgen secretion, and a slight blockage in the binding of androgens to their receptor. Although there is no evidence from controlled studies that the type of progestin makes a difference in outcome of hirsutism, the response of acne may be slightly affected. We favor the use of OCPs that contain a progestin with low androgenicity (e.g. norgestimate, desogestrel, ethynodiol diacetate) or an antiandrogenic progestin (e.g. drospirenone or cyproterone acetate) because of the relatively healthy metabolic biochemical profile that they yield. OCPs should be used in conjunction with cosmetic measures.

If hirsutism is severe or remains bothersome despite 6 or more months of monotherapy with an OCP, we suggest adding an antiandrogen. Spironolactone is an aldosterone antagonist that exhibits dose-dependent competitive inhibition of the androgen receptor as well as inhibition of 5α-reductase activity. Spironolactone is the most widely used antiandrogen in the US, with the maximum effect at 9–12 months, although there is considerable variation among individuals. Spironolactone should not be used without some form of contraception as it may cause decreased virilization in a male fetus. We advise against the use of the antiandrogen flutamide because of its potential hepatocellular toxicity.

The 5α-reductase inhibitor finasteride can be considered as an alternative to antiandrogens. Gonadotropin-releasing hormone agonist treatment with estradiol add-back is reasonable only for the rare women with a suboptimal response to the above therapies or sensitivity to the steroid doses in OCPs. There is little evidence to support a clinically significant improvement in hirsutism with the use of insulin sensitizers such as metformin or thiazolidinediones.

When to refer and to whom

If girls with hirsutism have hyperandrogenemia and clinical features suggesting a cause other than PCOS, referral to an endocrinologist is suggested.

✋ Patient/parent advice

- Many women will have some degree of sexual hair growth in a male pattern.
- Hormonal therapy requires about 9 months for the maximal effect to be seen.
- If hirsutism worsens, or other signs of virilization occur, further work-up should be pursued.

Further reading

Martin KA, Chang RJ, Ehrmann DA, *et al*. Evaluation and treatment of hirsutism in premenopausal women: An Endocrine Society clinical practice guideline. *J Clin Endocrinol Metab* 2008;93(4):1105–1120.

Rosenfield RL. Hirsutism. *N Engl J Med* 2005;353(24): 2578–2588.

Rosenfield RL. What every physician should know about polycystic ovary syndrome. *Dermatol Ther* 2008;21:354–361.

36 The breast

36.1 Breast concerns

Kaylene J. Logan and Eduardo Lara-Torre

Department of Obstetrics and Gynecology, Virginia Tech-Carilion School of Medicine, Roanoke, VA, USA

Between the ages of 7 and 13 years, female hormones will stimulate the development of breasts (thelarche). In African-American females, the average age of thelarche is 8.3 years; whereas in white females, it is 10.3 years. Estrogen stimulates the growth of fatty (adipose) tissue and lactiferous ducts, while progesterone stimulates the growth of lobules and alveoli. Menarche usually follows within 2 years after the onset of thelarche (see Figure 14.2 and Table 36.1.1).

Abnormalities in development of the adolescent breast

Thelarche is considered delayed if it has not begun by age 13 years and, classically, premature if before the age of 8 years (see Chapters 15 and 16). Breast development between the ages of 6 and 8 is common, and may not be pathologic. In addition, there can be abnormalities in the size, shape, location, and number of breasts (Table 36.1.2).

There is a spectrum of breast asymmetry, with some degree of normal asymmetry in all females. Mild asymmetry may be more pronounced in puberty as the breasts develop, especially if one breast bud appears before the other.

⚗ Science revisited

- In the fetus, breast tissue begins to form at 4 weeks' gestation. Two thickened ridges, known as the milk line, form from ectoderm, and extend initially from the axilla to the inguinal canal.
- Most of this tissue recedes, leaving only the thoracic component at the sites the breasts will develop.
- Between 10 and 20 weeks' gestation, the lactiferous ducts develop, and at 8 months, the nipple appears.
- Also in the third trimester, the mother's estrogen promotes canalization of the ducts.
- At birth, male and female breasts are indistinguishable.

☝ Patient/parent advice

- Breast asymmetry usually equilibrates, and requires reassurance only.
- Asymmetry may be due to a mass, cyst, abscess, or trauma, and the patient should always be evaluated if there is a concern.
- Developmental asymmetry may be conservatively managed with breast pads or prostheses, padded bras, or with surgical augmentation or reduction in an appropriate patient who has completed breast development.

Practical Pediatric and Adolescent Gynecology, First Edition. Edited by Paula J. Adams Hillard.
© 2013 John Wiley & Sons, Ltd. Published 2013 by John Wiley & Sons, Ltd.

Breast masses

Benign breast masses

The most common of all adolescent breast masses is the fibroadenoma. These are benign masses that average 2–3 cm in size, usually present as a single, round, painless mass, and are more common in African-American females and in late adolescence. Fibroadenomas may slightly enlarge during menses, showing most rapid growth in the first 6–12 months, then a growth plateau, and even regression 10% of the time. The diagnosis can be made by physical

> **✋ Caution**
>
> • Do not biopsy breast masses in a child or adolescent; the normal breast bud may be damaged or removed in the biopsy. Use ultrasound or fine needle aspiration (FNA) to aid in diagnosis if required.
> • Risks of breast surgery include infection, scars, and potential difficulty with breastfeeding. Appropriate candidates must give fully informed consent and surgery delayed until breast development is complete to prevent the need for re-operation.

Table 36.1.1 Tanner staging of breast development (see Figure 14.2)

1 Preadolescent stage; nipple elevation only
2 Breast bud stage; elevation of breast and nipple as small mound, with enlargement of areola diameter
3 Further enlargement of breast and areola; increased pigmentation of areola
4 Further areola enlargement and pigmentation; nipple and areola form secondary mound above level of breast
5 Mature stage; smooth contour; projection of nipple only with recession of areola to level of breast

> **✋ Caution**
>
> When evaluating breast masses in adolescents, the use of ultrasound, not mammography, is the imaging modality of choice. The high density of the breast during adolescence makes mammography a poor technique and it should be avoided.

Table 36.1.2 Developmental abnormalities

Abnormality	Etiology/comments	Tips for management
Amastia (complete absence) Hypomastia (underdevelopment of breast)	Complete involution of milk line Poland syndrome Malnutrition Crohn disease Trauma to breast bud Endocrine disorders	Surgical augmentation
Polymastia (accessory breast tissue) Polythelia [accessory nipple(s)]	Failure of milk line to recede Located anywhere along milk line, most commonly axilla or below normal breasts May enlarge during pregnancy and lactation	Usually asymptomatic; may be surgically removed if painful or causes discharge
Breast hypertrophy (macromastia, uncontrollable enlargement)	One or both breasts is excessively sensitive to estrogen May cause difficulty for adolescents socially or with participation in sports, as well as chronic back and neck pain	Observation Supportive garments Surgical reduction
Tuberous (or tubular) breasts (stalk-like breasts form when base of breast is underdeveloped and nipple–areola complex enlarged)	Exogenous hormones used to induce secondary sex characteristics Gonadal dysgenesis	Plastic surgery reconstruction and augmentation

exam, in which the mass may feel firm or rubbery, well-circumscribed, mobile, and be located in the upper outer quadrants. Management in most cases requires reassurance and observation. If the mass is persistent for years, even into adulthood, rapidly growing, or the diagnosis is uncertain, FNA or excisional biopsy is indicated.

Giant fibroadenomas are rare and tend to occur in slightly younger populations. They typically grow larger than 5 cm and may have a softer texture on exam, often mistaken for normal breast tissue. Dilated veins may also be seen on the surface of the breast. Often these require early excision to avoid significant asymmetry or deformity. A preoperative FNA is recommended to rule out a phyllodes tumor.

Mastalgia refers to breast pain that may be cyclic or noncyclic in nature. A common cause of adolescent mastalgia is fibrocystic changes, characterized by diffuse thickenings and lumps that demonstrate cyclic tenderness and enlargement. Ninety percent of all women will develop fibrocystic changes in their lifetime; however, only 50% may have clinical signs or symptoms. The character of fibrocystic changes may evolve over months, and serial observation is appropriate. Noncyclic mastalgia may be seen in early pregnancy, with initiation of combined oral contraceptive pills (OCPs), or with physical or emotional abuse. Nonbreast causes may include chostochondritis, rib fractures, and cervical radiculopathy. Treatment modalities are listed in Table 36.1.3.

Juvenile papillomatosis is a benign mass, usually unilateral and painless, comprised of multiple cystically dilated ducts and varying degrees of intraductal proliferation. This mass is significant because it may be a marker for increased risk of breast cancer. Treatment involves total resection, preserving as much normal breast tissue as possible.

✋ Patient/parent advice

- A poor fitting support garment is a common cause of mastalgia.
- Proper fitting by a store specialist can assist and resolve many cases of painful breasts, and teens should be encouraged to get fitted often, as their breasts change significantly throughout adolescence and early adulthood.

Table 36.1.3 Treatment of mastalgia

- Comfortable supportive bra; sports bra for athletics
- Acetaminophen, NSAIDs (oral or topical)
- Low-dose combined oral contraceptive (20 μg ethinyl estradiol) or lowering the dose if already on them
- 3-month trial of caffeine elimination: coffee, tea, soda, chocolate; smoking cessation, weight loss, and relaxation techniques
- Refractory cases (off-label use): danazol, toromifene, cabergoline, and bromocriptine

---

Montgomery's tubercles are small, projections at the edge of the areola, related to the glands of Montgomery. When these glands become obstructed, they can cause local inflammation and a mass. Associated symptoms include tenderness, swelling, and erythema. When compressed, the cyst may release a brownish discharge. Ultrasound can confirm the diagnosis. Treatment involves antibiotics and nonsteroidal anti-inflammatory drugs (NSAIDs) for a week, followed by observation and serial exams. Resection is indicated if the cyst does not spontaneously resolve in 2 years.

Other benign breast masses that require excision include hamartomas, adenomas, and erosive adenomatosis. Erosive adenomatosis may present with erythema, erosion, and crusting of the nipple. Breast trauma such as seatbelt injuries or a direct blow to the breast may also lead to fat necrosis, presenting as a solid mass. Mondor disease is a superficial thrombophlebitis with a palpable and visible fibrous cord which may result from trauma.

Malignant masses

Malignant breast masses are rare in the adolescent, but deserve attention due to their serious nature (Table 36.1.4). Metastatic disease to the breast (such as lymphoma) is the most common cause of breast cancer in adolescents. Primary breast cancer is extremely rare in this age group with only a few cases reported since the late 1800s. Risk factors for malignancy include prior chemotherapy or radiation therapy.

Reviewing pertinent symptoms, previous diagnoses, and surgical procedures, as well as determining the patient's and family's anxiety level should be the

Table 36.1.4 Malignant masses

	Presentation	Treatment
Phyllodes tumor (benign or malignant)	Large, painless, rapidly-growing, multilobular, mobile mass	Wide local excision with 2 cm margin and close follow-up
Carcinoma	Long-standing lump with or without pain, usually without nipple discharge	Excisional biopsy versus simple mastectomy, with or without adjuvant therapy

Table 36.1.5 Nipple discharge

Appearance	Differential diagnosis	Management
Purulent	Infection	Culture and antibiotics
Bloody	Mammary duct ectasia Chronic cystic mastitis Intraductal cysts Intraductal papillomas Chronic nipple irritation Cold trauma	Culture and cytology Antibiotics if appropriate
Sticky green/ brown	Mammary duct ectasia	Culture and antibiotics

initial steps in evaluating a breast mass. Ultrasound remains the primary imaging modality if malignancy is suspected. Persistent cystic masses may require FNA; if clear, the fluid may be discarded, but if bloody, cytologic analysis is required. A solid, non-mobile, enlarging mass should undergo biopsy or excision, sparing the areola when possible.

The counseling related to family history of *BRCA 1* and *2* mutations is still in evolution and is beyond the scope of this chapter.

Other breast conditions

Nipple discharge may be endocrine-related (galactorrhea; (see Chapter 36.2) or nonendocrine. Characteristics of nipple discharge and associated conditions are listed in Table 36.1.5 (see also Chapter 36.2).

Mammary duct ectasia is a benign dilation of the subareolar ducts, caused by obstruction, infection, abscess, or chronic inflammation. If the fluid is dark, the breast may appear blue over the mass. These fluid collections usually resolve spontaneously.

Intraductal papillomas are subareolar lesions caused by abnormal proliferations of mammary duct epithelium projected into a dilated lumen and may cause a bloody discharge. They are bilateral 25% of the time, and are treated by local excision, sparing the areola.

Nipple piercing is becoming increasingly common, whether as a personal statement, for fashion or acceptance, to boost self-esteem, or as a rite of passage. Nipple piercing may be a sign of high-risk behaviors,

Table 36.1.6 Etiology and treatment of breast infections

	Etiology	Treatment
Mastitis	Usually related to lactation Staph or strep enter through cracks in the nipples	Antibiotics, analgesics, breast support, continued breast feeding
Abscess	Periareolar shaving Hair plucking Nipple piercings Epidermal inclusion cysts	In addition to above, small abscesses may require needle aspiration; large abscesses may require incision and drainage

and should prompt immunization against tetanus and hepatitis B, and screening for other risk behaviors that could lead to HIV and hepatitis B and C. Patients with a strong family history of diabetes may benefit from screening to prevent complications associated with infection, if it were to occur. Other risks of piercing include bleeding, pain, abscess, hematoma or cyst formation, allergic reactions, and keloid formation. If infection develops, management includes good hygiene and warm compresses, keeping the piercing in or using a sterile replacement until the infection resolves. Antibiotics or incision and drainage may be required (Table 36.1.6).

✮ Tips and tricks

• The need for self and clinical breast examination in teens is currently a topic of debate. Given the low risk of malignancy in this age group and the unnecessary anxiety to patients and their parents of finding benign conditions of the breast, the time may be better spent counseling on more common risks of this age group such as sexuality.

• Creating breast self-awareness as the teens become young adults should be encouraged as part of their transition into their mid 20s.

Further reading

De Silva NK, Brandt ML. Breast disorders in children and adolescents. In: Sanfilippo J, Lara-Torre E, Edmonds K, Templeman C (eds). *Clinical Pediatric and Adolescent Gynecology*. New York: Informa Healthcare, 2009, pp. 195–211.

Laufer MR, Goldstein DP. The breast: Examination and lesions. In: Emans SJ, Laufer MR, Goldstein DP (eds). *Pediatric and Adolescent Gynecology*, 5th edn. Philadelphia: Lipincott Williams & Wilkins, 2005, pp. 729–759.

Wiebke EA, Niederhuber JE, Glasser GA. Breast diseases: benign and malignant. In: Carpenter SK, Rock JA (eds). *Pediatric and Adolescent Gynecology*, 2nd edn. Philadelphia: Lipincott Williams & Wilkins, 2000, pp. 463–487.

36.2   Breast discharge

Donald E. Greydanus[1] and Colleen Bryzik Dodich[2]

[1]Western Michigan University School of Medicine, Kalamazoo, MI, USA
[2]Oakland University-William Beaumont School of Medicine and Beverly Hills Pediatrics, Bingham Farms, MI, USA

Breast discharge can be due to nipple discharge or galactorrhea.

Nipple discharge

A number of factors and disorders can be etiologically linked with nipple discharge in the adolescent female (Table 36.2.1). The medical history considers any history of trauma (including self-manipulation, shaving or plucking), breast disorders, and/or menstrual dysfunction. Colored sweat secretion by peri-areolar apocrine glands defines apocrine chromhidrosis. You should ask about the color and amount of the discharge, as well as if it is unilateral or bilateral, while performing a careful breast examination that includes the nipple. Surgery may be necessary to remove a breast lesion such as an offending breast duct.

The Montgomery glands on the areola may secrete a clear to brownish discharge that can evolve over a period of weeks to months and may be associated with small subareolar lumps. This discharge is usually self-limited with no treatment needed; however, these glands can become blocked and infected, leading to the formation of an abscess. Infection is usually associated with lactation, but can also occur with breast manipulation, and is accompanied by breast swelling, erythema, and tenderness.

Treatment for breast abscess includes warm compresses and antibiotics to cover *Staphylococcus* and

> ### ⚗ Science revisited
>
> • The most common infectious organism in a breast abscess is *Staphylococcus aureus*, although other microbes have been implicated, including *Streptococcus pyogenes*.
> • Hyperprolactinemia can be due to a benign macroprolactinemia with increased amounts of oversized prolactin molecules that are immunologically, but not biologically, active.

Streptococcus species. If the infection is extensive and unresponsive to initial treatment or if a cyst persists, then incision and drainage may be necessary.

Galactorrhea

Galactorrhea is the secretion of breast milk not related to childbirth or abortion. The discharge can be clear, green, yellow, or white (milky). It can range from scant to copious. Most causes are either idiopathic (benign galactorrhea due to end-organ hypersensitivity to normal levels of prolactin), pharmacologic or such factors as hypothyroidism (rarely hyperthyroidism), suckling, self-manipulation, or pituitary prolactinoma (Table 36.2.2).

Practical Pediatric and Adolescent Gynecology, First Edition. Edited by Paula J. Adams Hillard.
© 2013 John Wiley & Sons, Ltd. Published 2013 by John Wiley & Sons, Ltd.

Table 36.2.1 Causes of nipple discharge

- Milky discharge:
  - Lactation
  - Breast cancer
  - Phenothiazine
  - Pituitary microadenoma
  - Elevated thyroid-stimulating hormone (hypothyroidism)
  - Acromegaly
- Yellow discharge:
  - Galactocele
  - Physiologic effects
- Serous, clear or greenish discharge: physiologic breast cyst
- Bloody discharge:
  - Cystic ductal hyperplasia
  - Intraductal papilloma
  - Cystosarcoma phyllodes
  - Papillary carcinoma
- Brownish discharge:
  - Montgomery's gland secretion
  - Intraductal papilloma
- Purulent discharge: mastitis or breast abscess

Reprinted from: Nova Science Publishers, Inc., *Pediatric and Adolescent Sexuality and Gynecology*, 306–7, 2010, Hatim A. Omar, Donald E. Greydanus, Artemis K. Tsitsika and Dilip R. Patel, with permission from Nova Science Publishers, Inc.

★ Tips and tricks

Sudan stain is helpful in revealing the presence or absence of fat globules to confirm galactorrhea.

✋ Caution

The pregnancy-induced increase in prolactin levels can be prolonged after miscarriage, abortion, or even delivery without nursing.

The medical history should look for headaches, visual disturbances (e.g. visual field loss due to optic chiasm compression), and menstrual dysfunction. A drug history is important. For example, use of an oral contraceptive may cause galactorrhea. You should be suspicious of dopamine receptor blockers (e.g. phe-

Table 36.2.2 Causes of galactorrhea

- Pregnancy, lactation
- Stress
- Exercise
- Recent pregnancy terminated by spontaneous or induced abortion
- Neurogenic:
  - Chest wall disorders:
    - Bronchiectasis and chronic bronchitis
    - Herpes zoster
    - Chronic crutch use
    - Thoracotomy or thoracoplasty
    - Burns to chest wall
    - Breast (nipple) manipulation or stimulation (sexual foreplay)
    - Chronic inflammatory disease or abscess of the breast
  - Psychogenic, including pseudocyesis and pseudonursing
  - Miscellaneous:
    - Hysterectomy or uterine tumors
    - Laparotomy
    - Spinal cord disorders and surgery
    - Idiopathic normoprolactinemia, with or without amenorrhea
- Central nervous system abnormalities:
  - Diffuse brain disease:
    - Coma
    - Pseudotumor cerebri
    - Encephalitis and sequelae
    - Uremia
  - Tumors, infiltrations, structural abnormalities:
    - Neurocutaneous syndromes
    - Craniopharyngioma
    - Pineal tumors
    - Other intracranial tumors, cysts, and masses
    - Histiocytosis X
    - Sarcoidosis
  - Pituitary:
    - Stalk section
    - Empty sella syndrome
    - Pituitary infarction and Sheehan syndrome
    - Hyperprolactinemia with or without prolactinoma
    - Other functional pituitary tumors
- Miscellaneous:
  - Hypothyroidism and hyperthyroidism
  - Hypogonadism
  - Adrenal tumors and hypernephromas
  - Nelson syndrome

(Continued)

Table 36.2.2 (Continued)

- ○ Testicular and ovarian tumors
- ○ Polycystic ovary syndrome (PCOS)
- ○ Starvation or re-feeding (including anorexia nervosa)
- ○ Cushing disease
- ○ Chronic renal disease
- ○ Cirrhosis
- ○ Acute intermittent porphyria
- ○ Oral contraceptive pills
- ○ Monoamine oxidase inhibitors
- ○ Amphetamines
- ○ Chlordiazepoxide
- ○ Meprobamate
- ○ Metoclopramide
- ○ Bromocriptine withdrawal
- ○ Cimetidine and ranitidine
- ○ Tamoxifen
- ○ Verapamil
- ○ Isoniazid
- ○ Estrogens
- ○ Opiates (including codeine and heroin)
- ○ Phenothiazines, thioxanthenes, other psychotropic drugs
- ○ Tricyclic antidepressants
- ○ Other chemotherapy drugs (cisplatin, cytosine arabinoside, adriamycin)
- ○ Others

Reproduced from Greydanus DE. Breast and gynecological disorders. In: Hofmann AD, Greydanus DE (eds). *Adolescent Medicine*, 3rd edn. Stamford, CT: Appleton Lange, 1997, p. 531, with permission from Elsevier.

nothiazines, butryophenones, or tricyclic antidepressants), lactotroph stimulators (e.g. verapamil, opiates, or high-dose estrogens), dopamine depletors (e.g. cocaine), or gastrointestinal dopamine antagonists (e.g. metoclopramide). Any relationship to heavy marijuana use remains anecdotal and controversial. Evaluate for conditions listed in Table 36.2.2. The hyperprolactinemia is usually less than 1750 mU/L in hypothyroidism or polycystic ovary syndrome (PCOS).

The evaluation can include a cytologic analysis of the discharge fluid, a thyroid screen and serum prolactin, as well as gonadotropins; you should consider a head MRI or CT. Management is based on the underlying etiology. For example, thyroid dysfunction should be corrected or a pituitary adenoma should be treated pharmacologically (e.g. dopamine agonists such as bromocriptine) or, if necessary, surgically. If there is an offending drug, stop it if possible and use an alternative medication that does not induce hyperprolactinemia.

✋ **Patient/parent advice**

Avoid any breast manipulation, as frequent checks to see if the discharge is still present may exacerbate the problem.

Further reading

Greydanus DE, Matytsina LA, Gains M. Breast disorders in children and adolescents. *Prim Care* 2006;33(2):455–502.

Greydanus DE, Tsitsika AK, Gains MJ. The gynecology system and the adolescent. In: Greydanus DE, Feinberg AN, Patel DR, Homnick DN (eds). *The Pediatric Diagnostic Examination*. New York: McGraw-Hill Medical Publishers, 2008, pp. 701–749.

Prabhakar VK, Davis JR. Hyperprolactinemia. *Best Pract Res Clin Obstet Gynaecol* 2008;22(2): 341–353.

37 Vaginal discharge

Seema Menon, Mandakini Sadhir, and Susan Jay

Medical College of Wisconsin, Children's Hospital of Wisconsin, Milwaukee, WI, USA

Adolescents often seek medical care secondary to vaginal discharge. While infectious etiologies should be the immediate focus, there are several noninfectious causes of vaginal discharge in this population. Diagnosis typically requires a thorough history, focused physical exam, and laboratory testing.

Physiologic vaginal discharge

Vaginal and cervical secretions increase 6–12 months prior to menarche. This discharge is comprised of mucoid endocervical secretions, sloughed epithelial cells, normal bacterial flora, and vaginal transudate. Physiologic discharge is hormone dependent and fluctuates with the menstrual cycle. Patients typically present secondary to the discharge, but deny pruritus or discomfort. Physical exam is notable for a lack of vulvar or vaginal erythema. The discharge itself is clear to white in color, has no offensive odor, and has a pH of less than 4.5. Abundant leukocytes and few polymorph nuclear leukocytes are seen on saline microscopy (Figure 37.1A). Patients should be reassured that this is a normal finding.

Differential diagnosis and management

Vaginitis

Vulvovaginal candidiasis (VVC), bacterial vaginosis (BV), and trichomoniasis are the three most common causes of vaginitis (Table 37.1).

VVC is one of the most common female genital tract infections (see Chapter 43.1). The causative organism is typically *Candida albicans*. Risk factors for VVC include immune suppression, antibiotics, and wearing tight-fitting garments. Thick discharge, vaginal and vulvar pain, swelling, pruritus, dyspareunia, and external dysuria are common presenting complaints.

BV is the most common cause of malodourous vaginal discharge in adolescents (see Chapter 43.2). This condition is polymicrobial and caused by a reduction of *Lactobacillus* species and overpopulation of normal vaginal flora such as *Gardnerella vaginalis*. The mechanism leading to alteration of vaginal flora is poorly understood. The condition is described as a *vaginosis* and not a *vaginitis*, as there is little or no inflammation. Risk factors include intercourse and use of feminine hygiene products. Patients with BV typically present with malodorous ("fishy") vaginal discharge, without pain or irritation.

Unlike VVC and BV, trichomoniasis is a sexually-transmitted infection (STI) caused by the flagellated protozoan, *Trichomonas vaginalis*. This organism can survive outside the body for a limited amount of time; therefore, nonsexual transmission is theoretically possible. No risk factors for this infection have been determined other than sexual activity. The common presentation of trichomoniasis is profuse vaginal discharge. Inflammation and erythema may be notable.

Microscopy is most commonly used to establish a diagnosis (Figure 37.1). When microscopy is indeterminate or unavailable, other laboratory tests are

Practical Pediatric and Adolescent Gynecology, First Edition. Edited by Paula J. Adams Hillard.
© 2013 John Wiley & Sons, Ltd. Published 2013 by John Wiley & Sons, Ltd.

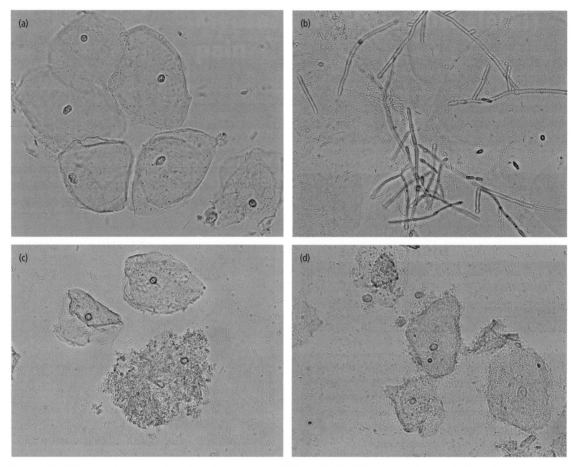

Figure 37.1 Microscopic examination of vaginal samples. (a) Normal cells; (b) pseudohyphae; (c,d) clue cells.

available. Amsel's criteria have been developed to improve the specificity of diagnosing BV and are listed in Table 43.2.2.

Culture may be performed to diagnose trichomonas and VVC. Culture is not helpful in BV diagnosis as this is a polymicrobial infection; Gram stain is the gold standard diagnostic test. Multiple molecular tests are available for the diagnosis of trichomonas and BV. These tests offer a higher sensitivity than microscopy when diagnosing trichomonas, and a comparable sensitivity to Amsel's criteria when diagnosing BV.

Specific CDC recommended treatment regimens are addressed in Chapters 43.1 and 43.2. Treatment of these infections leads to resolution of bothersome symptoms. In addition, both BV and trichomonas have been associated with increased acquisition of human immunodeficiency virus (HIV), highlighting another important reason for treatment. If a complicated VVC infection is suspected, a longer treatment course is recommended. If a non-*Candida albicans* VVC occurs, a non-fluconazole agent should be used.

Cervicitis

Chlamydia trachomatis
Chlamydia trachomatis is the most commonly reported sexually-transmitted disease (STD; see

Table 37.1 Diagnosis and treatment of common causes of vaginosis

	Vulvovaginal candidiasis	Bacterial vaginosis	Trichomonas
Physical exam findings of the external genitalia	Labial and vaginal edema Labial and vaginal erythema Perineal excoriations Satellite lesions of the intertriginous groin region	No signs of vulvitis or vaginitis	Mild vaginal inflammation Cervical punctuation/ petechiae ("strawberry" cervix) is rare
Gross appearance of discharge	Lack of offensive odor Thick, curd like, "cottage cheese" Milky white in color Adherent to vaginal walls	Thin Gray in color Homogenous Malodorous ("fishy")	Copious Frothy Profuse Watery Green or yellow, occasionally white or grey
Microscopy findings	Hyphae and pseudohyphae (Figure 37.1B) with saline and 10% KOH solution pH >4.5	Clue cells (Figure 37.1C,D) Malodor with addition of 10% KOH solution (+ whiff test)	Motile trichomonads with addition of saline Malodor may be detected with addition of 10% KOH
Treatment	Clotrimazole 2% cream 5 g intravaginally for 3 days or Clotrimazole 1% cream 5 g intravaginally for 7–14 days or Fluconazole 150-mg oral tablet, one tablet in single dose	Metronidazole 500 mg orally twice a day for 7 days* or Metronidazole gel 0.75%, one full applicator (5 g) intravaginally, once a day for 5 days	Metronidazole 2 g orally in a single dose or Tinidazole 2 g orally in a single dose

*Alternative regimens are available on the CDC website (www.cdc.gov); see also Table 43.2.3.

Chapter 44.3). Prevalence is highest in young females. Many chlamydial cervicitis infections are asymptomatic, but bothersome discharge may be noted. Physical exam findings vary from a normal appearing cervix, to a cervix that is friable (bleeds with gentle probing).

Diagnosis relies on collection of an endocervical swab, vaginal swab, or urine specimen. A variety of testing methods are available, but nucleic acid amplification testing (NAAT) offers the greatest sensitivity when using endocervical specimens and is FDA approved for urine specimens. Treatment is important to resolve symptoms, and to prevent ascending genital tract infections as well as further transmission.

Neisseria gonorrhea

Gonococcal infection is caused by Gram-negative intracellular diplococcal bacteria. Young females represent the demographic group with the highest prevalence (see Chapter 44.4). This infection is usually asymptomatic in women. The cervix may bleed easily during examination.

Laboratory testing methods includes NAAT, nucleic acid hybridization test, and culture. Gram stain is not appropriate for testing in females. NAAT is the only testing method approved for testing from vaginal swab and urine specimens. Culture and sensitivity testing is also available, but should be reserved for patients in whom resistance to first-line therapy is suspected. Treatment of this infection is imperative for symptom resolution, prevention of upper genital tract infection, and reduction of transmission.

> ### ✋ Caution
>
> - STD prevention education should be a focus if trichomonas, chlamydia or gonorrhea infection is diagnosed.
> - Sex partners should be treated and testing for other STDs should be encouraged.
> - Routine test of cure is not recommended.
> - Re-testing approximately 3 months after treatment should be done if symptoms are persistent, or if re-infection is suspected.

Pelvic inflammatory disease

Pelvic inflammatory disease (PID) describes upper genital tract infections (see Chapter 51). This infection is polymicrobial and can involve any of the microorganisms comprising normal vaginal flora, not just gonorrhea and chlamydia. In addition to vaginal discharge, abdominal and pelvic pain, fever, and nausea can be present. Physical exam findings include cervical motion tenderness, uterine and adnexal tenderness, and/or abdominal pain with or without rebound tenderness.

PID is typically diagnosed clinically. PID treatment should be implemented if all other causes of pain have been ruled out, and two of the following three criteria are present: abdominal pain, cervical motion tenderness, and adnexal tenderness. The presence of fever, leukocytosis, leukocytes in the discharge, elevated C-reactive protein, elevated sedimentation rate, and positive gonococcal and/or chlamydial tests strengthen the specificity of the clinical diagnosis.

Foreign body

Tampons are the most commonly retained foreign body in adolescents. Vaginal discharge with offensive odor is the typical complaint. Diagnosis is made by visual inspection of the vagina. Treatment is simply to remove the foreign body; antibiotic therapy is not required unless a concurrent infection is diagnosed. Placement of foreign objects into the vagina may occur during sexual assault. This possibility should be recognized and sensitively investigated.

Genital tract anomalies

Genital tract anomalies typically present with amenorrhea, pain, or difficulty identifying the vaginal introitus (see Chapter 46). An obstructing longitudinal or transverse vaginal septum leads to a hematocolpos when menstrual blood accumulates in the vagina. The obstructing septum can rupture, converting the previously sterile and uninfected hematocolpos into an infected cavity. Drainage from this infected pyocolpos can cause a purulent or malodorous vaginal discharge.

Radiologic studies, including ultrasound MRI and hysterosalpinogram, are helpful to clarify anatomy. Treatment of a genital tract obstruction requires surgical resection by a gynecologic surgeon experienced with these anomalies.

Oncology

Adenocarcinoma of the cervix and vagina are rare, but have been reported in the adolescent population. Abnormal vaginal discharge may be the presenting complaint of a cancerous lesion if it is erosive. Diagnosis is made by pathologic review of a tissue biopsy.

Certainly, this diagnostic possibility should not be immediately considered when evaluating an adolescent with vaginal discharge. However, if vaginal discharge is persistent and common causes have been ruled out, careful inspection for ulcerative lesions should be done.

Fistula

Rectovaginal, enterovaginal, and vesicovaginal fistulas can present with vaginal discharge. These typically occur after gynecologic surgery, or in developing countries, after a prolonged obstructed labor. While rare, this diagnosis must be considered as more adolescents undergo complex surgical procedures. Fistulous tracts causing vaginal discharge may also occur in patients with Crohn disease.

Imaging using CT, MRI, vaginography, or barium enema may be required to confirm the diagnosis. Ultimately, a surgical approach by an experienced surgeon is typically needed for treatment of a fistula.

Further reading

CDC. STD treatment guidelines 2010. http://www.cdc.gov/std/treatment/2010/

Emans SJ, Laufer MR, Goldstein DP. *Pediatric & Adolescent Gynecology*, 5th revised edn. Philadelphia: Lippincott Williams & Wilkins, 2004.

Neinstein LS. *Adolescent Health Care: A Practical Guide*, 5th edn. Philadelphia: Lippincott Williams & Wilkins, 2007.

38 Pelvic masses

Noam Smorgick-Rosenbaum and Elisabeth H. Quint

Department of Obstetrics and Gynecology, University of Michigan Health System, Ann Arbor, MI, USA

The pelvic mass in a teenager is usually diagnosed in one of two ways. The teen may present with symptoms such as pelvic pain, and physical exam or pelvic ultrasound demonstrates a pelvic mass. The second scenario is an adolescent who presents for a regular health visit and is found to have an asymptomatic mass on exam. The evaluation for each will be slightly different. The algorithm in Figure 38.1 will help to achieve the right diagnosis.

Diagnosis

The differential diagnosis for pelvic masses in adolescents is listed in Table 38.1.

The history and physical exam is described in Table 38.2.

Laboratory tests are listed in Table 38.3.

The first imaging tool is usually the pelvic ultrasound, being inexpensive, widely available, and non-invasive. The pelvic ultrasound is ideally performed via a transabdominal and transvaginal approach. The transabdominal approach, alone or combined with the transperineal/translabial approach, may be used for patients who are not sexually active or are uncomfortable with the vaginal probe. When malignancy is suspected, further information regarding tumor spread, such as ascites and lymphadenopathy, can be obtained from a computed tomography (CT) scan. Pelvic magnetic resonance imaging (MRI) is useful to further characterize uterine and obstructive anomalies of the reproductive tract.

> ### ☆ Tips and tricks
>
> • Remember to interview the patient in private for her confidential information and behaviors.
> • Asking the patient whether she is comfortable with tampon use may help determine the feasibility of performing an internal pelvic exam.
> • A virginal teen presenting with primary amenorrhea or dysmenorrhea may not easily tolerate a pelvic exam. When indicated, the patency and length of the vagina may be assessed with gentle insertion of a well lubricated small Q-tip. Care must be taken to avoid touching the hymen since this may cause significant discomfort to the patient.
> • An external genital exam and a rectoabdominal exam may provide information on vaginal and abdominal masses (particularly in cases of obstructive anomalies) and is usually well tolerated.

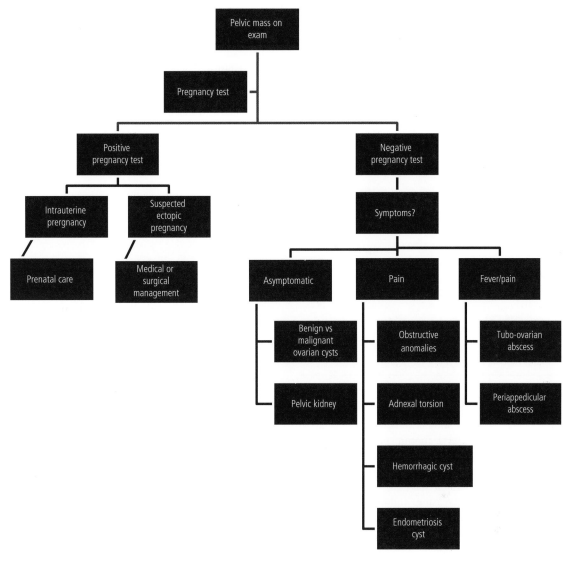

Figure 38.1 Approach to the evaluation of pelvic masses in adolescents.

Ovarian and tubal masses (see Appendices 1.15.1–1.15.3)

Adnexal masses are among the most commonly diagnosed pelvic masses in teens. The majority of *cystic* lesions are functional ovarian cysts such as follicular cysts and corpus luteum cysts. Nonfunctional benign cysts such as mature cystic teratoma, paratubal cysts, and, less frequently, benign epithelial tumors (e.g. cystadenoma) can present as a pelvic mass. *Solid* lesions are more suspicious for malignancy, although the risk of malignancy in adolescents with ovarian masses is low (about 4% of surgically removed masses). Among the malignant ovarian masses, germ cell tumors are the most common histology (see Chapter 48.2). Endometriomas are rare in teens.

The symptoms caused by ovarian masses depend on the cyst size and growth velocity, and include pelvic pain and urinary and gastrointestinal symptoms for large cysts. Acute abdominal pain associated

Table 38.1 Differential diagnosis of pelvic masses in adolescents

- Ovarian masses—cystic:
  - Follicular cysts
  - Corpus luteum cysts
  - Hemorrhagic functional cysts
  - Benign nonfunctional masses
  - Infectious masses
  - Malignant masses
- Obstructive genital lesions:
  - Imperforate hymen
  - Transverse vaginal septum
  - Obstructed uterine horn/remnants
- Uterine:
  - Leiomyoma
  - Adenomyosis
- Tubal:
  - Paratubal cysts
  - Infectious masses
- Urinary:
  - Full bladder
  - Pelvic kidney
- Gastrointestinal:
  - Appendiceal abscess

Table 38.2 Evaluation

History
- Detailed menstrual history
- Reproductive history
- Review of systems:
  - Abdominal pain
  - Abnormal bleeding
  - Vaginal discharge
  - Gastrointestinal symptoms
  - Urinary symptoms
  - Constitutional symptoms

Physical exam
- Tanner staging: breast and pubic hair
- Abdominal exam:
  - Abdominal/pelvic mass
  - Ascites
- Systemic tumor spread/adenopathy
- Signs of virilization
- External genital exam
- Rectoabdominal versus vaginal bimanual exam:
  - Size
  - Tenderness
  - Mobility
  - Regularity of cyst wall

with an ovarian cyst should warrant an evaluation for ovarian torsion, cyst rupture or a hemorrhagic cyst. Ovarian torsion may also present with nausea and vomiting, in addition to pelvic pain. Symptoms from a malignant ovarian mass are often nonspecific and may include increasing abdominal girth and nausea or vomiting. Large ovarian masses may be palpated on abdominal exam, while smaller ones may be palpated on bimanual or rectoabdominal pelvic exam.

The use of tumor markers should be considered in specific circumstances (see Table 38.3).

Functional cysts usually appear as simple or hemorrhagic cysts on ultrasound. Shadowing is suggestive of a mature benign teratoma. Growing ovarian masses and solid or complex ovarian masses should be evaluated for malignancy and the mass' characteristics may help with the index of suspicion. Color Doppler velocimetry may be applied when ovarian torsion is suspected, although this test is neither sensitive nor specific for this diagnosis and needs to be interpreted in combination with the symptomatology.

Table 38.3 Laboratory tests

- Pregnancy test: *always* indicated
- Complete blood count (CBC):
  - Anemia
  - Elevated WBCs
- Tumor markers: when malignancy is suspected; useful for diagnosis and follow-up:
  - Large, solid, or complex masses on imaging
  - Mass growing in size
- Renal function: for urinary tract masses
- STI testing

Ectopic pregnancy

In the US, the overall pregnancy rate in women aged 15–19 years is 10%, and about 75% of pregnancies are unplanned. Adolescents are at higher risk for ectopic pregnancy due to their higher age-specific incidence of sexually-transmitted infections (STIs) and pelvic inflammatory disease.

Adolescents may complain of missed periods or abnormal bleeding, but often the pregnant teen presents with vague symptoms. The clinician may need to ask (in private) about missed or abnormal periods, sexual activity, use of contraception, and specific symptoms of early pregnancy. Abdominal pain and/or vaginal bleeding should prompt an evaluation for an ectopic pregnancy (see Chapter 47). The gravid uterus can be palpated abdominally after 12 gestational weeks, while an enlarged and softened uterus is noted on bimanual exam after the sixth gestational week. Adnexal mass and/or tenderness in the setting of a positive pregnancy test could be the corpus luteum cyst of pregnancy or an ectopic pregnancy.

A low threshold for obtaining a urine pregnancy test is recommended in adolescents. In cases of suspected ectopic pregnancy, a quantitative β-human chorionic gonadotropin (β-hCG) titer is obtained and the results correlated with the last menstrual period (LMP) and the ultrasound findings.

A pelvic ultrasound is obtained to identify the presence of an intrauterine gestational sac and verify the gestational age. Ectopic pregnancy is often difficult to diagnose on ultrasound and the combination of the β-hCG level and the ultrasound will lead to the correct diagnosis.

Obstructive anomalies of the reproductive tract (see also Chapters 9 and 46)

Complete obstructive anomalies may present as a pelvic mass in an adolescent with primary amenorrhea, cyclical abdominal pain, and developed secondary sexual characteristics. The most common types of obstructive anomalies with this presentation are imperforate hymen and transverse vaginal septum, and the less common ones are vaginal atresia (failure of development of the distal part of the vagina), uterine remnants or cervical atresia. The diagnosis of incomplete obstruction (obstructed hemivagina with a septate uterus or uterus didelphis and non-communicating uterine horn with functional endometrium) is often delayed. These teenagers present with cyclical menstrual pain prompting the diagnosis and treatment of dysmenorrhea, with imaging studies later revealing the correct diagnosis. All obstructive anomalies may cause endometriosis due to retrograde flow.

In addition to pelvic pain, nausea and vomiting and pain with bowel movements may be present when the amount of trapped blood is very large. Rarely, the presentation may be of an infectious process as a pyocolpos. The bulging membrane of the imperforate hymen is easily seen on exam. In cases of transverse vaginal septum, the vagina appears short. In both cases, the hematocolpos should be readily palpated on rectoabdominal exam. If a vaginal bulge is not palpated on rectal exam, imaging is mandatory.

Imaging is usually recommended for evaluation of obstructive anomalies, except for the imperforate hymen when the diagnosis is obvious on visual and rectal exam. Ultrasound can be helpful, but MRI is the gold standard. MRI is used to measure the vaginal septum's thickness, to differentiate between transverse vaginal septum and partial vaginal atresia, and to describe uterine and cervical anomalies. Ultrasound and/or MRI may also be used to diagnose anomalies of the urinary tract, which are more common in these patients.

> ### ✋ Caution
>
> Not all patients with primary amenorrhea, abdominal and pain, and a vaginal opening not clearly identified on exam have an imperforate hymen. You should insure the diagnosis is correct by ordering imaging studies prior to taking the patient to the operating room. Consider the following:
> - If you can visualize a normal hymen, then the diagnosis is *not* imperforate hymen.
> - If you do *not* feel a vaginal bulge on rectal exam, the diagnosis is *not* imperforate hymen.

Tubo-ovarian abscess (see also Chapter 51)

Pelvic masses from an infectious process involving the adnexa may occur as a complication of pelvic inflammatory disease (PID) in sexually-active adolescents. Adolescents have the highest age-specific rates of PID, with almost 20% of cases in the US occurring in this age group.

Most patients will present with pelvic pain of some duration, as well as fever or foul smelling vaginal discharge. Other nonspecific symptoms include menstrual irregularities, dyspareunia, nausea, vomiting, diarrhea, constipation, dysuria, and urinary frequency. It is important to evaluate risk factors for PID and sexually-transmitted diseases, including unprotected intercourse, multiple sexual partners, and previous infections.

The vital signs give an indication of severity of the illness. The minimum requirements for the diagnosis of PID on exam are uterine tenderness or cervical motion tenderness. The abdomen is palpated to rule out significant peritoneal signs. The tubo-ovarian abscess (TOA) is often readily palpable as a tender and relatively fixed adnexal mass.

Cervical or urinary samples for *Neisseria gonorrhoeae* and *Chlamydia trachomatis* are obtained. Blood cultures are indicated for high fevers and generalized illness. Often, the systemic nature of the infectious process will be manifested in an elevated neutrophil blood count, erythrocyte sedimentation rate (ESR) and C-reactive protein (CRP). Elevated liver function tests may be present in perihepatitis (Fitz–Hugh–Curtis syndrome).

Pelvic ultrasound is very helpful as an adjunct to the pelvic exam in identifying the TOA. The TOA appears as a complex mass involving one or two ovaries and the fallopian tubes. If the diagnosis is unclear, a CT scan may be helpful.

Uterine masses

Although common in adult women, adenomyosis and leiomyomas are very rare in adolescents, with only about a dozen cases reported in the literature. All reported cases of adolescents with leiomyomas were benign on pathology.

The clinical presentation is variable according to the uterine size and myometrial location, and may include pelvic pressure, heavy uterine bleeding, abdominal girth enlargement, and urinary symptoms. Large leiomyomas are easily palpated on abdominal and/or pelvic exam. Typically, leiomyomas have a firm texture on exam.

Pelvic ultrasound is very helpful to define leiomyoma location and size.

Gastrointestinal conditions

Most cases of pelvic masses associated with the gastrointestinal tract in adolescents occur with late presentation of acute appendicitis leading to formation of an appendiceal abscess. Other causes of gastrointestinal tract pelvic masses in the pediatric population (e.g. duplication and congenital obstruction) are rare in adolescents.

Patients may present with the "classic" symptoms of acute appendicitis, including right lower quadrant abdominal pain, anorexia, fever, nausea, and vomiting. However, an atypical presentation with generalized malaise and various bowel symptoms is not uncommon.

A tender mass in the right lower quadrant is typically palpated, and signs of peritoneal inflammation may be elicited. In those cases the appendix is retrocecal or pelvic in location; the psoas sign and obturator sign (respectively) may be positive.

Systemic inflammatory signs are often present.

Ultrasound and CT scan readily identify the abscess, and are also used to guide percutaneous drainage when required.

Urologic conditions

Occasionally a very full bladder can masquerade as a central pelvic mass, especially in patients with decreased urinary sensation. A pelvic kidney is a rare cause of pelvic mass in adolescents. Other urinary tract anomalies as well as anomalies of the Müllerian system should be looked for in an adolescent diagnosed with an ectopic kidney.

Further reading

Gray-Swain MR, Peipert JF. Pelvic inflammatory disease in adolescents. *Curr Opin Obstet Gynecol* 2006;18:503–510.

van Winter JT, Simmons PS, Podratz KC. Surgically treated adnexal masses in infancy, childhood, and adolescence. *Am J Obstet Gynecol* 1994;170:1780–1786.

Wright KN, Laufer MR. Leiomyomas in adolescents. *Fertil Steril* 2011;95:2434.e15–17.

39.1 Pelvic and abdominal pain

Geri D. Hewitt

Nationwide Children's Hospital and Department of Obstetrics, Gynecology and Pediatrics, Ohio State University College of Medicine, Columbus, OH, USA

Chronic pelvic and abdominal pain

Chronic pelvic pain is a common complaint in adolescent women. It is defined as cyclic or noncyclic, intermittent or constant pain of at least 6 months' duration. Chronic pelvic pain often frustrates the patient, her parents, and her clinician, and can lead to significant functional problems, such as changes in family dynamics or school absenteeism. Many patients see multiple physicians including pediatricians, gynecologists, gastroenterologists, and emergency room doctors, trying to seek specific diagnoses, effective treatments, and relief of symptoms. As the time lengthens between the onset of symptoms and definitive diagnosis or relief of symptoms, patient frustration may increase, leading to doctor shopping and possible narcotic use. It is important to address the patient and her family's concerns regarding the pain in a prompt manner.

Potential etiologies for chronic pelvic pain in adolescent women are numerous and may be multifactorial (Table 39.1.1). Broadly, these may include psychosocial, gynecologic, urologic, musculoskeletal, and gastroenterologic causes. It is important to explore all potential etiologies, both organic and nonorganic, from the onset of the evaluation.

Patients and their families need education and support to understand that the problem has been longstanding and that they may have to invest some

> ★ **Tips and tricks**
>
> • Make sure you explore all possible etiologies of chronic pelvic pain form the onset of the diagnosis, including psychosocial factors.
> • The causes may be multifactorial and if health is not optimized in all areas, patients may not have optimal improvement of their symptoms.
> • Patients and their families will be more open to exploring psychosocial interventions if these are introduced early in the evaluation rather than only after a normal diagnostic laparoscopy.

time to complete diagnostic tests as well as to try therapeutic interventions. Sometimes families are reluctant to try medical intervention in the absence of a concrete etiology for the patient's pain. Diagnostic tests that are "normal" and eliminate a possible etiology should be interpreted as reassuring rather than frustrating. They may need education to understand that the goal of therapy is improvement of the patient's pain and return to normal function. While a specific etiology is often identified, sometimes the patient may reach that goal without a clear diagnosis.

Practical Pediatric and Adolescent Gynecology, First Edition. Edited by Paula J. Adams Hillard.
© 2013 John Wiley & Sons, Ltd. Published 2013 by John Wiley & Sons, Ltd.

Table 39.1.1 Etiologies of chronic pelvic pain

- Gynecologic causes:
  - Endometriosis
  - Pelvic inflammatory disease
  - Congenital anomalies
  - Pelvic adhesive disease
  - Ovarian masses
- Urologic causes:
  - Chronic urinary tract infections
  - Kidney stones
  - Interstitial cystitis
- Gastroenterologic causes:
  - Constipation
  - Irritable bowel disease
  - Lactose intolerance
  - Inflammatory bowel disease
  - Hernia
  - Chronic appendicitis
  - Abdominal migraines
- Musculoskeletal causes:
  - Trauma or old injury
  - Leg length discrepancy
  - Postural problems
  - Trigger points
- Psychosocial causes:
  - Depression/anxiety
  - School avoidance
  - Physical or sexual abuse
  - Eating disorders
  - Substance abuse

✋ Patient/parent advice

Patients and/or their parents are sometimes reluctant to initiate hormonal contraceptive pills to treat pain. Important points to emphasize include:

- Low-dose oral contraceptive pills (OCPs) are very safe in healthy young women without a personal or family history of blood clots.
- OCPs are not associated with weight gain.
- OCPs will have no negative impact on future fertility.
- OCPs do not cause cancer.
- OCPs actually lower the risks of ovarian and uterine cancer.

Diagnosis

Evaluation of the patient with chronic pelvic pain should begin with a thorough history with emphasis on the duration and frequency of symptoms, location and severity of pain, what causes exacerbation and improvement, as well as medications and therapies tried. A prospective pain calendar can be useful in obtaining the above information; the patient should also record her menses to include any cyclic component. School absences as well as other missed activities or responsibilities should also be recorded. It is important to understand the patient's lifestyle as well as her coping mechanisms. Major life events, real or perceived stressors, friendships, and romantic relationships should be explored.

Oftentimes information gained from the history will impact how the clinician moves forward with the evaluation. The gynecologic history should include age of menarche, cycle interval and flow, presence of dysmenorrhea, sexual activity, exposure to sexually-transmitted infections, cyclic component of the pain, and any pregnancies. Primary dysmenorrhea can often be diagnosed based on history alone, with the onset of cramping lower abdominal pain just prior to and during menses with resolution of symptoms when menses is completed (see Chapter 45). Concomitant headaches, nausea and vomiting, constipation and diarrhea, as well as musculoskeletal complaints during this time frame are common.

Important questions exploring potential gastroenterologic etiologies include dietary history, nausea, emesis, and bowel habits. Constipation is a very common contributor to chronic pelvic pain. Patients often will not want to discuss their bowel habits, but what they define as "normal for them" may actually be constipation.

Urinary frequency, dysuria, or hematuria may warrant more extensive urologic evaluation.

Clues that a musculoskeletal etiology may be involved include a history of pain worsening or improving with certain positions, activities, or movements. Musculoskeletal pain may be cyclic in nature as hormonal fluctuations often impact joints and soft tissues.

In the past medical history it is important to note any illnesses, surgeries, traumatic or sport-related injuries, scoliosis, mental health issues, eating disorders, and substance abuse. Family history should explore the prevalence of endometriosis, chronic pain, and mental health concerns.

The physical exam should start with the patient's overall appearance as well as her affect. Watching how the patient walks between the exam room and bathroom as well as her movement on the exam table can be informative. To screen for musculoskeletal causes of pain, the patient's posture should be examined, looking for evidence of lordosis, one-legged standing, or leg length discrepancy. The upper and lower back should be palpated while the patient is sitting. Once the patient is supine, leg flexion and head and leg raises should be done with abdominal wall palpation. The patient should be asked to point to the area of greatest pain on her abdomen. Diffuse migratory pain is less likely than specific focal pain to have a primarily organic etiology. The abdominal wall should be palpated, feeling for masses, evidence of constipation, or tender areas suggestive of trigger points (see Chapter 39.2).

The pelvic exam should focus on the gynecologic as well as urologic causes of pain. The urethra and bladder base should be palpated noting any specific tenderness. The pelvic floor muscles should be palpated to assess tenderness and spasm. The vaginal fornices and uterosacral ligaments should be palpated for tenderness or masses. The uterus and adnexa should be palpated on bimanual examination assessing for tenderness, fixed position, and enlargement.

A rectal examination is essential, especially if a gastroenterologic etiology or endometriosis is suspected. If a large mass of stool is detected, or if the patient has a wide rectal vault, constipation should be suspected.

Laboratory tests should be tailored to the patient's history and physical exam. Common laboratory tests include complete blood count (CBC) with differential, sedimentation rate, urinalysis, and urine culture. If a patient is sexually active, screening tests for gonorrhea and chlamydia as well as a pregnancy test are important. Other laboratory tests may be indicated based on the patient's symptoms, history, and physical exam.

Imaging studies can be very helpful, not only to confirm a diagnosis, but also to provide reassurance. A plain film of the abdomen can be very helpful if constipation is suspected. Not only can the clinician confirm the diagnosis, but also they can show the image to the patient and her family as concrete evidence of at least one area that needs to be addressed to help improve pain.

The majority of patients with chronic pelvic pain will undergo a pelvic ultrasound. The likelihood of finding a significant abnormality is small if the patient has a normal pelvic examination; however, it can be very important in patients with an abnormal or compromised exam. The reassurance provided by a normal pelvic ultrasound may be important to the patient and her family, who are often worried about underlying pathology contributing to her symptoms, such as large masses or tumors. Small, simple, ovarian cysts will often be identified on pelvic ultrasound; these common findings are unlikely contributors to chronic pelvic pain (see Chapter 48.1). Larger (>4 cm) or more complex adnexal masses, however, are potential etiologies. An abnormal pelvic ultrasound is highly predictive of similar pathology being identified at the time of laparoscopy. Obstructive uterine anomalies can also be identified by ultrasound and may contribute to both cyclic and chronic pelvic pain (see Chapter 46); pelvic ultrasound should be considered in patients with dysmenorrhea not relieved with hormonal contraceptives and NSAIDs for this reason. It is important to keep in mind that the pelvic ultrasound cannot diagnose endometriosis, pelvic inflammatory disease (PID), or adhesions. Thus a normal pelvic ultrasound should not necessarily be the endpoint in the evaluation of a young woman with chronic pelvic pain.

A CT scan of the abdomen and pelvis can be helpful when evaluating patients for gastroenterologic causes of pain such as chronic appendicitis and inflammatory bowel disease.

Laparoscopy has been shown to be safe in adolescents and has become an important diagnostic tool. Common indications for performing laparoscopy in this population include presence of a pelvic mass, progressive dysmenorrhea, dysmenorrhea unresponsive to hormonal contraceptives and NSAIDs, and any "diagnostic dilemma" such as suspected chronic PID or chronic appendicitis. The incidence of identifying pathology at the time of surgery varies by author and patient population; most, but not all, appropriately selected patients will have pathology. Common findings at the time of laparoscopy include endometriosis, pelvic adhesive disease, adnexa masses and torsion, appendicitis, uterine anomalies, and PID.

Laparoscopy has an important role in the management of chronic pelvic pain; its usefulness includes diagnosis, therapeutic intervention, as well as reassurance. Most abnormalities identified can be surgically treated at the time of diagnostic laparoscopy.

★ Tips and tricks

- The value of a negative laparoscopy in providing reassurance for the patient and her family should not be underestimated.
- Pictures of normal anatomy can be taken during surgery and shared with the patient and her family afterwards for optimal reassurance.
- This is particularly helpful in the patient with any psychosomatic component of her pain.

Acute pelvic and abdominal pain

Acute pelvic pain is also a relatively common complaint in young women; however, the symptoms are typically of much shorter duration and the differential diagnosis is not quite as broad. Many clinicians feel acute pelvic pain is a more easily managed clinical problem than chronic pain.

✋ Caution

- Remember that not all patients with chronic pelvic pain require a diagnostic laparoscopy.
- Laparoscopy is indicated for patients that have undergone a thorough evaluation of other causes and continue to have pain that limits their functional abilities.
- Laparoscopy should be considered in patients with abnormal imaging studies, dysmenorrhea despite a combination of hormonal contraceptives and NSAIDs, or in the case of diagnostic dilemmas.
- While most diagnostic laparoscopies in appropriately selected patients will reveal pathology, a negative laparoscopy can be very reassuring to patients and their families and help patients regain their optimal well-being by removing a focus on possible causes of pain such as endometriosis.

Common gynecologic problems presenting with acute pain include PID, ruptured ovarian cysts, hemorrhagic ovarian cysts, adnexal torsion, and ectopic pregnancy. Common urologic conditions are urinary tract infections, both cystitis and pyelonephritis. Kidney stones are much less common in younger women than adults. Gastroenterologic problems that may present with acute pelvic pain include appendicitis, constipation, irritable bowel syndrome, and viral illnesses.

History can be very helpful in developing the differential diagnosis. Important questions include onset, duration, location and severity of pain, as well as contributing or alleviating factors. The presence or absence of fever and chills as well as general malaise is important as well. Gynecologic information should include menstrual cycle history, including last menstrual period; sexual health history, including numbers of partners, most recent sexual contact, contraceptive method, and condom use; and presence of other gynecologic complaints such as irregular vaginal bleeding or discharge. Patients reporting sexual activity need to be evaluated for PID; it is an unlikely diagnosis in virginal women.

Dysuria, frequency, and hematuria are symptoms suggestive of urinary tract involvement. Gastroenterologic symptoms such as loss of appetite, nausea, vomiting, constipation, and diarrhea are important to explore. While nausea and vomiting can occur with an acute abdomen from a gynecologic concern, the presence of these symptoms may suggest a gastroenterologic cause. Anorexia is often an early symptom of appendicitis. Intermittent colicky pain should raise suspicion about adnexal torsion.

Whether the patient has had similar symptoms in the past and recent sick contacts are also important historical information. Past medical and surgical history, medications, and family history should be included, although these are usually less helpful with acute as compared to chronic pelvic pain.

Vital signs can be an important aspect of the physical exam to try to determine whether the patient has an infectious etiology (elevated temperature) and severity of illness (blood pressure abnormalities and tachycardia). The clinician should look carefully at the patient before the exam and try to get a sense of the severity of her pain and illness. Lungs should be auscultated since some patients with pneumonia can present with abdominal pain. A heart exam can confirm tachycardia. Testing for costovertebral angle tenderness is important in patients with an elevated temperature and urinary complaints to evaluate for pyelonephritis.

The abdominal exam is very important in determining whether the patient has a surgical abdomen, including the presence of tenderness, guarding, rebound on palpation, and absent or diminished bowel sounds on auscultation. A surgical abdomen can indicate the need for immediate surgery in the case of ovarian torsion, acute appendicitis, or ruptured ectopic pregnancy. Patients with a surgical abdomen can also require immediate medical as opposed to surgical intervention, with the diagnoses of PID or pyelonephritis.

A pelvic examination should look for the presence or absence of vaginal discharge, cervical motion tenderness, uterine tenderness, as well as adnexal masses or tenderness. Empiric treatment for PID should be considered if the patient has cervical motion, uterine, or adnexal tenderness. Other findings such as elevated temperature and vaginal discharge increase the likelihood of PID.

A rectal examination may be indicated to feel for masses in the cul-de-sac and to test the stool for the presence of blood.

Helpful laboratory tests include a CBC with differential (evaluate white blood cells for possible ovarian torsion or infectious etiology), and urinalysis and urine culture (to evaluate for urinary causes). In patients with known or suspected sexual activity, a urine or serum pregnancy test and urine or cervical screening for chlamydia and gonorrhea become important. A negative pregnancy test eliminates ectopic pregnancy from the differential. Negative screening tests for chlamydia and gonorrhea do not eliminate the diagnosis of PID, but positive testing helps confirm the diagnosis.

Patients with adnexal masses or tenderness require diagnostic imaging studies. Pelvic ultrasound is very helpful to evaluate both the adnexa and uterus. Etiologies of acute pain, such as large ovarian masses, hemorrhagic ovarian cysts, and tubo-ovarian abscesses can all be identified with ultrasound. Performing Doppler studies and demonstrating decreased blood flow to and/or from the adnexa suggests torsion, which may occur even in the absence of an adnexal enlargement. Identifying free peritoneal fluid can sometimes suggest a recently ruptured ovarian cyst or raise concern about intra-abdominal bleeding. Abdominal–pelvic CT scan is recommended if there is a concern for appendicitis.

Laparoscopy may be required for either diagnostic or therapeutic reasons. Patients with suspicion of adnexal torsion require diagnostic laparoscopy. Delay in diagnosis (with subsequent "detorsing") can lead to ovarian necrosis and decreased fertility. Other emergent situations requiring laparoscopy include hemoperitoneum secondary to a suspected gynecologic etiology, such as a ruptured hemorrhagic corpus luteum or ruptured ectopic pregnancy. Larger or complex adnexal masses may be the source of pain and require laparoscopy for both confirmation and conservative surgical removal (see Chapter 48.1). Laparoscopy can also be very helpful to confirm an unclear diagnosis. Many etiologies of pain will present with very similar symptoms, physical findings, laboratory results, and imaging studies. PID and acute appendicitis can have very similar presentations and evaluations and may require diagnostic laparoscopy for absolute diagnosis.

Summary

Both chronic and acute pelvic pain are relatively common conditions in young women. A careful history and physical exam, thoughtful interpretation of laboratory results and imaging studies, and the judicial use of diagnostic laparoscopy can lead to the appropriate diagnosis and facilitate the initiation of a treatment plan to help the patient return to her normal state of health.

Further reading

American College of Obstetricians and Gynecologists. Endometriosis in adolescents. ACOG Committee Opinion No. 310. *Obstet Gynecol* 2005;105:921–927.

Economy KE, Laufer MR. Pelvic pain. *Adolesc Med* 1999;10(2):291–304.

Hewitt GD, Brown RT. Acute and chronic pelvic pain in female adolescents. *Med Clin North Am* 2000;84(4): 1009–1025.

39.2 Myofascial (musculoskeletal) pain

John Jarrell

University of Calgary, Calgary, AB, Canada

Myofascial pain syndrome is a disease of muscle that causes local and referred pain. It is characterized by a motor abnormality (a taut or hard band within the muscle) and by sensory abnormalities (tenderness and referred pain). It is classified as a musculoskeletal pain syndrome that can be acute or chronic, regional or generalized. It can be a primary disorder causing local or regional pain syndromes, or a secondary disorder that occurs as a consequence of some other condition.

Causes are:

• **Injury.** Myofascial pain can occur in any skeletal muscle of the body. In most cases, the condition is associated with an injury to the muscle either through direct trauma or muscle overload, such as a seatbelt lap-restraint injury. Among adolescents, this is an uncommon cause of abdominal pain.

• **Visceral disease.** The most common form of myofascial pain in the pelvis is associated with pain-related disorders of the viscera of the pelvic organs.

Diagnosis

The recognition of myofascial pain requires several steps. Initially, it is helpful to identify the presence or absence of cutaneous allodynia.

By gently examining this area of allodynia, you can usually identify one or more small nodules that when

> ### ⚙ Science revisited
>
> • The concept of visceral disease resulting in somatic presentation of pain and tenderness was first identified in the early 1900s.
>
> ○ Henry Head mapped out the so-called Head zones that demonstrated the well-known referral patterns from myocardial ischemia, cholecystitis, and appendicitis; these were the precursors of the dermatomes.
>
> ○ In the early 1900s, James MacKenzie demonstrated there were tender areas as a result of visceral disease, located on the abdominal wall.
>
> • More recently, the concept of central sensitization has been recognized.
>
> ○ This indicates that severe pain from the pelvic organs (dysmenorrhea, endometriosis) can under certain circumstances generate changes in the dorsal horns of the spinal cord.
>
> ○ A persistent outpouring of glutamate into the synaptic cleft results in persistent efferent discharge, causing clinical symptoms of persistent and continuous pain, painful bowel function, urinary frequency, myofascial trigger points, and areas of cutaneous allodynia surrounding the trigger points (a case history is described in Figure 39.2.1).

Practical Pediatric and Adolescent Gynecology, First Edition. Edited by Paula J. Adams Hillard.
© 2013 John Wiley & Sons, Ltd. Published 2013 by John Wiley & Sons, Ltd.

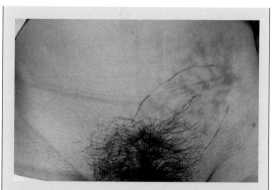

Figure 39.2.1 Case history: A 17-year-old presents with persistent left lower quadrant pain that has been present for about 1 year. Her menarche was at 14 years and she has been plagued by severely painful menses ever since. The pain is sharp and is described as a knife-like sensation that never goes away. She notes that her bowel movements have become severely painful. She has developed urinary frequency that results in several episodes of nocturia each night. She has lost many days at school while lying in a fetal position in her bed for days. On examination, there is evidence of a hot water bottle pigmentation on the left lower quadrant. An area of cutaneous allodynia can be demonstrated in the area of the pigmentation. Within this area of allodynia, there are several nodular areas identified as a trigger points (see markings).

☆ Tips and tricks

Testing for cutaneous allodynia
- A Q-tip is gently drawn down the anterior abdominal wall in the mid-clavicular line.
- A sudden change in the response to this stimulus from nonpainful to painful or sharp represents allodynia; usually this occurs in the region of the T11–L1 dermatome.

---

pressed reproduce the pain. The pain is described as knife-like or sharp. It does not have the characteristics of neuropathic pain (burning, electric shocks, pins and needles). When pressed, the pain can radiate across the abdomen, into the chest or back or pelvis. The pain is relieved by releasing the pressure.

The same process can be applied to the perineum among adolescents who have difficulty with penetrative sexual function. Cutaneous allodynia is apparent in the S3 dermatome and gentle examination of the perineum will reveal a trigger point that is severely tender. If a single digit examination is undertaken, similar painful bands on the levator ani muscles with identify the trigger points.

Management

Although the above signs indicate the presence of visceral disease, their presence should not immediately direct the clinician to operative intervention, e.g. laparoscopy. Many cases are the direct result of dysmenorrhea and the laparoscopic destruction of minimal endometriosis is thought, potentially, to aggravate the development of the chronic pain state.

The mainstay of treatment of these young women is menstrual suppression. The major reason is that menstrual bleeding is a major pain generator and makes the expression of the viscerosomatic pain much more severe. Menstrual suppression (see Chapter 29.3) can be achieved with continuous oral contraceptives, the progestin medicated intrauterine device (IUD), depot medroxyprogesterone acetate, or the contraceptive vaginal ring; if these are either unacceptable or ineffective, gonadotropin-releasing hormone (GnRH) agonists with add-back estrogen may be used.

Other medications that are useful include the neuroleptics (gabapentin and pregabalin). Low-dose amitriptyline (lower doses than are used to treat depression) are also helpful for the management of chronic pain.

Direct treatment of the trigger points is best managed by the adolescent herself. Stretching exercises directed at the release of the trigger point can be done by the patient or with a trained physiotherapist. Injection of the abdominal trigger points with 1% xylocaine can be helpful in reinforcing the abdomen as a source of pain, but is usually of limited benefit if the patient is able to perform the appropriate exercises.

The same conservative approaches are of help in the perineum as well. In addition to the above, botulinum toxin 100IU can be injected into the perineum and both levator ani muscles. Injection into the obturator internus muscles can be helpful for women with trigger points in these muscles.

★ Tips and tricks

- Botulinum toxin is injected at the lowest point of the perineum into the perineal body. The tip of the needle is swung laterally to access the levator muscles, avoiding the Bartholin ducts.
- When injecting botulinum toxin into the perineum, apply lidocaine 2% should be applied for a full 10 minutes to reduce unnecessary pain.
- Pain associated with orgasm usually indicates severe myofascial dysfunction in the obturator internus muscles.

✋ Caution

Botulinum toxin should not be injected into the abdominal wall as it can migrate to the hip and result in severe weakness of the hip.

⬡ Science revisited

- Botulinum toxin requires approximately 7–10 days to take effect.
- It generally lasts 3 months.
- A positive effect is the change in the consistency on palpation of the pelvic muscles from that of "a well done steak" to a steak just purchased fresh from the butcher.

Prognosis

The condition does improve for most adolescents with simple physiotherapeutic approaches of stretching. Incremental intervention can be undertaken as indicated above.

It is typically the exception that a persistent nociceptive source of viscerosomatic pain remains and laparoscopic diagnosis and management may be required.

Further reading

Jarrell J. Demonstration of cutaneous allodynia in association with chronic pelvic pain. *J Vis Exp* 2009;28(ii):1232.

Jarrell J. Endometriosis and abdominal myofascial pain in adults and adolescents. *Curr Pain Headache Rep* 2011; 15(5):368–376.

Jarrell J, Giamberardino MA, Robert M, Nasr Esfahani1 M. Bedside testing for chronic pelvic pain: discriminating visceral from somatic pain. *Pain Res Treat* 2011;2011:692102.

Nasr-Esfahani M., Jarrell J. Cotton-tipped applicator test: validity and reliability in chronic pelvic pain. *Am J Obstet Gynecol* 2013;208(1):52.

Acknowledgements

The Calgary Health Trust provided funding for the study entitled "Cutaneous manifestations of chronic pelvic pain."

Amenorrhea

Melanie Nathan and Andrea L. Zuckerman

Tufts Medical Center, Boston, MA, USA

Amenorrhea, or the absence of menses, in the adolescent is a common presenting complaint to primary care physicians and gynecologists. Like many disorders, this is a problem that can occur due to a variety of etiologies. Often, clinicians differentiate between primary (never had a menses) and secondary (has undergone menarche) as a means to determine the etiology (Table 40.1). However, there are many diagnoses that overlap between the two. A better way to categorize amenorrhea is to examine the state of the gonads (ovaries): the ovaries may be producing estrogen with normal gonadotropin levels (eugonadal), or they may be hypoestrogenic with low or elevated gonadotropin levels (hypogonadal) (Table 40.2).

Amenorrhea is variably defined as:
- No menses for 6 months after menarche
- No menses for three times the normal cycle length, or
- Development of normal secondary sexual characteristics and no menses by age 15 years (2 SD above the mean) or by age 16 years (3 SD).

Women are normally amenorrheic during times in their lives such as prepubertally, postmenopausally, and during pregnancy and lactation.

> ### Science revisited
>
> **Embryology**
> - During development, both males and females initially have two pairs of genital ducts known as the mesonephric and the paramensonephric ducts.
> - With the presence of a Y chromosome, the testes produce Müllerian inhibiting substance (MIS) which inhibits the development of the paramesonephric ducts.
> - In the absence of the Y chromosome and with two X chromosomes present, ovaries develop and MIS is not produced, causing the paramesonephric ducts to develop and the mesonephric ducts to regress.
> - The superior end of these ducts open into the future peritoneal cavity as fallopian tubes, while the lower ends fuse to become the uterus and upper vagina.
> - The lower part of the vagina develops from the urogenital sinus.

Eugonadal amenorrhea

Congenital anomalies

Anatomic or congenital anomalies (see Chapter 46) are causes of eugonadal amenorrhea. Patients have ovaries that function normally. Congenital reproductive tract anomalies that result in complete blockage of the outflow tract result in primary amenorrhea, often not diagnosed until adolescence. An imperforate hymen occurs in 1 in 1000 to 1 in 10 000 births

Practical Pediatric and Adolescent Gynecology, First Edition. Edited by Paula J. Adams Hillard.
© 2013 John Wiley & Sons, Ltd. Published 2013 by John Wiley & Sons, Ltd.

and may present with cyclic pelvic pain and a mass on exam from a hematocolpos (a collection of menstrual blood in the vagina behind the imperforate hymen). This problem is managed surgically with resection of the hymenal tissue, thereby allowing the blood collection to drain. A transverse vaginal septum, though very rare, may present very similarly to an imperforate hymen; however, the blockage is more proximal in the vagina and may not be visualized as easily on exam. This problem is also more difficult to manage surgically and care must be taken to avoid scarring or strictures.

Vaginal agenesis is another anomaly that can result in primary amenorrhea. Mayor–Rokitansky–Kuster–Hauser syndrome (MRKH) is the congenital absence of the uterus and the upper two-thirds of the vagina in women, normal development of secondary sexual characteristics, and a normal 46, XX karyotype. It is found in about 1 in 5000 women and is the second most common cause of primary amenorrhea. Most cases are associated with uterine agenesis or the presence of a nonfunctioning uterine horn. In about 7–10% of cases, a normal or rudimentary uterus is found with functional endometrial tissue; the absence of the vagina will cause a blocked outflow tract (hematometra) and may present very similarly to an imperforate hymen or transverse vaginal septum. Other associated malformations with this syndrome include renal and skeletal anomalies as well as hearing defects. Treatment is the creation of a neovagina. The preferred method is nonsurgical, using dilators to create a neovagina at the patient's own pace. Other more intricate surgical procedures can be done after extensive counseling the patient about proper postoperative care to prevent scarring.

Androgen insensitivity and other XY disorders

Receptor abnormalities and enzyme disorders can also cause amenorrhea in the adolescent. Complete androgen insensitivity syndrome is an X-linked recessive disorder and is characterized by a 46,XY karyotype and a female phenotype. The cause of this disorder is a defect in the androgen receptor that makes it resistant to the influence of testosterone. It can be partial (patients have some axillary and pubic hair) or complete (no axillary or pubic hair). The external genitalia are female with underdeveloped labia minora and a small blind vaginal pouch; testes are also present due to the Y chromosome. The testes during development produce Müllerian-inhibiting substance and therefore the upper third of the vagina, the uterus, and the fallopian tubes are all absent. During puberty, breast development occurs as excess androgens are converted to estrogen.

Table 40.1 Causes of primary and secondary amenorrhea

Primary amenorrhea	Secondary amenorrhea
Congenital anomalies	
Polycystic ovary syndrome (PCOS)	PCOS
Congenital adrenal hyperplasia (CAH)	CAH
Androgen insensitivity, 5-alpha reductase deficiency, Swyer syndrome	
Turner syndrome	Turner syndrome
Primary ovarian insufficiency (POI)	POI
Hyperprolactinemia	Hyperprolactinemia
Hypothalamic causes	Hypothalamic causes

Table 40.2 Causes of amenorrhea classified according to the state of the gonads (ovaries)

Eugonadal	Hypergonadal hypogonadism	Hypogonadal hypogonadism
Congenital anomalies	Turner syndrome	Hyperprolactinemia
Polycystic ovary syndrome	Primary ovarian insufficiency	Hypothalamic causes
Congenital adrenal hyperplasia		
Androgen insensitivity, 5-alpha reductase deficiency, Swyer syndrome		

5-Alpha-reductase deficiency is another enzyme deficiency disorder with a 46, XY karyotype; however, the phenotype with this disorder is either completely female or with ambiguous genitalia. In this condition, the enzyme converting testosterone to dihydrotestosterone (DHT), its more potent metabolite, is missing and therefore the female phenotype presides. However, due to the increase in testosterone production at the time of puberty, virilization does tend to occur at this time of life.

Swyer syndrome (a form of gonadal dysgenesis) is another condition that presents with 46, XY karyotype but with female phenotype. These patients are missing Müllerian-inhibiting substance and thus develop normal female external genitalia, uterus and fallopian tubes; however, the gonads are testicular in nature.

✋ Caution

Any female patient with a karyotype containing a Y cell line needs to have her intra-abdominal gonads resected as they are at risk for undergoing malignant transformation. This is more difficult in patients with streak gonads as there may be gonadal tissue at the pelvic brim down into the pelvis. All gonadal tissue in these patients needs to be removed.

Polycystic ovary syndrome

Polycystic ovary syndrome (PCOS) (see Chapter 50) is a common spectrum of disorders that includes oligomenorrhea, hirsutism, chronic anovulation, and metabolic disorders that include impaired glucose tolerance. The ovaries often appear polycystic with multiple small cysts under the ovarian cortex. The diagnosis of PCOS is difficult, as no one test is confirmatory. This condition is characterized by a metabolic disorder resulting in dysregulation of glucose and insulin metabolism; estrogen levels are elevated thereby, with ovarian dysfunction and irregular menses. This disorder is also characterized by symptoms of hyperandrogenism such as acne and facial hair growth. Treatment is medical, with progestin therapy, either alone or in a combination oral contraceptive pills. Addition of metformin has also been shown to help restore normal ovulatory cycles. Lifestyle modification is also important in improving outcomes.

Congenital adrenal hyperplasia

Late-onset congenital adrenal hyperplasia (CAH), although uncommon, also presents in adolescence and must be differentiated from PCOS by enzyme studies. This disorder is characterized by overproduction of androgens due to enzyme deficiencies in the complicated steroidogenesis pathway. Most cases of CAH result from 21-hydroxylase deficiency and are diagnosed by a morning blood draw of 17-hydroxyprogesterone. Stimulation tests are also often done to confirm the diagnosis. Treatment of CAH is similar to PCOS, although in cases of severe enzyme deficiency, patients also need salt replacement in times of stress.

Hypergonadotropic hypogonadal amenorrhea

Primary ovarian insufficiency

When estrogen levels are low, it is important to determine whether the gonadotropin levels [follicle-stimulating hormone (FSH) and luteinizing hormone (LH)] are elevated. In cases of elevated gonadotropin levels, levels should be repeated several weeks apart to confirm the diagnosis of primary ovarian insufficiency (POI). Epidemiologically, chromosomal abnormalities are by far the most common cause of primary amenorrhea (about 50% of cases).

Turner syndrome

Gonadal dysgenesis is the single most common cause of primary amenorrhea, the most common type being Turner syndrome. It occurs in 1 in 2500 to 1 in 3000 live-born girls. Turner syndrome is caused by an absent X chromosome or the absence of a part of the X chromosome, and is characterized by ovaries that are mainly replaced by fibrous tissue called streak gonads. The remainder of the genital tract develops normally. Patients can exhibit mosaicism with 46,XX cells and other cell lines that may include part of a Y cell line. At least 40 cells need to be karyotyped to rule out a Y cell line. If any Y cell lines are present, the gonads need to be removed to decrease the risk of malignant transformation of the gonads.

Patients with Turner syndrome may present with delayed puberty or may have undergone pubertal development and present with amenorrhea. Other common characteristics are short stature, high arched palate, and a webbed neck. Cardiac anomalies are also common, including coarctation of the aorta, bicuspid aortic valve, and dissection of the aortic root. Hypertension, diabetes mellitus, and thyroid disease are all also common, as are renal anomalies.

Other etiologies

Other etiologies of POI include exposure to chemotherapy and radiation for the treatment of childhood malignancies. Chemotherapy changes to the ovary include ovarian fibrosis and follicle destruction. The age at exposure and the type of chemotherapy and/ or radiation administered are important factors in the development of POI. The prepubertal ovary is the most resistant to the effects of both. Patients who undergo cranial radiation may also develop ovarian hypofunction due to pituitary and hypothalamic dysfunction.

Associated autoimmune disorders include thyroid disease, parathyroid disease, diabetes mellitus, and adrenal disorders. Ovarian function in these patients may wax and wane. Evaluation includes thyroid function tests, morning cortisol levels, calcium, phosphorous levels, and an antinuclear antibody (ANA).

Hypogonadotropic hypogonadal amenorrhea

Pituitary disorders

Pituitary disorders can cause amenorrhea, most commonly hyperprolactinemia. Elevated levels of prolactin may be caused by a microadenoma (<1 cm mass), macroadenoma (>1 cm mass), or medications, and may be associated with galactorrhea (clear or milky discharge noted from the breasts). Prolactin levels are influenced by many factors and should be assessed in the morning, on two different occasions if elevated, to consider this a cause of amenorrhea. Falsely elevated prolactin levels may be caused by exercise, breast stimulation, and late day variation of prolactin secretion. If truly elevated, a brain MRI should be obtained to assess for pituitary adenoma. Hypothy-

roidism is another disorder stemming from the pituitary that if present can result in amenorrhea. It is important to ask in the history about other symptoms such as cold intolerance and weight gain.

Hypothalamic suppression

Hypothalamic causes of amenorrhea, a diagnosis of exclusion, include stress, intensive exercise, chronic illness, eating disorders, congenital gonadotropin-releasing hormone (GnRH) deficiency (Kallman syndrome if in conjunction with anosmia), or constitutional delay of puberty. Levels of FSH and LH are low to normal. Examination reveals a hypoestrogenic state by vaginal maturation index.

Evaluation

The key to diagnosing the cause of amenorrhea starts with taking a good history. First, you should determine whether or not the patient has completed other stages of puberty such as thelarche and pubarche. If this has not occurred, the etiology is more likely to be a global one, such as pituitary failure, karyotype abnormalities, or ovarian failure (Table 40.3). It is also important to ask about family history, focusing on other members with similar issues. You should ask about symptoms of virilization as many of the disorders that may result in amenorrhea can also be associated with androgen excess. Changes in stress levels, weight or diet should be addressed, especially in patients who otherwise have met their pubertal milestones. A thorough medication/drug history needs to be elicited as certain medications can cause hormonal abnormalities that may result in amenorrhea. Questions such as galactorrhea, fatigue, and heat or cold intolerance can lead to further endocrine evaluation.

The physical exam (Table 40.4) focuses on assessment of breast and pubic hair development with Tanner staging of both, and observation of signs of androgen excess or pituitary dysfunction. Height, weight, and BMI % for age will define under or overweight. A careful skin exam looking for hirsutism, acne, and striae is important. If hirsutism is not present on the exam, this does not mean it does not exist. Many women today, even young girls, will wax and shave these areas prior to seeking medical

Table 40.3 Clues to possible etiology of amenorrhea in the history

Pertinent history	Possible etiology
Menarche/menstrual history	Primary vs secondary amenorrhea
Cyclic pain/bleeding	Congenital obstructive anomaly
Changes in stress, weight, exercise levels	Hypothalamic amenorrhea
Signs of androgen excess acne, hair growth Medication/drug history	PCOS, CAH, testosterone-secreting tumor
Galactorrhea	Prolactinoma, medications
Short stature/other congenital anomalies	Turner syndrome
Signs and symptoms of thyroid disorder	Hypo/hyperthyroidism

Table 40.4 Physical exam

• Height/weight: BMI
• Skin exam: hirsutism, acne, striae
• Breast exam: assess development with Tanner staging
• External genitalia: pubic hair development, clitoral size, hymenal anomalies
• Internal genital exam: assess for uterus, tubes, and ovaries (can be deferred)
• Imaging: pelvic US/MRI to assess uterus, tubes, and ovaries

treatment. An external genital exam should be done to assess for clitoral size and hymenal anomalies. An internal vaginal exam to assess vaginal depth and presence or absence of a cervix and uterus is not always necessary, particularly in young teens. Imaging with an initial pelvic ultrasound and subsequent pelvic MRI if needed, can be used to further assess these structures.

Directed laboratory/imaging work-up help to further assess the cause of the amenorrhea. If the patient has delayed puberty along with the amenorrhea, an endocrine work-up should be initiated and should include thyroid function tests, prolactin levels, FSH, and LH. In a patient with amenorrhea, normal pubertal development, and a uterus, the most important initial test is a pregnancy test. If negative, you

should proceed with a further evaluation. Assessment of the bone age can be useful, because if the bones are also lagging behind there might be a thyroid disease, growth hormone deficiency, or constitutional delay. If LH and FSH levels are elevated, you should obtain a karyotype as the most common reason for this is Turner syndrome. If FSH and LH levels are low, you should obtain a head MRI to rule-out pituitary tumor or disease of the hypothalamus causing amenorrhea.

Other studies may include imaging of the genital organs with ultrasound or MRI to establish whether or not a uterus is present.

If everything is normal on the work-up, it is reasonable to give the patient a progesterone challenge test. If the patient has a withdrawal bleed, then the amenorrhea is likely caused by anovulation. If there is no withdrawal bleed, it may indicate that there is also not enough estrogen around to create a uterine lining to bleed. This patient may need to be treated initially with estrogen and then undergo a progesterone challenge test to induce a withdrawal bleed as she has hypothalamic suppression. If the patient has symptoms of hirsutism, testosterone, dehydroepiandrosterone sulfate (DHEAS), and 17-OH progesterone should be drawn to evaluate for PCOS, testosterone-producing tumors in the ovary or adrenals, and adult-onset CAH.

If the uterus and/or the vagina is abnormal on imaging, a karyotype will differentiate between Müllerian agenesis and androgen insensitivity.

✋ Patient/parent advice

For patients and families with unexpected and uncommon diagnoses such as Müllerian anomalies, Turner syndrome, or androgen insensitivity, the introduction of a "buddy" who has a similar diagnosis and who has already gone through treatment can be helpful.

Summary

Work-up and evaluation of patients with amenorrhea include a complete history and physical exam. Lab tests are also helpful, as are some radiographic studies. Treatment depends on the etiology of the amenorrhea.

Further reading

Fritz MA, Speroff L. *Clinical Gynecologic Endocrinology and Infertility*. New York: Lippincott Williams & Wilkins, 2010.

Katz VL, Lobo RA, Lentz G, Gershenson D. *Comprehensive Gynecology*, 5th edn. Philadelphia: Mosby, 2007.

Reindollar RH, Byrd JR, McDonogh PG. Delayed sexual development: a study of 252 patients. *Am J Obstet Gynecol* 1981;140:371–380.

41 Abnormal uterine bleeding

Jennifer E. Dietrich and Jennifer L. Bercaw-Pratt

Division of Pediatric and Adolescent Gynecology, Department of Obstetrics and Gynecology, Baylor College of Medicine, Houston, TX, USA

Abnormal uterine bleeding (AUB) is a common reason that adolescents present to a physician. In order to understand what constitutes abnormal uterine bleeding, the practitioner must be familiar with what is normal (see Chapter 29.2) Menstrual cycles in young females usually last 7 days or less and typically occur 21–45 days apart (see Appendix 1.10). During the average cycle, the young woman may use three to six pads or tampons per day. The first 3 years of menses after menarche are often anovulatory. Following 3 years of menses, a young woman should expect her cycles to occur every 21–34 days.

Some common terminology used in the description of abnormal bleeding is defined in Table 41.1. It has been suggested that these commonly used terms be discarded in favor of more easily understood and defined terms (Table 41.2).

> ### ★ Tips and tricks
>
> Common questions used to take a good menstrual history are:
> - "How old were you when you had your first period?"
> - "Do you have monthly periods? If not, are they too close together? Or too far apart?"
> - "How many days does you period last?"
> - "How many pads/tampons do you typically use each day?"
> - "Do you pass blood clots? Size of clots?"
> - "Do you ever bleed through your pad/tampon onto your clothes?"
> - "Do you have cramps with your menstrual period?"

Evaluation

When a young woman presents to her physician for abnormal bleeding, it is very important to take a comprehensive history, including a menstrual history.

A current list of medications is also important to review since medications such as tricyclic antidepressants, antipsychotics, valproic acid, and warfarin can influence the menstrual cycle. It is important to establish if the patient is currently using any hormone therapy, since this can affect bleeding. An extensive social history is important and should be obtained from the adolescent in private, as this will establish the adolescent's risk for pregnancy or sexually-transmitted infections (STIs). Family history is also useful to determine risk for coagulation disorders. Finally, attention must be paid to recent changes in weight; neurologic symptoms such as migraine headaches with aura, vision changes or syncope; hematologic symptoms such as bleeding gums or nose

Practical Pediatric and Adolescent Gynecology, First Edition. Edited by Paula J. Adams Hillard.
© 2013 John Wiley & Sons, Ltd. Published 2013 by John Wiley & Sons, Ltd.

Table 41.1 Common terms used in the description of abnormal bleeding

Polymenorrhea	Regular menstrual cycles occurring <21 days apart
Menorrhagia	Loss of >80 mL of blood per cycle
Metrorrhagia	Noncyclic bleeding
Oligomenorrhea	Menstrual cycles that are between 45 days to 6 months apart
Secondary amenorrhea	No menstrual cycle for 6 months
Dysfunctional uterine bleeding	Abnormal uterine bleeding that is not the result of structural or systemic disease

Table 41.2 Menstrual descriptions

Cycle regularity	Irregular, regular, or absent
Frequency of menstruation	Frequent, normal, or infrequent
Duration of menstrual flow	Prolonged, normal, or shortened
Volume of menstrual flow	Heavy, normal, or light

Reproduced with permission from Fraser IS, *et al. Fertil Steril* 2007;87:466–476. Elsevier.

bleeds; and dermatologic symptoms such as acne or hirsutism.

A complete physical exam should be performed. Vital signs include pulse, blood pressure, and body mass index (BMI). An exam should look for acanthosis nigricans, acne, hirsutism, petechiae, or bruising. The thyroid should be palpated. Pubertal staging includes an exam of the external genitalia. A speculum exam is required if the patient is sexually active or there is a reason based on history to suspect trauma, a foreign object or tumor. When a speculum exam is done, any vaginal discharge, vaginal lesions, or cervical lesions should be noted.

A pelvic ultrasound (transabdominal or transvaginal in the sexually-active female) can determine if any uterine or ovarian anomalies exist. Rarely, a pelvic

MRI may be indicated if anomalies are detected on pelvic ultrasound.

Initial laboratory analysis includes a pregnancy test along with a complete blood count. If the patient is sexually active, evaluation for STIs is required. When the bleeding is excessive, a coagulation panel and a work-up for von Willebrand disease should be considered. If the abnormal bleeding is irregular in timing, evaluation for causes of anovulation are appropriate, including checking for hyperprolactinemia, thyroid dysfunction, abnormal ovarian function, or elevated androgen hormone levels.

Differential diagnosis

The differential diagnosis of abnormal bleeding in adolescents is extensive (Table 41.3). Generally, abnormal bleeding can be divided into two categories:

Table 41.3 Differential diagnosis for abnormal timing of menstrual bleeding in adolescents

- Pregnancy
- Endocrine causes:
  - Thyroid dysfunction
  - Polycystic ovarian syndrome
  - Premature ovarian failure
  - Poorly controlled diabetes
  - Late-onset congenital adrenal hyperplasia
- Infection:
  - Vaginitis
  - Cervicitis
  - Endometritis
- Uterine anomalies:
  - Endometrial polyps
  - Uterine fibroids
- Tumors:
  - Ovarian tumors such as a granulosa cell tumor
  - Adrenal tumors
  - Prolactinoma
- Acquired conditions:
  - Stress-related hypothalamic dysfunction
  - Exercise-induced amenorrhea
  - Eating disorders (both anorexia and bulimia)
- Intrauterine device (IUD)
- Foreign objects
- Trauma

irregular timing versus excessive flow. With excessive blood loss, the differential includes von Willebrand disease, thrombocytopenia, and liver disease.

Management

Treatment depends on the underlying etiology. The most common reason for AUB remains immaturity of the hypothalamic pituitary axis in adolescents; therefore, hormone imbalance becomes the focus of treatment. Excluding pregnancy, infection, or anatomic sources is paramount to treatment success. Treatment for bleeding unrelated to pregnancy can be divided into three categories: acute, chronic, and transitioning to a maintenance phase to avoid bleeding.

> ✋ **Caution**
>
> - Medical therapy is first-line therapy.
> - Surgical intervention should be undertaken only when absolutely necessary to preserve fertility and avoid unnecessary hospital admissions or transfusions.
> - Management depends on patient stability and the presence of mild, moderate or severe anemia.

Acute bleeding (Figure 41.1)

In the setting of acute bleeding, it is most important to establish whether hemodynamic instability is

Acute Abnormal Bleeding

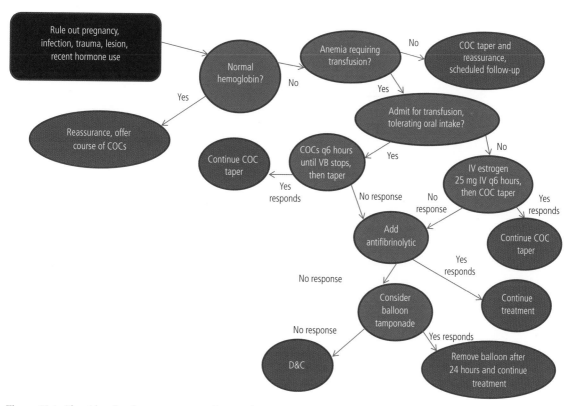

Figure 41.1 Algorithm for the management of acute abnormal bleeding.

present. Even the stable patient may become hemo-dynamically unstable if heavy bleeding is not addressed quickly. Two large-bore intravenous lines are critical to begin the resuscitation process for an orthostatic patient. In the absence of orthostasis, IV access may still be important for medications or blood products, depending on coagulopathy or if anemia is present.

Treatment options for heavy bleeding including IV conjugated estrogen (for patients unable to tolerate oral intake), high dose or low-dose combined oral contraceptive (COC) pills or high-dose progestins (Table 41.4). Antiemetic medications may be pre-scribed prophylactically to increase oral hormone tolerability. A careful review of the patient's medical history is important to establish whether a patient is a candidate for estrogen-containing medications. In patients in whom a coagulopathy is suspected, col-laboration with a hematologist may be helpful, since hemostatic agents such as DDAVP or clotting factor concentrates may be required in addition to hormonal therapy to control severe acute bleeding episodes. Finally, in the setting of severe bleeding unresponsive to medical treatment, the use of a 30-mL intrauterine Foley balloon may be necessary.

As maintaining fertility is paramount in this population, D&C or irreversible surgery, such as endometrial ablation or hysterectomy, should be avoided and utilized only in the setting of failed medical management.

Table 41.4 Options for treatment of acute abnormal uterine bleeding

Treatment	Dosage	Contraceptive benefit?
IV conjugated estrogen	25 mg IV every 4–6 hours until bleeding stops, then transition to COC	No initially; yes when on COC
Combined oral contraceptives (COCs)	Traditionally, any COC with 30, 35 or 50 μg ethinyl estradiol with high dose, tapering to lower dose, e.g. one tablet every 8 hours for 7 days, then every 12 hours for 7 days, then once per day thereafter, and ultimately allowing withdrawal bleeding to shed dys-synchronous endometrium	Yes
High-dose progestins	Norethindrone acetate 5–10 mg every 4 hours until bleeding stops, then every 6 hours for 4 days, then every 8 hours for 3 days, then every 12 hours for 2–14 days, then once per day thereafter or Medroxyprogesterone 10 mg (and up to 80 mg maximum) every 4 hours until bleeding stops, then every 6 hours for 4 days, then every 8 hours for 3 days, then every 12 hours for 2–14 days, then once per day thereafter	Possible-dependent on dose and type of progestin and consistency of use
Antifibrinolytics	Aminocaproic acid: 5–30 g orally/day divided every 3–6 hours for 5–7 days or 4–5 g IV over 60 minutes (maximum 30 g/day). Use every 8 hours or until bleeding is controlled, then taper to oral Tranexamic acid: 650 mg orally three times per day for 5–7 days or 10 mg/kg IV every 6–8 hours for 2–8 days	No
NSAIDs	Any NSAID with scheduled dosing for 3–5 days	No
Doxycycline	100 mg twice a day for 10 days	No

Chronic bleeding (Figure 41.2)

Many patients with chronic AUB may be managed in the outpatient setting. Fortunately, there are currently many hormonal combinations available. High-dose COC regimens that taper to a lower dose can control acute AUB episodes. Non-hormonal options are available as well (Table 41.4). To improve adolescents' compliance with hormonal therapy, it is important to review with them how to properly take these medications in addition to discussing the use, anticipated side effects, and expected length of treatment.

✋ Caution

• Hormonal therapies containing estrogen should be avoided in adolescents with risk factors for cardiovascular disease or thromboembolic disease.
• Consider progestin-only methods in these patients.

✋ Patient/parent advice

• Hormonal therapies require consistent use and long-term follow-up.
• Initial breakthrough bleeding can occur even with correct use, and should not be a reason to discontinue the therapy.

Maintenance phase therapies

Once an initial treatment plan has been successful in controlling an adolescent's AUB, it is important to establish a plan to prevent both emergent bleeding and unscheduled bleeding episodes. Hormonal options for young females include COCs, the transdermal patch, vaginal ring, and progestin-only options, including depot medroxyprogesterone acetate, progestin-only pills, the contraceptive subdermal implant, and the levonorgestrel intrauterine device (see Chapters 34.2–34.5). Other options

Chronic Abnormal Bleeding

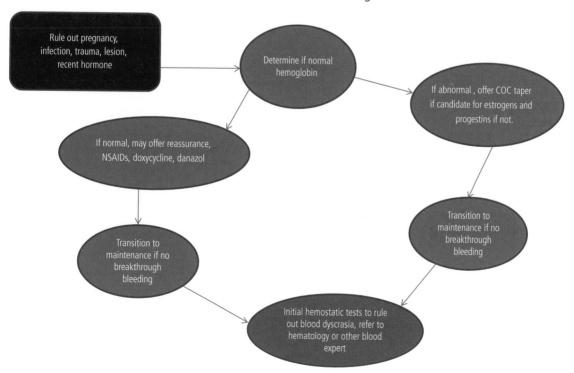

Figure 41.2 Algorithm for the management of chronic abnormal bleeding.

include a gonadotropin-releasing hormone (GnRH) agonist or danocrine, although side effects of the latter limit use. Adolescents may choose to cycle monthly, bimonthly or quarterly depending on their needs.

✋ Caution

- For adolescents with AUB, it is *imperative* to rule out pregnancy as hormonal therapy will be ineffective.
- With acute hemorrhage, hemodynamic stability must be established.
- With hemodynamic instability and a positive pregnancy test, ectopic pregnancy must be considered (see Chapter 47).

Special management considerations

One in four teens will contract a STI. It is important to rule out infection as a source for AUB. Rarely, bleeding in adolescents may be associated with vaginal or vulvar lesions such as condyloma, an endometrial polyp, or uterine leiomyomas.

Evidence at a glance

Nonhormonal treatment (Table 41.4)
- Evidence supports the use of NSAIDs for decreasing AUB compared to placebo.
- Doxycycline has shown some benefit in small studies among women with implant-related dysfunctional bleeding episodes. The generalizability of this treatment is not known with regard to other types of abnormal bleeding unrelated to the implant.
- Antifibrinolytics have shown the most promise in addressing AUB episodes, although there are limited data in the adolescent population.

Summary

Management of AUB in adolescents is dependent on the cause. Ruling out other conditions such as pregnancy or bleeding disorders is important to ensure success with hormonal or nonhormonal treatments. It is helpful for providers to consider the presentation, whether emergent or nonemergent, and the presence or absence of anemia, to guide treatment decisions. Both hormonal and nonhormonal options exist for the management of chronic abnormal uterine bleeding. Finally, there are many options for the maintenance phase of treatment.

Further reading

American College of Obstetricians and Gynecologists. Menstruation in girls and adolescents: using the menstrual cycle as a vital sign. ACOG Committee Opinion No. 349. *Obstet Gynecol* 2006:1323–1328.

Benjamins LJ. Practice guidelines: evaluation and management of abnormal vaginal bleeding in adolescents. *J Pediatr Health Care* 2009;23(3):189–193.

LaCour DE, Long DN, Perlman SE. Dysfunctional uterine bleeding in adolescent females associated with endocrine causes and medical conditions. *J Pediatr Adolesc Gynecol* 2010;23(2):62–70.

42 Premenstrual syndrome/premenstrual dysphoric disorder and mood disorders

Michael Dobbs and Paula Braverman

Division of Adolescent Medicine, Cincinnati Children's Hospital Medical Center, Cincinnati, OH, USA

Premenstrual syndrome (PMS) describes a set of physical, behavioral, and cognitive symptoms that occur in 75–80% of postmenarchal women during the luteal phase of the menstrual cycle and resolve quickly once menstruation begins. Premenstrual dysphoric disorder (PMDD), which affects 2–8% of reproductive-age women, is a distinct entity in the mental health field and is characterized by severe premenstrual emotional and behavioral symptoms that interfere with daily functioning on multiple levels, including social, work/school, and quality of life. Although strict DSM IV criteria exist for the diagnosis of PMDD (see Table 42.2), the American College of Obstetricians and Gynecologists (ACOG) has provided less stringent criteria for PMS, since studies involving adult women show that 20–40% describe premenstrual symptoms that interfere with daily functioning. One recent study utilizing the Premenstrual Symptoms Screening Tool revised for adolescents demonstrated that approximately one-third had severe PMS or PMDD.

The relationship between PMS and PMDD is under debate; some argue that the two represent differing degrees of severity for the same clinical entity, while others maintain that they are distinct entities with differing pathophysiology. The exact etiology for PMS/PMDD is unknown, but is thought to be related to enhanced responsiveness to the cyclic changes in normal serum levels of sex steroids (estrogen and progesterone) and their interaction with neurotransmitters.

> ## ⚕ Science revisited
>
> • The development of premenstrual symptoms is thought to be related to interactions between sex steroids and neurotransmitters such as serotonin, γ-aminobutyric acid (GABA), glutamate, and beta endorphins.
> • Twin studies suggest possible heritable factors in PMS/PMDD, including genes for the serotonergic 5HT1A receptor and the estrogen receptor alpha gene (*ESR1*).

Diagnosis

Over 200 affective and physical premenstrual symptoms have been described. The six core symptoms are: anxiety/tension, mood swings, aches, food cravings, cramps, and decreased interest in activities. Since many women with retrospective complaints of PMS/PMDD have symptoms that extend beyond the luteal phase, it is critical that the diagnosis be made prospectively. Whether utilizing the ACOG or DSM IV criteria, documentation of luteal-phase perimenstrual

---

Practical Pediatric and Adolescent Gynecology, First Edition. Edited by Paula J. Adams Hillard.
© 2013 John Wiley & Sons, Ltd. Published 2013 by John Wiley & Sons, Ltd.

Table 42.1 Adapted diagnostic criteria for PMS

1. At least one affective and one somatic symptom must be present in the prior three menstrual cycles during the 5 days before the onset of menses
2. The symptoms must resolve within 4 days of the onset of menses
3. Symptoms must be present using prospective recording for at least two cycles
4. The symptoms must adversely affect social or work activities

Affective symptoms	Somatic symptoms
Depression	Headache
Anxiety	Breast tenderness
Irritability	Abdominal bloating
Angry outbursts	Extremity swelling
Social withdrawal	
Confusion	

Reproduced with permission from American College of Obstetricians and Gynecologists. *Premenstrual Syndrome.* ACOG Practice Bulletin No. 15. 2000. Adapted from Mortola JF, Girton L, Yen SS. Depressive episodes in pre-menstrual syndrome. *Am J Obstet Gynecol* 1989;161:1682–1687. Lippincott Williams & Wilkins.

symptoms that significantly interfere with daily activities over several menstrual cycles is key to the diagnosis (Table 42.1).

The American Psychiatric Association's DSM IV-TR has laid out specific diagnostic criteria for PMDD. At least five of the symptoms listed in Table 42.2, one of which one must be a *major* symptom, must have been present in most menstrual cycles in the preceding year. Additionally, these symptoms must significantly interfere with social or work functioning, cannot be an exacerbation of other disorders, and must also be prospectively recorded. Many diagnostic tools for PMS/PMDD are available.

In some cases, there may be menstrual exacerbation of an underlying psychiatric or medical problem. Other diagnoses that must be considered include psychiatric diagnoses such as depression, anxiety, dysthymia, personality disorder, substance abuse, and bipolar disorder; and medical diagnoses such as autoimmune disorders, hypothyroidism, anemia, and endometriosis. There are no specific physical findings or laboratory tests that can be used to make the diagnosis of PMS/PMDD.

Table 42.2 PMDD symptoms

Major symptoms
- Affective lability
- Increased anxiety/tension
- Depressed mood or affect
- Persistent anger or interpersonal conflicts

Minor symptoms
- Changes in appetite
- Changes in sleep patterns
- Lethargy or fatigue
- Decreased interest in activities
- Difficulty with concentration
- Feeling overwhelmed or out of control
- Physical symptoms such as bloating, weight gain, headache, or breast tenderness

Based on data from The American Psychiatric Association. *Diagnostic and Statistical Manual of Mental Disorders, Fourth Edition, Text Revision.* Washington, DC: American Psychiatric Association, 2000, pp. 717–718.

> ✱ **Tips and tricks**
>
> - Use prospectively recorded symptoms over several menstrual cycles when making the diagnosis of PMS/PMDD.
> - Symptoms must occur during the luteal phase and resolve shortly after menses start.
> - Using a menstrual calendar to record symptoms in relation to menses can aid in making the diagnosis.

> ✋ **Patient/parent advice**
>
> - Menstrual-related symptoms are very common and do not necessarily represent PMS or PMDD.
> - Understanding the common symptoms associated with normal menstrual periods can help allay anxiety.
> - Diagnostic surveys are available to assist in the diagnosis.

Management

There are no universally accepted treatments for PMS/PMDD, especially in adolescents. Nevertheless, some treatment modalities have demonstrated efficacy in adult women and interventions should be targeted to specific symptom profiles.

Nonpharmacologic management

Lifestyle changes, including the establishment of regular exercise and stress management, appear to be effective at reducing the severity and frequency of symptoms. Other techniques include education regarding the normal menstrual cycle and cognitive behavioral therapy for more severe cases. Dietary changes with increased complex carbohydrates may be helpful by raising tryptophan, which is a precursor to serotonin.

Although there are a multitude of claims for the use of vitamins, minerals and supplements, very few well designed studies exist. There is evidence that calcium carbonate (1200 mg/day) can reduce physical and emotional symptoms and that herbal preparations containing vitex agnus-castus (which lower prolactin levels) or ginko biloba are effective.

Pharmacological management

Although antianxiolytics and antidepressants have been utilized symptomatically; as a class of drugs, selective serotonin reuptake inhibitors (SSRIs) have been well studied in adults and found to be effective for treatment of severe PMS/PMDD. SSRIs improve both physical and affective symptoms and can be considered a first-line option in patients with severe mood symptoms. Treatment does not need to be continuous; using the drugs only during the luteal phase is just as effective for mood symptoms. However, somatic symptoms may respond better to continuous dosing. Symptoms improve within 1–2 days and there is no "ramp up" time as there is with the treatment of depression. Because use is intermittent, there is little risk of developing SSRI withdrawal effects. Low doses can be used and side effects are usually minimal.

There are a paucity of studies on the use of SSRIs for PMS/PMDD in adolescents, but the recommended dose of fluoxetine is 20 mg/day, which would be applicable to this age group. Prescribers should be familiar with the 2004 FDA "black box" warning regarding the use of antidepressants in children and adolescents, which describes increased suicidal thoughts and attempts related to initiation of SSRIs.

Evidence at a glance

- SSRIs are well studied for the treatment of PMS/PMDD in adult women and have been found to be safe and effective.
- Most research indicates intermittent use of SSRIs during the luteal phase is as effective as continuous use, though some patients benefit from continuous use.

Suppression of hormonal cycling and ovulation with oral contraceptive pills (OCPs) or medroxyprogesterone acetate has also been widely used for the treatment of menstrual-related symptoms and are considered first-line therapy by some authors. Gonadotropin-releasing hormone (GnRH) agonists are also very effective, but are a last resort in adolescents because of issues related to bone density. Data on the effectiveness of OCPs are mixed, as some women report worsening of symptoms, and physical symptoms are more effectively treated than affective symptoms. Studies have suggested that shortening the hormone-free period and extended cycling may be more effective than traditional monthly cycling. An OCP formulation containing the newer synthetic progestin, drospirenone, has shown promise. Specifically, the formulation, containing 20 µg of ethinyl estradiol in a 24/4 cycling regimen has been shown to significantly improve both somatic and mood symptoms of PMDD in placebo-controlled trials. It is postulated that the antialdosterone and antiandrogenic effects of this novel progestin may contribute to its efficacy.

✋ Caution

Although all estrogen containing hormonal contraceptives have an increased risk of venous thromboembolism (VTE), recent reports have found evidence that third-generation progestins, including drospirenone, may be associated with a higher risk of VTE than OCPs with older generation progestins.

Initially, all patients with mild PMS symptoms should be offered nonpharmacologic therapy. Those with persistent symptoms after 2–3 months and those diagnosed with severe PMS or PMDD should be offered pharmacologic therapy. SSRIs are the initial recommended treatment modality for patients with PMDD. Since SSRIs will primarily improve mood symptoms, if there are significant somatic symptoms, suppression of ovulation with OCPs should also be considered as well as use of spironolactone or nonsteroidal anti-inflammatory drugs for specific somatic symptoms.

Follow-up

Following up 2–3 months after starting therapeutic intervention is recommended to assess clinical response. Use of diagnostic PMS/PMDD survey tools may be useful as objective measures of response.

The use of GnRH agonists in the case of severe symptoms is beyond the scope of this text and consultation with a gynecologist is recommended.

♀ Pearls

- Because premenstrual symptoms are very common, prospective evaluation in relation to the menstrual cycle is essential to the diagnosis of PMS/PMDD.
- Pharmacologic intervention utilizing OCPs containing drosperinone or intermittent SSRIs is appropriate and effective for moderate to severe PMS/PMDD.

Further reading

Cunningham J, Yonkers KA, O'Brien S, *et al.* Update on research and treatment of premenstrual dysphoric disorder. *Harvard Rev Psychiatry* 2009;17(2):120–137.

Freeman EW, Halberstadt SM, Rickels K, *et al.* Core symptoms that discriminate premenstrual syndrome. *J Womens Health* 2011;20:29–35.

Steiner M, Peer M, Palova E, *et al.* The Premenstrual Symptoms Screening Tool Revised for Adolescents (PSST-A): Prevalence of severe PMS and premenstrual dysphoric disorder in adolescents. *Arch Womens Mental Health* 2011;14:77–81.

43.1 Yeast/candida

Sofya Maslyanskaya and Elizabeth Alderman

Albert Einstein College of Medicine, Children's Hospital at Montefiore, Bronx, NY, USA

Common symptoms of vulvovaginal yeast infections include: pruritus, external dysuria, vaginal soreness, and dyspareunia. The most specific symptom is pruritus, but this only occurs in 38% of patients. Vaginal discharge varies in amount and consistency, from watery to a "cheesy" thick, white discharge (see Figure 10.1.9). Signs include vulvar edema, erythema, fissures, excoriations, and thick white curdy vaginal discharge. Three in every four women will have at least one episode of vulvovaginal candidiasis (VVC) in their lifetimes, and 40–45% will have two or more episodes. Recurrent VVC is defined as at least four episodes in 1 year, and occurs in less than 5% of women.

> ### ✋ Caution
>
> *Candida albicans* vulvovaginitis is uncommon in prepubescent girls and occurs mostly in association with a recent course of antibiotics, diabetes mellitus, immunodeficiency, or wearing of occlusive clothing or diapers.

Diagnosis (Table 43.1.1)

VVC exacerbations usually occur the week before menses or after a course of antibiotics or corticosteroids.

> ### ⚛ Science revisited
>
> • *Yeast blastosphores* are responsible for vaginal transmission and asymptomatic colonization.
> • *Hyphae* are chains of cells produced by germinated yeast and are found most commonly in symptomatic vaginitis.

Predisposing factors are listed in Table 43.1.2. Indicated or helpful diagnostic tests are:
• Perform wet preparation with saline and 10% KOH, and assess vaginal pH. 10% KOH improves visualization of yeast by disrupting its cellular matrix. Visualization of yeast, hyphae, pseudohyphae on wet prep (Figure 43.1.1) or Gram stain, or culture positive for a *Candida* species, is diagnostic. Discharge is associated with normal pH (4.5).
• Gram stain also shows a normal number of polymorphonuclear leukocytes.
• Fungal cultures are expensive and not readily available and should only be performed if wet prep or Gram stain is negative and the patient is symptomatic, despite first-line treatment.
• The differential diagnosis of vaginal discharge includes *Trichomonas vaginalis*, bacterial vaginosis, and physiologic leukorrhea (see Chapter 43.2). A

Practical Pediatric and Adolescent Gynecology, First Edition. Edited by Paula J. Adams Hillard.
© 2013 John Wiley & Sons, Ltd. Published 2013 by John Wiley & Sons, Ltd.

Table 43.1.1 Assessment

History
- Symptoms:
  ◦ Vaginal discharge
  ◦ Pruritus
  ◦ Dyspareunia
  ◦ External dysuria
  ◦ Vaginal pain
  ◦ Vulvar rash
- Duration of symptoms
- Relationship to menses
- Previous sexual activity
- Contraceptive use
- Pregnancy
- Recent course of antibiotics or steroid medications

Review of systems
- Symptoms of diabetes mellitus: polyuria, polydipsia, and polyphagia
- Immunologic deficiency: fevers, rashes, infections, hospital admissions for evaluation, and treatment of infections
- HIV: high-risk sexual behaviors, prior testing, and results

Physical exam
- There are rarely systemic signs of infection unless the patient is immunocompromised
- External genital examination:
  ◦ Vulvar edema
  ◦ Erythema
  ◦ Fissures
  ◦ Excoriations
  ◦ Thick white curdy vaginal discharge
  ◦ Pustulopapular peripheral skin lesions

DNA probe-based test, Affirm VP III, evaluates for *Trichomonas vaginalis, Gardnerella vaginalis,* as well as *C. albicans.* The test has a sensitivity greater than 83% and a specificity of greater 97%, and results are available within 45 minutes.

> ### ⚠ Caution
>
> 10–20% of women have vaginal colonization with *Candida* species and other yeasts.

Table 43.1.2 Predisposing factors for candida vaginitis

Genetic	Mannose-binding lectin polymorphism
Behavioral	Intercourse frequency/regularity
	Receptive orogenital sexual activity
	Inconsistent evidence regarding oral contraceptive pill
Dermatologic	Eczema
	Lichen sclerosus
HIV positive	More likely to have non-albicans *Candida* species
	Prophylaxis not recommended unless recurrent VVC
Medical conditions	Diabetes mellitus
	Immunodeficiency
	Recent course of antibiotics

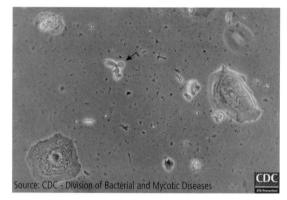

Source: CDC - Division of Bacterial and Mycotic Diseases

Figure 43.1.1 Wet prep with yeast buds.

Management

Vaginal cultures should be considered if a woman is symptomatic and physical exam is suggestive of vulvovaginal candidiasis or has significant risk factors, such as immunodeficiency or diabetes mellitus, and the wet prep is negative. Empiric treatment should be considered if vaginal cultures cannot be performed.

Self-diagnosis of VVC is not accurate and women who use over-the-counter medications for a presumptive diagnosis of candidiasis should seek medical attention if there is no resolution of symptoms within 7 days after treatment.

Treatment varies based on diagnosis of uncomplicated or complicated VVC. Severity of VVC is based on the presence of vulvar erythema, edema, excoriations, and fissures.

- **Uncomplicated VVC:** infrequent or mild to moderate in severity or likely caused by *C. albicans*.
- **Complicated VVC:** recurrent (at least four infections a year), or in a patient with immunosuppression, uncontrolled diabetes or severe VVC, or caused by non-albicans *Candida*.

> ★ **Tips and tricks**
>
> Consider sending a culture to assess for non-albicans *Candida* if a patient has recurrent VVC.

> ⚛ **Science revisited**
>
> - 85–95% of VVC is caused by *C. albicans*.
> - 5–15% is caused by *C. glabrata, parapsilosis*, and *krusei*, which are more resistant to treatment.

Uncomplicated vulvovaginal candidiasis

Therapy for uncomplicated VVC is described in Table 43.1.3.

> ✋ **Caution**
>
> Fluconazole is a pregnancy category C drug.

> ★ **Tips and tricks**
>
> Most patients prefer the convenience of oral administration, particularly those who are not sexually active or who have not used tampons.

> ✋ **Patient advice**
>
> Creams and suppositories are oil-based and may weaken latex condoms and diaphragms, compromising effectiveness (refer to condom product labeling).

Table 43.1.3 Recommended treatments for uncomplicated VVC

Over-the-counter	Prescription
Butoconazole 2% cream 5 g intravaginally for 3 days	Butoconazole 2% cream 5 g intravaginally for 1 day
Clotrimazole 1% 5 g intravaginally for 7–14 days	Nystatin 100 000-Unit vaginal tablet intravaginally for 14 days
Clotrimazole 2% cream 5 g intravaginally for 3 days	Terconazole 0.4% 5 g intravaginally for 7 days
Miconazole 2% cream 5 g intravaginally for 7 days	Terconazole 0.8% 5 g intravaginally for 3 days
Miconazole 4% cream 5 g intravaginally for 3 days	Terconazole 80 mg vaginal suppository; one suppository intravaginally for 3 days
Miconazole 100 mg vaginal suppository; one suppository intravaginally for 7 days	Fluconazole 150 mg tablet once; consider this method strongly if not sexually active and has not used tampons
Miconazole 200 mg suppository; one suppository intravaginally for 3 days	
Miconazole 1200 mg suppository; one suppository intravaginally for 1 day	
Tioconazole 6.5% ointment; 5 g intravaginally in a single application	

> ⚛ **Science revisited**
>
> Azoles work by inhibiting cytochrome p450 oxidase-mediated synthesis of ergosterol, an essential component of the fungal cytoplasmic membrane.

Complicated vulvovaginal candidiasis

Patients with complicated VVC should be treated with a longer course of antifungals, either 7–14 days

✋ Patient/parent advice

Side effects

• **Topical azoles:** usually no systemic side effects; infrequent local vaginal burning or irritation.

• **Oral azoles:** nausea, abdominal pain, headache, and altered palate; rarely abnormal elevations of liver enzymes.

• **Boric acid:** vulvovaginal burning and male partner dyspareunia if intercourse occurs after recent treatment.

• **Lactobacilli:** gastrointestinal disturbances in those with lactose intolerance and lactobacillemia in women who are immunosuppressed.

of topical or three doses (taken every third day: day 1, 4, and 7) of oral fluconazole in an attempt to produce clinical remission prior to initiating maintenance therapy.

If vaginal culture is indicative of *C. glabrata*, then a non-fluconazole azole should be used for treatment. If the infection recurs, then treatment with 600 mg of vaginal boric acid daily for 2 weeks should be initiated.

Maintenance treatments for patients with complicated VVC may be considered:
• Oral fluconazole weekly for 6 months
• Oral ketoconazole 100 mg daily for 6 months
• Clotrimazole 500 mg suppository once weekly for 6 months.

Follow-up

Patients should return if symptoms persist or if they recur within 2 months of the initial onset of symptoms. Cultures are negative in 80–90% of women after the course of treatment is completed. Avoidance of tight clothing and noncotton underwear to reduce moisture may help to prevent recurrences.

Further reading

Centers for Disease Control and Prevention. Sexually transmitted disease treatment guidelines. 2010. *MMWR Morb Mortal Wkly Rep* 2010;59:61–63.

Sobel JD. Vulvovaginal candidosis. *Lancet* 2007;369:1961–1971.

Van Kessel K, Assefi N, Marrazzo J, Eckert L. Common complementary and alternative therapies for yeast vaginitis and bacterial vaginosis: a systematic review. *Obstet Gynecol Surv* 2003;58:351–358.

43.2 Bacterial vaginosis

Jennifer Louis-Jacques and Rebecca Flynn O'Brien

Division of Adolescent/Young Adult Medicine, Children's Hospital Boston, Harvard Medical School, Boston, MA, USA

Bacterial vaginosis (BV) is a common cause of vaginal discharge that in some women can be chronic and recurrent. BV is found in 4–15% of college students, 10–25% of pregnant women, and 30–37% of women attending sexually-transmitted infection (STI) clinics. It is the result of both replacement of normal vaginal flora (*Lactobacilli* spp.), an increased concentration of *Gardnerella vaginalis*, and an overgrowth of anaerobic bacteria. With newer molecular techniques many new organisms have been identified to be associated with BV, termed BV-associated bacteria. Disruption of the normal acidic vaginal environment from extrinsic factors (e.g. douches, sexual intercourse, bacteriophages) results in alteration of the vaginal pH and resultant reduction in the native lactobacilli population. This ultimately allows other bacteria to populate the vagina, leading to the symptoms associated with BV.

> ### ☆ Science revisited
>
> - *Lactobacilli* spp. constitute the normal flora of the lower genital tract of women.
> - *Lactobacilli* spp. metabolize glycogen produced by the vaginal mucosa under the influence of estrogen, resulting in lactic acid production.
> - Lactic acid in combination with hydrogen peroxide production produces the normal acidic environment of the vagina.

BV is characterized by a thin, homogenous white, yellow or gray discharge, usually with a fishy/amine odor that smoothly adheres to the vaginal wall. BV is a sexually-*associated* infection occurring primarily in women of reproductive age. Associated risk factors are listed in Table 43.2.1. Half of women with BV have no symptoms. It is important to obtain a thorough sexual history, as BV can increase risk for infection with other STIs, pelvic inflammatory disease, and complications in pregnancy.

> ### ✋ Caution
>
> - Although BV is typically associated with sexual activity, BV can occur in virginal females.
> - The diagnosis should not be excluded in school-age girls if the right clinical scenario is present.

Diagnosis

Diagnosis of BV is typically made by microscopy using Amsel's criteria (Table 43.2.2); presence of three of the four criteria fulfills the diagnosis (Figure 43.2.1). However, even having two of the four criteria can be sufficient, with elevated vaginal pH and positive whiff test being the most sensitive and specific

Table 43.2.1 Risk factors for bacterial vaginosis

- Ethnicity (black race)
- Cigarette smoking
- New or multiple sex partners
- Intrauterine device
- Early age of sexual intercourse
- Oral sex
- Frequent douching (>1x/week)
- Sex during menses
- Sexual activity with other women (?shared sex toys)

Table 43.2.2 Amsel's criteria for clinical diagnosis of bacterial vaginosis

Three of the following four signs or symptoms to be present:
- Homogenous, thin, white adherent vaginal discharge
- Presence of clue cells (see Figure 37.1) on saline wet smear
- Positive whiff test [amine (fishy) odor of vaginal discharge with addition of 10% -KOH]
- Vaginal pH >4.5

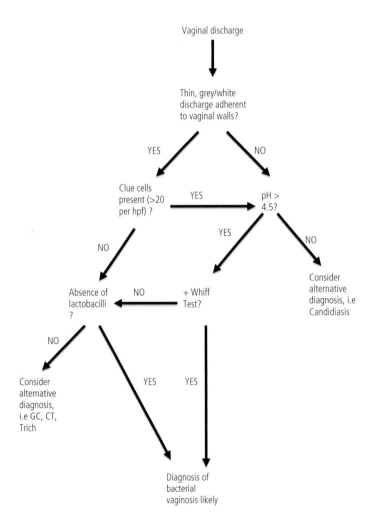

Figure 43.2.1 Algorithm for diagnosis of bacterial vaginosis.

criteria. Point of care tests can be used when microscopy is not available. Diagnosis by Pap smear or cultures for *G. vaginalis* is not recommended.

✭ Tips and tricks

- While the presence of clue cells (Figure 43.2.2) is one of the Amsel's criteria for diagnosis of BV, the absence of lactobacilli on normal saline wet prep can be supportive of the diagnosis.
- Elevated pH, malodorous vaginal discharge, and lack of increased white blood cells can help distinguish BV from trichomoniasis, a vaginitis also associated with elevated pH.

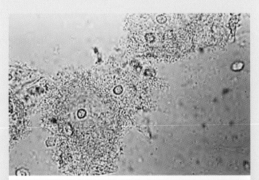
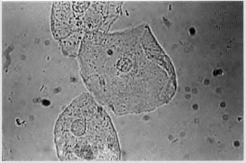

Figure 43.2.2 Bacterial vaginosis microsopy: Clue cells. ©Seattle HIV/STD Training Center. *Source*: University of Washington

Management

Treatment is indicated for any symptomatic patient, especially pregnant women, for whom BV is associ-

ated with increased risk of spontaneous miscarriages and preterm birth. For nonpregnant women, untreated BV is associated with increased risk of STI acquisition and postabortive endometritis. Treatment of sexual partners is not indicated, as it is not associated with reduced recurrences, although use of condoms may decrease recurrences. Standard treatment of BV involves either oral or intravaginal agents (Table 43.2.3). Patients should be encouraged to avoid douching and refrain from sexual intercourse during treatment. However, if unable to abstain they should be encouraged to properly use condoms.

Evidence at a glance

- Numerous studies have investigated nonantibiotic forms of treatment.
- Research is mixed with respect to intravaginal or oral probiotic use in conjunction with or in place of antibiotics.
- Some studies show superiority of probiotics while others show no difference compared to standard care.
- Attempts to re-acidify the vagina with intravaginal application of H_2O_2 found high clinical failure rates as well as undesirable side effect of local irritation.

✋ Patient advice

- Avoid douching.
- Condom use is recommended for all sexually-active young women and may prevent risk of recurrent BV.

Once treated, further follow-up is not necessary, but recurrences within the following year are common. It still unclear what leads to recurrences, but there is some thought that it is a result of persistence of anaerobic organisms and failure of lactobacilli to re-colonize the vagina. Unfortunately, an adequate treatment regimen to prevent recurrences has not emerged.

Table 43.2.3 Treatment of bacterial vaginosis

Treatment Regimen	Nonpregnant Women	Pregnant Women
Metronidazole 500 mg PO BID x 7 days	x	x
Metronidazole 0.75% gel, intravaginal daily x 5 days	x	
Clindamycin 2% cream, intravaginal bedtime x 7 days	x	
Tinidazole 2 g PO daily x 2 days*	x	
Tinidazole 1 g PO daily x 5 days*	x	
Clindamycin 300 mg PO BID x 7 days*	x	x
Clindamycin 100 mg ovules, intravaginal bedtime x 3 days*	x	
Metronidazole 250 mg PO TID x 7 days		x

*Alternative regimen.
Based on 2010 CDC STD treatment guidelines.

Further reading

Berlan ED, Emans SJ, O'Brien RF. Vulvovaginal complaints in the adolescent. In: Emans SJ, Laufer MR (eds). *Pediatric & Adolescent Gynecology*, 6th edn. Philadelphia: Lippincott Williams & Wilkins, 2012.

Donders G. Diagnosis and management of bacterial vaginosis and other types of abnormal vaginal bacterial flora: A review. *Obstet Gynecol Surv* 2010;65:2010.

Workowski KA, Berman S; Centers for Disease Control and Prevention. Sexually transmitted diseases treatment guidelines, 2010. *MMWR* 2010;59(12):1–110.

44.1 Genital herpes

Terri Warren
Westover Heights Clinic, Portland, OR, USA

Genital herpes is the most prevalent (and the third most incident) sexually-transmitted infection (STI) in the US. It can be caused by either herpes simplex virus type 1 or type 2, but HSV 1 is more common in teens and young adults.

> ### ⚛ Science revisited
>
> • HSV, an alphaherpesvirus, has an incubation period, from infection to symptoms, of 2–14 days, most commonly about 5 days.
> • Many first infections are completely asymptomatic, or symptoms are confused with some other condition.
> • 80% of those infected with HSV 2 do not know they are infected.

If symptoms are present, they may include sores in the genital area, dysuria, and flu-like symptoms, including myalgia, headache, light sensitivity, achiness, pain down the back of the leg, and lymphadenopathy. First infections commonly appear in the genital area (including the anus even without anal exposure) but recurrences can appear anywhere in the boxer shorts area (the area innervated by the sacral ganglia). Genitally, HSV 2 recurs on average four to six times per year, and HSV 1 far less often, about once every other year. About half of infected people experience something called a prodrome. Symptoms of the prodrome include tingling, skin sensitivity, and a crawling under the skin feeling that heralds an outbreak. Because of the receptive nature of intercourse, more females than males are infected with herpes. For reasons that are not completely clear, African-Americans are almost twice as likely to be infected with HSV 2 as Caucasians.

Diagnosis

Since herpes is a lifelong, highly-stigmatizing infection, getting the diagnosis right is essential. The Centers for Disease Control and Prevention (CDC) in its 2010 STD treatment guidelines states that HSV diagnosis should be made by lab test, not examination alone. It also states that any test for HSV, be it swab or antibody test, needs to be capable of making the distinction between HSV 1 and HSV 2. There are two ways to diagnose herpes using lab tests: swab tests from lesions and antibody tests from blood.

Though HSV culture is still commonly used, gene amplification tests [such as polymerase chain reaction (PCR)] are considered now to be the most sensitive and specific swab tests available. Collection media for culture and PCR are usually the same. The distinction is simply what is requested on the lab form. Type-specific IgG tests in those older than 12 years are quite

Practical Pediatric and Adolescent Gynecology, First Edition. Edited by Paula J. Adams Hillard.
© 2013 John Wiley & Sons, Ltd. Published 2013 by John Wiley & Sons, Ltd.

Evidence at a glance

- Genital herpes caused by HSV 2 in people aged 14–19 years is on the decline. Only 2% of this US group had HSV 2 infection in 2010.
- Though we know that the vast majority of people with HSV 2 antibody are infected genitally, it is far less clear how many people infected with HSV 1 have it genitally. The old adage that everything below the waist is HSV 2 and everything above is HSV 1 has been laid to rest.
- As oral sex becomes more and more common in sexual practice, so is the transmission of HSV 1 from the mouth to the genital area. This can occur both when a cold sore is present and when one is not, through asymptomatic viral shedding or unrecognized infection.
- Several studies have demonstrated the high rate of HSV 1 infection in young people (78% of new genital infections were HSV 1 in a study at the University of Wisconsin in Madison).
- Making the distinction between HSV 1 and HSV 2 genitally is important:
  ○ HSV 1 recurs far less often than HSV 2 genitally (0.7 vs 4–6 recurrences per year).
  ○ There is a strong link between the acquisition of HIV and having HSV 2 infection, but no such link exists for HSV 1 and HIV.

person who has had a cold sore would suggest that the infection is only oral.

✋ Caution

- Diagnosis by physical exam alone is not recommended by the CDC for the diagnosis of genital herpes:
  ○ A diagnosis of HSV based on visual exam alone in the absence of lab tests is wrong 20% of the time
  ○ Typing of the virus (HSV1 vs HSV2) by visual exam is not possible, as lesions caused by both types look identical.
- Serologic antibody tests in children younger than 12 years are not recommended due to high rates of false positives.
- There are also a significant number (50%) of false-positive HSV 2 results in people who have an index value of between 1.1 and 3.5 on the type-specific antibody test. People who test in this range need a confirmatory test, preferably a Western blot.

Teens may be less likely to get tested for herpes than older adults (Table 44.1.1).

Management

All first infections (or suspected first infections) should be treated with antivirals.

specific and sensitive if enough time has passed between infection and testing (4 months is recommended). Blood antibody tests do not indicate whether the infection is oral or genital, only that it is present. Thus, antibody tests are less useful in diagnosing HSV genital infection in teens, since their genital infections are often due to HSV 1. Another problem is that serologic testing for HSV 1 is not as sensitive as serologic testing for HSV 2 (91% vs 98%). For the teen with a history of cold sores, a positive HSV 1 antibody test would most accurately reflect that oral infection. Infection with the same type in a new location of the body after infection in another location has been well established (i.e. a history of cold sores since childhood is extremely unlikely). So, an HSV 1 positive antibody test in a

Table 44.1.1 Factors associate with a greater likelihood of HSV testing

- Older age
- Female
- White
- STD clinic attendees
- Test is free
- Short wait time for appointment
- Lots of STD knowledge
- No fear of judgment by healthcare provider
- Feel vulnerable to infection

Table 44.1.2 Recommended doses for first infection

Acyclovir (Zovirax)	Valacyclovir (Valtrex)	Famciclovir (Famvir)
400 mg three times a day for 7–10 days or 200 mg five times a day for 7–10 days	1000 mg (1 g) twice a day for 7–10 days	250 mg three times per day for 7–10 days

Reproduced from CDC.

★ Tips and tricks

- Begin antiviral therapy at the first sign of suspected infection; it is not necessary to have labs back to start treatment.
- If the patient has something other than herpes, the medicines will be excreted unchanged, as they require the presence of viral enzymes to be activated.
- It also is not necessary to know for sure if this is first infection or a recurrence.
- Treat as if a first infection regardless of its initial presentation because people with a new infection often get a second more severe round of sores about 5 days after the first ones.

The CDC recommended doses for first infection of genital herpes are given in Table 44.1.2. (Many people require another 10 days of treatment for resolution of symptoms, so be sure to write for a refill.)

After the first infection has passed, it is necessary to decide if the patient should take daily therapy, episodic therapy or no therapy.

- **Daily (or suppressive) therapy.** Appropriate for people who:
  ○ Concerned about transmission to a sex partner
  ○ Prefer to have fewer outbreaks
  ○ Are immunosuppressed
  ○ Are particularly susceptible to HIV infection due to their selection of sex partners
  ○ Are having difficulty with the psychological impact of herpes.
- **Suppressive therapy.** The options are given in Table 44.1.3. All of these medicines work equally well when

Table 44.1.3 Suppressive therapies

Acyclovir (Zovirax)	Valacyclovir (Valtrex)	Famciclovir (Famvir)
400 mg twice a day	500 mg if patient has nine or fewer outbreaks per year or 1000 mg (1 g) if 10 or more outbreaks a year	250 mg twice a day

Table 44.1.4 Doses for episodic therapy

Acyclovir	Valacyclovir	Famciclovir
400 mg three times a day for 5 days or 800 mg orally twice a day for 5 days or 800 mg orally three times a day for 2 days	500 mg twice a day for 3 days or 1000 mg (1 g) orally once a day for 5 days or 2000 mg (2 g) twice a day for 1 day	1000 mg twice a day for 1 day or 125 mg orally twice daily for 5 days

taken as directed. The differences between them are cost, likelihood of insurance coverage, and frequency of dosing.

- **Episodic therapy.** This means taking the antiviral medicines only during outbreaks. This may be appropriate for people with infrequent outbreaks (possibly genital HSV 1), someone with a partner who is also infected so transmission is not an issue, and people who are reluctant to take daily pills. Episodic therapy does very little, if anything, to reduce transmission to a sex partner. Most transmissions occur when symptoms are *not* present. Possible doses for episodic therapy are given in Table 44.1.4. Resistance and side effects are uncommonly seen with this class of drugs.

🖐 Caution

- Though daily therapy reduces transmission by almost half, shedding can still occur.
- Patients should still disclose their herpes status to sex partners for ethical and legal reasons.

Evidence at a glance

Duration of therapy

• Many clinicians are unsure of how long patients can safely remain on daily therapy.
• Both safety and efficacy of acyclovir have been demonstrated over more than 20 years of use.
• No hepatic or renal toxicity has been demonstrated.
• Dosing may need to be adjusted with renal impairment.

Psychological implications

Though the medical implications of having herpes are minor, the psychological impact can be devastating. Teens diagnosed with genital herpes encounter similar problems to adults, though the problems may be magnified. Anxiety and depression are common initials reactions to the diagnosis of herpes, but in teens this may be particularly difficult because, developmentally, they are in the process of acquiring self-certainty as opposed to self-consciousness and self-doubt; in addition, they are developing the ability to anticipate achievement rather than being paralyzed by feelings of inferiority. The identification and acceptance of a lifelong highly-stigmatizing STI can be challenging.

✋ Caution

Possible reactions to the diagnosis of HSV among adolescents

• Fear that parents will find out they have herpes
• Fear of rejection and discovery in a college/school society
• Fear they will never have a good and normal sex life
• Fear they will infect someone else
• Fear they will not fit in anymore with their social group
• Depression from having to live with a life-long highly-stigmatizing STI
• Depression because they see themselves as forever different from others, not quite as good

Prompt and effective communication from the healthcare provider can make a long lasting, positive impact on patient adjustment. Simple statements, coming from a trusted source like the clinician, can make a big difference.

✋ Patient advice

• You are still the same person you were before. Herpes does not define you.
• You can still safely have children and a family.
• You can still have sex, though with some alterations including condoms.
• You can transmit virus between outbreaks, even when you have no symptoms at all.
• There are effective treatments for herpes, and they are affordable and safe.
• Give yourself time to feel better. Most people are feeling much better in about 4 months or sooner.
• You can come back to talk to me anytime – my door is open.

Further reading

Gupta R, Warren T, Wald A. Genital herpes. *Lancet* 2007;370(9605):2127–2137.

Johnston C, Saracino M, Kuntz S, *et al.* Standard-dose and high-dose daily antiviral therapy for short episodes of genital HSV-2 reactivation: three randomised, open-label, cross-over trials. *Lancet* 2012;379(9816):641–647.

Roberts C. Genital herpes in young adults: changing sexual behaviours, epidemiology and management. *Herpes* 2005; 12(1):10–14.

44.2 Human papillomavirus and condyloma

Lea E. Widdice and Jessica A. Kahn

Division of Adolescent Medicine, Cincinnati Children's Hospital Medical Center, Cincinnati, OH, USA

Genital human papillomavirus (HPV) infection is most often subclinical; however, infection may cause anogenital cancers, genital warts (condyloma acuminata), or recurrent respiratory papillomatosis (RRP).

> ### ⚛ Science revisited
>
> Over 140 HPV types can infect human epithelium.
>
> - HPVs are classified based on their tropism for cutaneous or mucosal epithelium.
> - Cutaneous HPVs cause common warts, e.g. plantar warts.
> - Over 40 HPVs infect the mucosal epithelium, including oral, respiratory, and genital epithelium.
>   - Mucosal HPVs are further categorized based on epidemiologic evidence linking certain HPV types to cervical cancer and anogenital warts.
>   - Thirteen mucosal HPV types are considered oncogenic.
>   - Persistent infection with oncogenic, or high-risk, HPV is a necessary, but insufficient, cause of cervical cancer. The reasons some high-risk HPV infections persist and others clear is not completely understood. There is no standard definition of persistence. The longer an HPV virus is detectable, the higher the risk of cervical cancer.
> - Approximately 70% of cervical cancers are caused by HPV 16 and HPV 18.
>   - HPV 16 is also associated with 50% of vulvar cancers, 65% of vaginal cancers, 95% of anal cancers, and 65% of oropharyngeal cancers (cancers of the back of the throat, including the base of the tongue and tonsils).
> - HPV 6 and HPV 11 cause approximately 90% of genital warts. HPV 6 and HPV 11 also cause recurrent respiratory papillomatosis (RRP).

Symptoms of HPV-related disease vary. Cervical dysplasia is asymptomatic. Cervical cancer may present with abnormal vaginal bleeding or dyspareunia. Anal cancer may present with discharge, painful defecation, or a palpable lump. Genital warts usually present as painless papules of varying size in the anogenital region, and may be found on the perineum, perianal area, vulva, vagina, cervix, urethra, and anus.

The prevalence of HPV is high. In the US, the prevalence of cervical HPV is 45% among 20–24 year olds. Nearly one-quarter (24%) of 14–19 year olds are infected with cervical HPV. Some high-risk ado-

Practical Pediatric and Adolescent Gynecology, First Edition. Edited by Paula J. Adams Hillard.

lescent populations have prevalence rates of 70–80%. HPV infections are less common in adult women compared to adolescents. About one-quarter of older women are infected, with the rate of infection generally decreasing in older age groups. If high-risk HPV is detected in an adolescent, it is less likely to represent a persistent infection compared to an HPV infection detected in an older woman.

Accurate assessments of the incidence and prevalence of genital warts are difficult to determine. The prevalence of genital warts among sexually-active adults in the US is about 1%. Genital warts occur in adolescents but the prevalence is highest among women in their 20s.

In adolescents, HPV infections are most often transient; the majority are cleared by the immune system within 7–10 months. Seventy percent of infections will clear by 1 year and 90% by 2 years.

Low-grade squamous intraepithelial lesions (LSILs) are the cytologic manifestation of HPV infection. They are diagnosed with Pap testing, currently recommended to begin at age 21 years. As with HPV infection, rates of clearance are high. The rate of LSIL regression to normal cytology is highest among adolescents. In adolescents, 90% of LSILs will regress to normal by 3 years.

HPV is most often transmitted by sexual intercourse; however, it can also be transmitted through nonpenetrative sexual contact such as finger–genital contact. In children, HPV infections, including genital warts, can be transmitted perinatally, through nonsexual contact from caregivers, or by autoinoculation.

✋ Caution

- Children who are diagnosed with genital warts should undergo evaluation for sexual abuse, but genital warts are not diagnostic for abuse.
- The incubation period of HPV in children with perinatal transmission has not been conclusively determined, but ranges from 6 months to approximately 3 years.

Risk factors for HPV infection include early sexual debut, number of sexual partners, having a new sexual partner, inconsistent condom use, immunosup-

pression, a history of Chlamydia or herpes simplex 2, and smoking. Squamous metaplasia of the cervical transformation zone may increase adolescents' vulnerability to HPV infection. Risk factors for persistent HPV infection include older age, immunosuppression, smoking, infection with multiple HPV types, and presence of other sexually-transmitted infections (STIs).

Evidence at a glance

- HPV infections often occur soon after first sexual intercourse.
- Longitudinal studies have shown 40% of women become infected with cervicovaginal HPV within 2 years of first sexual intercourse.
- Fifty percent are infected within 3.5 years of first sexual intercourse.

Persistent infection with high-risk HPV is the primary risk factor for developing high-grade cervical intraepithelial neoplasia and cervical cancer. Other risk factors for cervical cancer include a history of not having had cervical cancer screening, smoking, immunosuppression, oral contraceptive use for longer than 5 years, and multiparity (more than 3 children). Condom use is associated with increased clearance of low-grade cervical dysplasia.

Risk factors for genital warts include smoking, multiple sexual partners, and early sexual initiation. Patients who are immunosuppressed, such as organ transplant recipients and those infected with HIV, are at elevated risk for HPV-related diseases. Warts in immunosuppressed individuals may grow rapidly, becoming large and difficult to treat. Condom use reduces the risk of transmission of HPV and genital warts. However, transmission may occur at sites not protected by condoms.

Two inherited disorders are associated with an increased risk of HPV-related disease. Epidermodysplasia verruciformis is a rare autosomal recessive disorder associated with a defect in the cell-mediated immune system leading to increased susceptibility to condyloma and squamous cell carcinomas of sun-exposed skin. Fanconi anemia is a rare autosomal recessive disorder associated with congenital malformations, bone marrow failure, and increased risk of cancers, including HPV-associated squamous cell carcinomas.

Diagnosis

It is important to assess a patient's sexual and gynecologic history, including sexual risk factors (see Appendices 1.11.1 and 1.11.2); genital lesions with or without bleeding, pain or pruritus; and abnormal vaginal bleeding. Medication history should include assessment of immunosuppressive therapy and medications or products used in the genital area. Social history should include an assessment of condom use, history of sexual abuse, and potential barriers to cervical cancer screening, follow-up, and treatment for genital warts. Dysplasia and genital warts may present or worsen during pregnancy. Urethral and meatal warts may cause reduced urinary flow or urinary obstruction.

Genital warts are most often painless. If symptoms do occur, warts may be pruritic or can cause discomfort if they are large or located in a sensitive anatomic location.

The physical examination should include inspection for oral lesions and evaluation of hoarseness, or respiratory distress. Genitalia should be examined for condylomata and other lesions. HPV infections do not cause a systemic immune reaction; therefore, lymphadenopathy and other systemic signs are not associated with infection.

Diagnosis of warts is based on physical exam findings. A bright light is often helpful in diagnosing lesions; acetic acid application is no longer recommended. Genital warts appear as pearly, filiform, fungating, or cauliflower-like papules or plaques. Filiform projections tend to coalesce at the base. They can appear smooth or lobulated. They can be skin colored, erythematous, or hyperpigmented. Multiple lesions are more common than single lesions.

★ Tips and tricks

- Multiple areas can be affected by genital warts.
- If genital warts are diagnosed in one area, an examination of the entire genital area, including the perianal and periurethral areas, is warranted.

Lab tests to detect HPV DNA are available to clinicians. However, these should be used only in the context of cervical cancer screening protocols. Current guidelines indicate that cervical cytology testing (Pap test) should begin at age 21 years in most healthy adolescents (see Chapter 30.2). In women 30 years and older, HPV DNA testing in combination with Pap testing is recommended. HPV DNA testing is not recommended for routine STI screening, because in adolescents and young adults HPV infections most often resolve without causing disease and the infectivity and transmissibility of infections detected with these tests in the clinical setting is unknown. It is not appropriate to use HPV DNA detection tests in the diagnosis of genital warts. If the diagnosis of condyloma is uncertain, referral to a specialist or biopsy is indicated. In addition, biopsy may be indicated for condylomata if lesions are pigmented, indurated, fixed, bleeding, ulcerated, or not responding to treatment, in order to rule out vulvar intraepithelial neoplasia. Exophytic cervical lesions should be managed by a specialist and considered for biopsy to assess for high-grade squamous intraepithelial lesions prior to treatment.

Colposcopy is used to evaluate abnormal cytology results in individuals aged 21 years and older, and to direct biopsies for histologic diagnosis of precancerous lesions (cervical intraepithelial neoplasia 2, 3), carcinoma *in-situ*, and invasive cancer (which are rare in young adults).

Molluscum contagiosum is a diagnosis that can be mistaken for genital warts; it is a viral infection causing smooth, pink or erythematous, waxy papules (see Chapter 10.1). Molluscum is notable for central umbilication of the papules. Vestibular papillomatosis may also be mistaken for condyloma. These are 1–2 mm, soft, pearly, flesh-colored papules located linearly and symmetrically along both sides of the inner labia minora. Grouping of the papules may occur, but the bases remain discrete. Condylomata lata (a manifestation of secondary syphilis), prominent sebaceous glands, skin tags, and seborrheic keratosis may also be mistaken for condylomata.

Management

Two HPV vaccines, a quadrivalent and a bivalent vaccine are currently available for prevention (see Chapter 24). Completion of the three HPV vaccine doses prior to initiation of sexual activity provides the most protection from all HPV types covered by the vaccine. However, sexually-experienced men and women can still benefit from vaccination and should be vaccinated. HPV DNA testing prior to vaccination is not indicated.

> ### ★ Tips and tricks
>
> - Provider recommendation for HPV vaccination is consistently associated with patient acceptance of HPV vaccine.
> - Multiple professional medical organizations support recommendations for routine immunization against HPV infection.

Cervical cancer screening guidelines exist for adolescents (see Chapter 30.2), adult women, and women with HIV. Screening guidelines are the same for women with and without genital warts. No recommended clinical guidelines exist for the use of anal cytology for anal cancer screening.

Treatment is not recommended for asymptomatic HPV infection, but is directed toward the specific clinical manifestations of HPV infection. Guidelines for the management of abnormal cytology and histology in young adults have been published. A range of treatment options exists for genital warts. These include topical patient-applied therapies, topical provider-applied therapies, and surgical excision (Table 44.2.1). No over-the-counter treatments are available for genital warts. The main goal of therapy

Table 44.2.1 Treatment options for genital warts

Treatment	Mechanism of action	General directions
Patient applied		
Podofilox 0.5% solution or gel	Antimitotic agent	Applied to visible genital warts twice a day for 3 days followed by 4 days of no therapy Repeat for up to four cycles Total wart area treated should not exceed $10\,cm^2$ The total volume of podofilox should be limited to 0.5 mL per day
Imiquimod 5% cream	Stimulates production of interferon and other cytokines	Apply at bedtime, three times a week for up to 16 weeks Must be washed off with soap and water 6–10 hours after application
Sinecatechins 15% ointment	Unknown	Applied three times daily until complete clearance of warts Should not be continued for longer than 16 weeks Should not be washed off after use
Provider-administered		
Cryotherapy, liquid nitrogen or cryoprobe	Cytolysis	Application of liquid nitrogen until the wart turns white
Podophyllin resin 10–25% in a compound tincture of benzoin	Antimitotic agent	Applied and allowed to air-dry Treatment can be repeated weekly Application should be limited to <0.5 mL of podophyllin or a wart area of $<10\,cm^2$ per session Do not apply on or around open lesions or wounds Must be washed off 1–4 hours after application
Trichloroacetic acid (TCA) or bichloroacetic acid (BCA) 80–90%	Cell protein coagulation	Applied only to warts and allowed to dry Treatment can be repeated weekly for up to 6 weeks
Surgical removal		Requires substantial clinical training and additional equipment

---

✋ Caution

Cervical cancer screening must be continued in all women regardless of HPV vaccination status.

---

is to improve cosmetic appearance and decrease discomfort. The impact of therapy on transmissibility is not known.

✋ Caution

- The safety of podofilix, imiquimod, podophyllin, and sinecatechins during pregnancy has not been established.
- Imiquimod and sinecatechins may weaken condoms and diaphragms.

Treatment decisions depend on patient preference, provider experience, and the size and location of warts. Management algorithms lead to improved outcomes for genital wart treatment. Treatment options should be discussed with patients to determine if the patient understands and can comply with instructions.

✯ Tips and tricks

Young patients concerned about confidentiality may have difficulty following through on instructions to wash off provider-applied treatments either because they may not anticipate where they will be or they may not foresee a lack of privacy 1–4 hours after their appointment. Patients may need prompting from the provider to plan how and where they will wash off provider-applied therapies.

Follow-up

Genital warts are generally benign lesions. Warts may regress without treatment, may remain unchanged, or may progressively enlarge.

✋ Patient advice

- Teens and young adults diagnosed with HPV-related diseases should notify their partners.
- Partners should be assessed for HPV-related diseases and screened for other STIs.

When to refer/to whom

- Patients with intra-anal warts may have warts on the rectal mucosa. Referral to a provider with expertise in anoscopy is warranted.
- Patients with vaginal warts should be managed by a provider experienced with treatments other than cryoprobe because of the risk of perforation or fistula formation with the use of cryoprobe on vaginal tissue.
- Women with exophytic cervical warts should be managed by a specialist who can perform a biopsy.
- Patients with warts at the urethral meatus may have intra-urethral warts. Referral to a specialist for examination of the urethra is appropriate.
- Children with genital warts must be evaluated for sexual abuse; genital warts are not diagnostic, but may be a sign, of sexual abuse.

Further reading

Jayasinghe Y, Garland SM. Genital warts in children: what do they mean? *Arch Dis Child* 2006;91(8):696–700.

Kahn JA. Human papillomavirus infection and anogenital warts. In: Neinstein LS (ed). *Adolescent Health Care: A Practical Guide*, 5th edn. Philadelphia: Lippincott Williams & Wilkins, 2008, pp. 842–849.

Workowski KA, Berman S; Centers for Disease Control and Prevention. Sexually transmitted diseases treatment guidelines, 2010. *MMWR Recomm Rep* 2010;59(RR-12): 1–110.

44.3 Chlamydia

Taraneh Shafii[1] and Gale R. Burstein[2]

[1]Division of Adolescent Medicine, University of Washington School of Medicine, Seattle, WA
[2]Erie County Department of Health, and The State University of New York at Buffalo School of Medicine and Biomedical Sciences, Buffalo, NY, USA

Chlamydia trachomatis (CT) is the most common bacterial sexually-transmitted infection (STI) in the US with the highest prevalence rates occurring amongst adolescent and young adult females.

⚛ Science revisited

Chlamydiaceae family

Species (genus)	Diseases
C. trachomatis (two biovars)	
Non-LGV (A-C, D-J)	Cervicitis, urethritis, pelvic inflammatory disease, trachoma, conjunctivitis, infant pneumonia
LGV (L1-L3)	Lymphogranuloma venereum (LGV)
C. pneumoniae	Pharyngitis, bronchitis, pneumonia
C. pisttaci	Psittacosis

Microbiology of *Chlamydia trachomatis*
- An obligatory intracellular bacterium
- Infects the columnar epithelium
- Two forms in the life cycle: elementary body and reticulate body
- Survives by replication that causes cell death

Symptoms and signs of chlamydia infection may include report of vaginal discharge and evidence of cervicitis on examination. However, since the majority of female chlamydia infections are asymptomatic, annual screening of all sexually active females aged 25 years or younger is the standard of care. Adolescent females are at increased risk for acquiring chlamydia infection due to the physiologic immaturity of the vagina and cervix, higher prevalence of CT infection in peer sexual partners, inconsistent condom use, and poor healthcare services utilization. If untreated, chlamydia infection may progress to pelvic inflammatory disease (PID) and the associated morbidities of ectopic pregnancy, infertility, and chronic pelvic pain.

Diagnosis

Obtaining an accurate sexual health history is essential to diagnosing STIs in adolescent females (Table 44.3.1; see also Appendix 1.11.3). All adolescents are entitled to private time with their provider, i.e. without a parent or guardian, for some portion of *all* medical visits to build rapport with the medical provider, foster healthcare independence in the young woman, and to ensure confidentiality and accuracy of the health information provided by the patient. In all 50 states, minors are legally entitled to access confidential STI healthcare services, although age minimums vary by state. When provided with a safe,

---

Practical Pediatric and Adolescent Gynecology, First Edition. Edited by Paula J. Adams Hillard.
© 2013 John Wiley & Sons, Ltd. Published 2013 by John Wiley & Sons, Ltd.

Table 44.3.1 Confidential sexual history

Ask about:
- All types of sexual behaviors including oral, vaginal, and anal intercourse
- Gender of sex partners
- Number of sex partners in the past 2 and 12 months
- New partners in the past 2 months
- Contraception use
- Condom use
- Difficulty with condom use (e.g. breakage, slippage)
- Negotiating condom use with partners
- Quality of relationships with partners (e.g. safety)
- Pregnancy history
- Past STI testing or infections

Table 44.3.2 Review of systems

Ask about:
- Change in vaginal discharge including:
  - Amount,
  - Character,
  - Color,
  - Odor;
- Vulvar discomfort, irritation, and pruritus
- Genital sores or lesions
- Dysuria
- Intermenstrual bleeding
- Bleeding with sexual intercourse
- Pain or discomfort with sexual intercourse
- Abdominal or pelvic pain

☆ Tips and tricks

- **Establish rapport.** Greet the adolescent first, her family members second. Start with small talk, save the most personal questions for last, so the adolescent has time to get comfortable with you. Interview her fully dressed and try to keep her covered as much as possible during the exam.
- **Promise confidentiality with a caveat.** "What we talk about today is confidential, which means I am not going to tell your family unless I am worried that someone has been hurting you; you have been or are thinking about hurting yourself or hurting someone else."
- **Include parents/guardians, then ask them to leave.** Parents/guardians offer valuable health information and are a source of support for the patient and provider, but all adolescents need time alone with their healthcare provider. Ask parents/guardians about their concerns and once heard, advise them: "I spend some time talking alone with all adolescent patient, so if you would step out to the waiting room I will come get you when we are finished."

Paper or electronic surveys that include questions on sexual health may be useful to obtain detailed and accurate sexual histories from patients in busy clinic settings.

✋ Caution

- Never ask an adolescent about sex in front of their parents/guardian as you may not get accurate information. Always interview your patient alone when taking a sexual history.
- Adolescents are concrete thinkers so avoid asking, "Are you sexually active?" They may think you are asking if they had sex today or this week. Instead ask, "Have you ever had sex?"
- Pay attention to the "hidden agenda." A female adolescent complaining of abdominal pain may actually be worried that she is pregnant, but may be too embarrassed or nervous to say this and needs you to broach the subject.

The review of systems is described in Table 44.3.2.

A pelvic exam is recommended for all females with genital symptoms (Table 44.3.3). Asymptomatic females may not require a pelvic exam and may be screened for chlamydia infection using urine specimens or self-collected vaginal swabs. For females engaging in receptive anal intercourse, rectal swab specimens may be obtained.

Nucleic acid amplification tests (NAATs) are the most sensitive CT tests and are licensed for use

nonjudgmental atmosphere and ensured confidentiality of their responses, adolescents will provide accurate information when asked. The key here is: *if you want to know the answer you must ask the question.*

Table 44.3.3 Physical exam

External genital exam:
- Check for findings suggestive of an STI, such as:
  - Inguinal lymphadenopathy
  - Presence of vaginal discharge
  - Vulvar irritation
  - Vulvar lesions

Speculum exam
Allows for visualization of the cervix to assess for diagnostic signs of cervicitis including:
- Mucopurulent endocervical exudate and
- Endocervical friability
- (Both of these may be observed through use of endocervical cotton swab specimen to identify mucopurulent or bloody discharge respectively on the swab)

Bimanual exam
- Adnexal tenderness
- Uterine tenderness
- Cervical motion tenderness
- The presence of any one of these is clinically diagnostic for PID in the absence of other abdominal or pelvic pathology

with urine, vaginal, or endocervical specimens. Adolescent females often prefer urine or self-collected vaginal swab specimens over provider-collected specimens. Vaginal specimens are preferred over urine due to slightly improved performance, although urine remains an acceptable specimen for CT NAATs. Having these options available may increase compliance with STI screening. Although NAATs sensitivity is superior to culture for detecting rectal chlamydia infections, NAATs are not FDA-approved for chlamydia testing of rectal swab specimens. NAATs may be used to test rectal swabs for chlamydia in laboratories that have obtained Clinical Laboratory Improvement Amendments (CLIA) approval to perform these tests.

Other infectious etiologies for cervicitis include *Neisseria gonorrhoeae*, and less commonly *Trichomonas vaginalis* and primary infections with herpes simplex virus 2.

Management

Prompt treatment of chlamydia infection is important to prevent PID and transmission to sexual partners.

To enhance compliance, the simplest treatment regimens are preferred for adolescents and, when possible, single dosing, directly observed therapy is ideal. Centers for Disease Control and Prevention (CDC) recommended regimens found to be equally efficacious are azithromycin 1 g orally in a single dose *or* doxycycline 100 mg orally twice daily for 7 days (www.cdc.gov/std/treatment). Patients are advised to abstain from sexual activity for 7 days after they and their sexual partners are treated to ensure adequate antibiotic coverage and prevent reinfection.

All sexual partners from the preceding 60 days need to be treated for chlamydia infection. If last sexual intercourse was more than 60 days prior to diagnosis, the patient's last partner should be treated. Since health departments are not able to routinely offer partner services for chlamdyia, expedited partner therapy (EPT), the clinical practice of treating the sex partners of patients diagnosed with chlamydia or gonorrhea by providing prescriptions or medications to the partner without the healthcare provider first examining the partner, is an effective public health strategy to increase partner treatment and decrease re-infection rates. In patient-delivered partner therapy (PDPT), the method of EPT most commonly used, healthcare providers give the index patient the medication or a written prescription for the medication to deliver to their partners. All partners should be encouraged to seek medical care for examination and complete STD testing. As of August, 2012, 32 states have legalized EPT (www.cdc.gov/std/ept).

Follow-up

Test of cure or repeat testing 3 weeks after treatment is no longer recommended except during pregnancy or for cases of poor compliance, persistent symptoms or re-infection. Chlamydia NAATs may continue to be positive if repeated less than 3 weeks after treatment due to residual DNA or RNA. Due to high rates of re-infection from untreated partners or new infection from new partners, follow-up testing is recommended 3 months after treatment or whenever persons next present for medical care in the 12 months following initial treatment.

When to refer/to whom

In cases of patients with multiple infections, contact your local health department to assist with partner services, or if treatment failure is suspected, report to your local health department or the CDC.

Prevention

Beyond abstinence, condoms are the most effective method to prevent transmission and acquisition of chlamydia. Young women should be encouraged to use condoms with every partner and with every sexual encounter. To facilitate successful condom use, clinicians should provide to their patients condoms and information on how to use condoms effectively, including techniques, and how to negotiate condom use with partners. Other strategies to reduce infection risk include STD testing with new partners prior to initiating sexual activity and choosing lower risk partners (e.g. partners with fewer number of sex partners).

✋ Patient/parent advice

Patients
• **Get tested.** Most people infected with STIs do not know they are. You cannot tell just by looking at your partner if they are "clean" or not.
• **Use condoms.** Practice using condoms before you need one so you can use them in the "heat of the moment." Unroll one down two fingers or try a banana!
• **Know your partners.** How many people have they had sex with before you? Do they have other sex partners now in addition to you? Are they willing to use condoms with you? Do they treat you well?

Parents
• **Talk to your teens.** Talking about sex does not give teens the "green light" to do it. Sharing your values on sexuality is powerful and helps them make good choices.
• **Take them to the doctor.** Helping your teen access sexual health services before they need it is the first step in keeping them healthy.

• **Ask them where they are and who they are with.** How old is their partner? Do they feel safe? Who else is around when they are together?

✋ Patient/parent advice

Websites
• Advocates for Youth
http://www.advocatesforyouth.org/
• The American Social Health Association
http://www.iwannaknow.org
• Campaign for Our Children
http://www.cfoc.org/
• The Center for Young Women's Health (CYWH)
http://www.youngwomenshealth.org/
• Similar site for males at: http://youngmenshealthsite.org/
• Children Now
http://www.talkingwithkids.org/
• Columbia University's Health Promotion Program "Go Ask Alice" website for adolescents and young adults
http://www.goaskalice.columbia.edu/
• Rutgers, the State University of New Jersey, teen sexual health
http://www.sexetc.org/
• MTV collaboration with Kaiser Family Foundation
http://www.itsyoursexlife.com/
• Planned Parenthood Teens
http://www.teenwire.com/
• Society of Obstetricians and Gynecologists of Canada
www.sexualityandu.ca
• Nemours teen health
http://teenshealth.org/
• Wired Kids, Inc
http://www.wiredkids.org/
• The American Academy of Pediatrics
http://www.healthychildren.org/English/Pages/default.aspx

Further reading

CDC 2010 STD Treatment Guidelines http://www.cdc.gov/std/treatment/

The Center for Young Women's Health (CYWH) http://www.youngwomenshealth.org

The Guttmacher Institute http://www.guttmacher.org

44.4 Gonorrhea

Bree Weaver and J. Dennis Fortenberry

Indiana University School of Medicine, Indianapolis, IN, USA

Gonorrhea is a bacterial sexually-transmitted infection (STI) of the urethra, cervix, fallopian tubes, rectum, and pharynx. Clinical signs and symptoms are the same for adolescent and adult women (Table 44.4.1). STIs disproportionately affect adolescents and young adults. Among adolescents, STIs disproportionately affect racial minorities. Gonorrhea is the second most commonly reported STI after chlamydia.

Risk factors for genital gonorrhea infection are both behavioral and biologic (Table 44.4.2).

✋ Caution

- Gonococcal infections can be asymptomatic.
- Many adolescents and young adults may not think of oral sex as a risk for an STI.
- Sequelae of untreated gonococcal infections can be severe.
- Patients with STIs should be tested for HIV and counseled on contraception.
- Gonorrhea is a reportable disease in most areas.

Patients with clinical syndromes compatible with gonorrhea or with positive gonorrhea tests should be tested for other STIs, such as chlamydia, trichomoniasis, syphilis, and HIV.

✋ Patient/parent advice

- Adolescents can consent for their own STI screening and treatment; no parental consent is needed.
- Providers are not required to tell parents about test results.
- Confidentiality may inadvertently be breeched if parents get an explanation of benefits (EOB) from their insurance company that reveals the types of testing that were done.

Gonorrhea transmission by nonsexual contact (i.e. from hands or fingers or contact with countertops or toilet seats) has not been documented; the organism dies quickly when exposed to oxygen or dry, cool surfaces. Gonococcal infection in a person who is not sexually-active is indicative of sexual abuse.

Diagnosis

Patients should be asked about genital, rectal, and pharyngeal symptoms, as well as fever, abdominal pain or dysuria.

Many infections will not have specific physical exam findings. Pelvic exam is not necessary to diagnose gonorrhea. Urine or patient-collected vaginal

Practical Pediatric and Adolescent Gynecology, First Edition. Edited by Paula J. Adams Hillard.
© 2013 John Wiley & Sons, Ltd. Published 2013 by John Wiley & Sons, Ltd.

Table 44.4.1 Symptoms of gonorrhea infection

Genital infection	Pharyngeal gonorrhea	Anorectal gonorrhea	Disseminated gonococcus
Vaginal itching	Asymptomatic (most)	Anal itching	Tenosynovitis of small joints
Dyspareunia	Signs and symptoms of bacterial pharyngitis	Purulent discharge	Pustular dermatitis
Vaginal discharge		Pain with defecation	Polyarthralgias
			Fever and chills + purulent arthritis

Table 44.4.2 Risk factors for genital gonorrhea

Behavioral risk factors	Biological risk factors	Risk factors for disseminated gonococcus
New sexual partners	Cervical immaturity/ectopy	Recent menstruation
Multiple sexual partners	Lower local antibody (IgA) response	Recent or current pregnancy
Partners with multiple partners	Insertion of IUD with infection	Systemic lupus erythematosis
Substance use	No specific genetic predisposition	Complement deficiencies (disseminated gonococcus may suggest complement deficiency, especially with history of other *Neisseria* infections)
Inconsistent condom use		

swabs can be tested for gonorrhea and other STIs, making a speculum exam unnecessary for sample collection. If a speculum exam is performed, a clinician may see mucopurulent discharge in the vagina or the cervical os, and a normal appearing, or inflamed and friable cervix. Bimanual exam is necessary to assess for signs of pelvic inflammatory disease (PID).

Pharyngeal gonorrhea infections may manifest as pharyngeal erythema, cervical lymphadenopathy,

---

★ **Tips and tricks**

The 5 Ps of sexual history taking
- **P**artners:
  - "Do you have sex with men, women, or both?"
  - "In the past 2 months, how many partners have you had sex with?"
  - "In the past 12 months, how many partners have you had sex with?"
  - "Is it possible that any of your sex partners in the past 12 months had sex with someone else while they were still in a sexual relationship with you?"
- **P**revention of pregnancy:
  - "What are you doing to prevent pregnancy?"
- **P**rotection from STDs:
  - "What do you do to protect yourself from STDs and HIV?"
- **P**ractices:
  - "To understand your risks for STDs. I need to understand the kind of sex you have had recently."
  - "Have you had vaginal sex, meaning 'penis in the vagina sex'?" If yes, "Do you use condoms never, sometimes or always?"
  - "Have you had anal sex, meaning 'penis in the rectum/anus sex'?" If yes, "Do you use condoms never, sometimes or always?"
  - "Have you had oral sex, meaning 'mouth on the penis or vagina'?"
- **P**ast history of STDs:
  - "Have you ever had an STD?"
  - "Have any of your partners had an STD?"

tonsillar exudates, and fever. Anorectal gonorrhea infections may cause purulent rectal discharge. Patients with disseminated gonoccocal infection have fever, swelling and tenderness of the wrist, knees, ankle, fingers, or toes, and pustules on the skin, which may be few in number.

The Centers for Disease Control and Prevention (CDC) publish evidence-based STD Treatment Guidelines regarding the diagnosis, treatment, and prevention of STIs. These guidelines recommend at least annual screening of all sexually active females younger than age 25 years. Higher risk groups, such as incarcerated or pregnant adolescents, should be screened more often. Females with urinary complaints, such as dysuria and urinary frequency, should be tested for STIs. Some experts suggest screening regardless of reported sexual activity, as there may be inaccuracies in reporting or the patient may not feel comfortable disclosing sexual activity.

Various lab tests for gonorrhea are available, including Gram stain, culture, nucleic acid hybridization tests, and nucleic acid amplification tests (NAATs). There is no blood test for gonorrhea. Some tests are FDA approved only for certain anatomic sites.

Gram staining of endocervical, pharyngeal, or rectal specimens is not sufficient to detect infection and is not recommended for diagnosing gonorrhea in women. Culture may be performed and offers the advantage of antibiotic susceptibility testing on isolates. Nucleic acid hybridization testing and NAAT are more sensitive than culture.

A variety of commercially available NAATs are now widely used, and are recommended by the CDC for diagnosis. Sensitivity varies slightly by NAAT types. NAAT are FDA approved for urine, endocervical or vaginal swabs (clinician or patient collected). NAAT on vaginal and cervical swabs are equivalent; urine NAAT testing in females is less sensitive than vaginal/cervical testing. NAATs are not FDA approved for use on rectal or pharyngeal specimens. However, individual labs can conduct validation tests to meet Clinical Laboratory Improvement Amendment (CLIA) requirements, and could subsequently use NAAT for these specimens.

The differential diagnosis for gonorrhea should include other STIs with similar clinical presentations, such as chlamydia and trichomonas, though the latter

is more common in older women. Patients should be tested for other STIs, including HIV.

Uncomplicated gonococcal infections should be distinguished from complicated infection, such as PID or tubo-ovarian abscess, as the management will differ.

Management

Penicillin, doxycycline, and fluroquinolones are no longer recommended for treatment. The cepha-

---

⚛ Science revisited

- Cephalosporin treatment failures have been reported in Europe and Asia.
- In the US, decreased cephalosporin susceptibility, defined as an elevated minimal inhibitory concentrations (MIC; the lowest concentration of an antibiotic that inhibits visible growth of the bacteria) to cephalosporins, has been reported.
- Decreased susceptibility can precede the emergence of resistance.
- The Gonococcal Isolate Surveillance Project (GISP) is a CDC-sponsored surveillance system to monitor antibiotic susceptibility of gonorrhea isolates:
  ○ Approximately 4% of all reported gonorrhea cases in males are included each year
  ○ Percentage of isolates with elevated MIC to cephalosporins:
    – For cefixime: 0.2% in 2000 → 1.4% in 2010
    – For ceftriaxone: 0.1% in 2000 → 0.3% in 2010
- Overall, there is a low prevalence of isolates with decreased cephalosporin susceptibility in the US.

From Centers for Disease Control and Prevention. Cephalosporin susceptibility among *Neisseria gonorrhoeae* isolates – United States, 2000–2010. *MMWR* 2011;60 (26);873–877.

Table 44.4.3 Recommended management

Uncomplicated gonococcal infections of the cervix, urethra, and rectum
- Ceftriaxone 250 mg in a single intramuscular dose

plus
- Azithromycin 1 g orally in a single dose

or
- Doxycycline 100 mg orally twice daily for 7 days*

Alternative regimens

If ceftriaxone is not available:
- Cefixime 400 mg in a single oral dose

plus
- Azithromycin 1 g orally in a single dose

or
- Doxycycline 100 mg orally twice daily for 7 days*

plus
- Test-of-cure in 1 week

If the patient has severe cephalosporin allergy:
- Azithromycin 2 g in a single oral dose

plus
- Test-of-cure in 1 week

Uncomplicated gonococcal infections of the pharynx
- Ceftriaxone 250 mg in a single intramuscular dose

plus
- Azithromycin 1 g orally in a single dose

or
- Doxycycline 100 mg orally twice daily for 7 days*

Disseminated gonococcal infection
- Hospitalization is recommended for initial therapy
- Recommended treatment: ceftriaxone 1 g IM or IV every 24 hours

Alternative regimen
- Cefotaxime 1 g IV every 8 hours

*Because of the high prevalence of tetracycline resistance among Gonococcal Isolate Surveillance Project isolates, particularly those with elevated minimum inhibitory concentrations to cefixime, the use of azithromycin as the second antimicrobial is preferred.
From the CDC Sexually Transmitted Diseases Treatment Guidelines, 2012; From del Rio, C *et al*; *MMWR* 2010; 59:RR-12 and 2012;61(31):590–594.

losporins are the only class to which the organism remains susceptible (Table 44.4.3). There is emerging evidence of decreased susceptibility to cephalosporins in Asia. Most isolates remain susceptible to doxycycline and azithromycin, but these are not recommended to be used alone for treatment. Current recommendations endorse the addition of azithromycin or doxycycline to the cephalosporin even with negative chlamydia testing results, to provide dual antibiotic treatment of gonorrhea and potentially hinder development of drug resistance.

Evidence at a glance

- NAAT using a vaginal swab is recommended for diagnosis of genital infection.
- Fluoroquinolones are not recommended for treatment.
- A cephalosporin plus azithromycin or doxycycline is recommended for treatment.

Follow-up

If symptoms persist and treatment failure is suspected, a patient should be retested for gonorrhea with culture and susceptibility testing. Many suspected treatment failures will actually be re-infection from an untreated partner or a new partner. Patients should be retested 3 months after treatment to assess for re-infection.

Sequelae of gonorrhea include PID; gonorrhea causes an estimated 40% of all PID.

Prevention strategies include identifying and treating asymptomatic infections to decrease the duration of infection and transmission. All patients should be counseled about behaviors that might carry higher risk for infection, including sex without condoms, drug use, and multiple partners.

When to refer/to whom

Any patient with documented treatment failure should be referred to an infectious diseases specialist for assistance with management. Isolates with decreased cephalosporin susceptibility should be reported locally and to the CDC.

Further reading

Centers for Disease Control and Prevention. *Sexually Transmitted Disease Surveillance 2009*. Atlanta: U.S. Department of Health and Human Services, 2010.

Centers for Disease Control and Prevention. Guidelines for the laboratory diagnosis of gonorrhea, chlamydia and syphilis. http://www.aphl.org/aphlprograms/infectious/std/Pages/stdtestingguidelines.aspx

Centers for Disease Control and Prevention. Sexually transmitted diseases treatment guidelines, 2010. *MMWR* 2010;59(RR12):1–110. www.cdc.gov/std/treatment/2010/default.htm

44.5 Trichomonas

Samantha E. Montgomery and Jill S. Huppert
Cincinnati Children's Hospital Medical Center, Cincinnati, OH, USA

Trichomonas vaginalis (TV) was first described in 1836 as a microorganism present in the vaginal discharge of symptomatic women. Originally viewed as a minor nuisance, it was first classified as a sexually-transmitted pathogen in the late 1930s after infection was recognized in soldiers.

> ### ⬡ Science revisited
>
> • TV is a pear-shaped, motile, flagellate parasitic protozoan that adheres to the vaginal epithelium.
> • Once attached, TV releases cysteine proteinases which cause inflammation, breakdown of the epithelium, and an elevation of the vaginal pH.
> • TV is an obligate parasite that phagocytoses bacteria, vaginal epithelial cells, and erythrocytes.

TV is the most common nonviral sexually-transmitted infection (STI), with 8–10 million new cases annually in the US. In a national sample of adolescent women, the prevalence of TV was 2.5%, compared to 3.9% for chlamydia and 1.3% for gonorrhea. TV is more prevalent in black women compared to Asian and white women, a difference that may arise from social factors such as low socioeco-nomic status, lack of access to care, lower condom use, and douching. TV is underestimated for three reasons: widespread use of insensitive diagnostic methods, lack of reporting requirements, and the largely asymptomatic nature of infection.

TV infection increases the likelihood of infection with other STIs, likely due to increased susceptibility due to breakdown of the vaginal mucosal barrier. In cross-sectional studies, adolescent women with TV were two to four times more likely to have bacterial vaginosis, chlamydia, gonorrhea, herpes, or cervical intraepithelial neoplasia than women without TV. Women with TV appear to have an increased risk of pelvic inflammatory disease (PID) and preterm birth. In longitudinal studies, TV doubles the risk of persistent human papillomavirus (HPV) infection, as well as the risk of acquiring human immunodeficiency virus (HIV).

In population studies, 85–90% of women with TV are asymptomatic. When symptoms are present, the most common are vaginal discharge and foul odor, followed by abnormal bleeding, postcoital spotting, and urinary symptoms. Signs of trichomonas infection may include vulvar erythema, vaginal pH greater than 4.5, vaginal leukocytes, and a positive "whiff" test on a KOH prep due to the presence of amines. Only 10% of women have the frothy-green discharge classically attributed to TV and only 2% will have the punctuate hemorrhages characteristic of "strawberry cervix".

Practical Pediatric and Adolescent Gynecology, First Edition. Edited by Paula J. Adams Hillard.
© 2013 John Wiley & Sons, Ltd. Published 2013 by John Wiley & Sons, Ltd.

Evidence at a glance

- Trichomonas-mediated breakdown of the vaginal mucosal barrier facilitates the transmission of HIV in two ways:
  - Increases viral shedding in HIV-positive women
  - Increases susceptibility to infection in HIV-negative women.
- Trichomonas also increases the viral load, thereby increasing the infectivity of HIV-positive women.
- In African studies, trichomonas infection conferred a 1.5–3-fold increase in HIV transmission.
- In women with trichomonas and HIV infection, treatment of the trichomonas infection with a standard dose of metronidazole decreased the level of HIV RNA in vaginal secretions.
- By reducing viral shedding, the diagnosis and treatment of trichomonas may play a significant role in reducing the spread of HIV.

Risk factors for adolescents that contribute to exposure to trichomonas include multiple partners, older partners, previous history of an STI, and douching. Because of this, providers who care for at-risk teens should consider screening of asymptomatic women for TV, and all adolescent women with genitourinary symptoms should be screened for STIs including chlamydia, gonorrhea, and trichomonas.

Diagnosis

The most widely used method to diagnose TV is wet mount microscopy due to its ability to make an immediate diagnosis. Other diagnostic methods include culture, rapid antigen, ribonucleic acid (RNA) probe, and nucleic acid amplification tests (NAATs). Table 44.5.1 highlights the test characteristics of each method, compared to NAAT. Most methods can be performed on patient- or physician-collected vaginal swabs. Because of the poor sensitivity of wet mount, many experts recommend further testing if the wet mount is negative.

☆ Tips and tricks

- Pelvic exam is not a requirement for TV screening.
- For any diagnostic method, self-collected vaginal swabs are an effective means of sampling.
- Teens should be instructed to insert the swab 1–2 inches into the vagina, rotate it for 20 seconds, and then place it in the collection container.
- Urine testing is not available.

Management

Initial therapy for TV is a single 2-g dose of oral metronidazole, which has a greater than 90% cure rate; however the definition of "cure" is changing with increasingly sensitive diagnostic methods. Untreated TV may persist for months to years, and some infections may resolve without treatment. Side effects of metronidazole include nausea, vomiting, metallic taste, gastrointestinal upset, and an antabuse/disulfiram reaction with alcohol. All sexual partners within the last 60 days should be informed and treated.

Table 44.5.1 Comparison of diagnostic tests for *Trichomonas vaginalis*

Diagnostic test	Sensitivity (%)	Specificity (%)	Cost	Time	Availability
Wet mount	51–60	100	$	Minutes	High
Rapid antigen	85–90	100	$$	Minutes	Medium
Culture	85–90	100	$$$	Days	Low
RNA probe	63	100	$$$	Hours	Low
NAAT	98	98	$$$$	Days	Rare

Approximately 2.5–5% of TV infections are metronidazole resistant. A 2-g oral dose of tinidazole is more expensive than metronidazole and has a 92% cure rate. It may work in cases where metronidazole has failed for two reasons: the half-life of tinidazole is longer and levels in genitourinary secretions are higher than metronidazole. Most clinically resistant infections will respond to higher doses of metronidazole (2 g daily for 10–14 days) or tinidazole (2 g PO daily for 5 days). If infection persists, the patient should be referred to an expert for susceptibility testing and ongoing management.

✋ Caution

- Control of TV in the adolescent population depends on screening of asymptomatic patients.
- Trichomonas has a high rate of asymptomatic carriage, which has important consequences for the spread of disease because affected patients remain unaware that there is a problem.
- The risk of spread is compounded by a failure to screen and treat sexual partners.
- Since re-infection is common, and TV is thought to have a recurrence rate of about 30%, treated patients should be rescreened 3 months following treatment.

Pregnancy

Trichomonas infection in pregnancy has been associated with preterm delivery, premature rupture of membranes, and low birth weight. Treatment during pregnancy has not been shown to improve pregnancy outcomes. Metronidazole has not been shown to be carcinogenic or teratogenic in humans. Screening of asymptomatic women in pregnancy is not currently recommended, but treatment of symptomatic women with TV is warranted.

✋ Patient/parent advice

- Trichomonas in adolescents is as common as chlamydia.
- Infection with trichomonas often has no symptoms.
- Trichomonas infection may have serious health consequences.
- It is critical that partners are notified and treated.

Further reading

Forhan SE, Gottlieb SL, Sternberg MR, *et al.* Prevalence of sexually transmitted infections among female adolescents aged 14 to 19 in the United States. *Pediatrics* 2009; 124;1505–1512.

Johnson V, Mabey D. Global epidemiology and control of *Trichomonas vaginalis*. *Curr Opin Infect Dis* 2008;21: 56–64.

Wendel K, Workowski K. Trichomoniasis: Challenges to appropriate management. *Clin Infect Dis* 2007;44: S123–129.

44.6 HIV

Anita Radix[1] and Donna Futterman[2]

[1]Callen-Lorde Community Health Center, New York, NY, USA
[2]Montefiore Medical Center, Albert Einstein College of Medicine, Bronx, NY, USA

Gynecologists, pediatricians, family physicians, and other clinicians who care for adolescents play an important role in the detection, treatment, and care of human immunodeficiency virus (HIV)-infected adolescents.

In 2009, approximately 1670 young women aged 13–24 years were newly diagnosed with HIV infection in the US. Most new infections in women (about 90%) occur through heterosexual contact.

Adolescents are at increased risk for HIV and sexually-transmitted infections (STIs) because of the interplay between behavioral, biologic, and socioeconomic factors. During adolescence, risk-taking and experimentation are normative, and many sexually active adolescents fail to take appropriate prevention precautions.

Since 2006, the Centers for Disease Control and Prevention (CDC) has recommended that all people aged 13–64 years be screened for HIV. In addition, those with HIV risk behaviors (including sex without a condom) presenting for treatment of STIs, or with signs and symptoms consistent with HIV infection, should be offered HIV testing.

Several gynecologic conditions are attributed to or complicated by HIV infection, such as persistent or recurrent vulvovaginal candidiasis. Acquired immunodeficiency syndrome (AIDS) indicator conditions include invasive cervical carcinoma and chronic ulcers (>1 month) due to herpes simplex.

> ### ⬡ Science revisited
>
> **Biologic factors that contribute to heightened risk of HIV**
> - During puberty the single-layer columnar epithelium of the immature cervix may be more vulnerable to infection.
> - Male-to-female transmission of STIs is much more efficient than female-to-male transmission given the larger surface area of the lower female genital tract.
> - STIs may be asymptomatic, increasing the chance they will go untreated, and increasing susceptibility to HIV.
> - Semen remaining in the vagina and rectum for prolonged periods after sexual intercourse increases the period of HIV exposure.

A comprehensive sexual health history (see Appendices 1.11.1 and 1.11.2) should be obtained on all HIV-infected adolescents. Baseline lab tests should be obtained to screen for other STIs. Nucleic acid amplification tests (NAATs) are preferred for chlamydia and gonorrhea screening and should be obtained from all sites of sexual activity. STI screening tests should be repeated annually and more frequently (e.g. at 3–6-month intervals) for high-risk sexual activity,

★ Tips and tricks

Providers often have difficulty incorporating HIV testing into their clinical encounters. ACTS (Advise–Consent–Test–Support) is a streamlined approach to facilitate routine testing http://www.adolescentaids.org/healthcare/acts.html):

- **Advise** patients to get an HIV test, ask if patients are ready to be tested today, and if they are not, answer the patient's concerns and then encourage testing.
- **Consent** patients according to applicable state law; an increasing number of states are moving away from requirements for specific written consent to an opt-out approach, in which HIV testing is included under general consent for care, as encouraged by the CDC.
- **Test** with rapid or conventional HIV test.
- **Support** patients after testing HIV positive or negative.

Evidence at a glance

Gynecologic conditions associated with HIV infection

Offer HIV testing for the following:
- Persistent or recurrent vulvovaginal candidiasis
- Severe or persistent bacterial vaginosis
- Idiopathic genital ulcers
- Moderate/severe cervical dysplasia (CIN 2–3)
- Pelvic inflammatory disease (PID)
- Gonorrhea
- Chlamydia
- Chronic or persistent herpes simplex ulcers (>1 month)
- Invasive cervical carcinoma

papillomavirus (HPV) vaccination to HIV-infected females between the ages of 9 and 26 years.

★ Tips and tricks

Baseline STI testing should be obtained on all newly HIV-diagnosed clients:
- Syphilis serology (e.g. RPR or VDRL)
- Trichomonas
- Gonorrhea cervical, rectal[1], pharyngeal[2] NAAT
- Chlamydia cervical, rectal[1] NAAT
- Hepatitis B and C serology (if hepatitis B negative, vaccinate)

[1]History of receptive anal sex.
[2]History of receptive oral sex.

☙ Caution

- Guidelines for cervical cancer screening differ for HIV-infected adolescents due to higher rates of infection with oncogenic HPV types and cervical dysplasia.
- Start cervical cancer screening after onset of sexual activity (do not wait until age 21 years).
- Papanicolaou (Pap) tests should be obtained at baseline and again in 6 months.
- If the results are normal, Pap tests should be obtained annually.
- Refer women with ASCUS, ASCH, LSIL, HSIL, and atypical glandular cell Pap test results for colposcopy rather than observation or relying on reflex HPV testing.

Evidence at a glance

- There are insufficient data to recommend use of HPV DNA testing as part of management of ASCUS in HIV-infected women.
- Most guidelines recommend that Pap abnormalities, including (ASCUS), atypical squamous cells, cannot exclude HSIL (ASCH), LSIL, HSIL, and atypical glandular cells need follow-up colposcopy and biopsy for further evaluation.

including sex without a condom, multiple sexual partners, sex work, and substance use. Pregnancy testing should be performed when indicated by history or exam findings, but should always be considered with missed menses, abnormal bleeding, or pelvic pain. Clinicians should offer hepatitis B vaccination to those without immunity, as well as human

Reproductive health needs, including contraception, should be discussed with all HIV-infected adolescents.

✋ Caution

Contraception

Several contraceptives commonly prescribed to adolescents have significant interactions with antiretroviral medications that can affect contraceptive efficacy or frequency of side effects, including:

- Combined estrogen/progestin contraceptives, especially when used with antiretroviral classes such as the protease inhibitors and non-nucleoside reverse transcriptase inhibitors (NNRTIs).
- No significant interactions have been found between oral contraceptives and integrase inhibitors, CCR5 antagonists or nucleoside reverse transcriptase inhibitor (NRTI) classes.
- Clinicians may consider switching to progestin-only methods, such as DMPA/Depo-Provera, which provide effective and longer-term contraception.
- There are few data on interactions between the contraceptive ring and antiretrovirals; however, these ensure improved compliance rates compared with pills.
- All methods of contraception should be paired with condom use (female or male condoms) and education provided on effective (consistent and correct) use.

✋ Patient advice

- Always use a condom; it could save your life.
- It is risky to have sex with someone who has shared needles.
- You often cannot tell whether your partner has been infected with an STD.
- If you are not sure about yourself or your partner, you should choose not to have sex at all.
- If you do have sex, be sure to use a condom for vaginal, anal, and oral sex.
- If you think you and your partner should be using condoms but your partner refuses, you should say *no* to sex with that person.

The NNRTI efavirenz has been associated with risk of birth defects and is therefore usually avoided in young women. Before use, a pregnancy test should be obtained and clients given education and effective contraception.

Young women who are considering pregnancy should receive extensive preconception counseling, including the use of antiretrovirals to reduce mother-to-child transmission of HIV. Pregnant women should be comanaged by an obstetrician with expertise in HIV disease as well as an HIV specialist. The use of antiretroviral therapy, avoidance of breastfeeding, and preventive antiretrovirals for the newborn after delivery have successfully reduced mother-to-child transmission of HIV.

Further reading

Aberg JA, Kaplan JE, Libman H, *et al*. Primary care guidelines for the management of persons infected with human immunodeficiency virus: 2009 update by the HIV Medicine Association of the Infectious Diseases Society of America. *Clin Infect Dis* 2009;49(5):651–681.

Henry-Reid L, Martinez J. Care of the adolescent with HIV. *Clin Obstet Gynecol* 2008;51(2):319–328.

Kaplan JE, Benson C, Holmes KH, *et al*. Guidelines for prevention and treatment of opportunistic infections in HIV-infected adults and adolescents: recommendations from CDC, the National Institutes of Health, and the HIV Medicine Association of the Infectious Diseases Society of America. *MMWR Recomm Rep* 2009;10;58:1–207.

44.7 Other sexually-transmitted diseases

Ellen S. Rome

Center for Adolescent Medicine, Cleveland Clinic Children's Hospital, Cleveland, OH, USA

Syphilis

The incidence of syphilis has shown an uphill trend since 1980, paralleling the increase in illicit drug use and human immunodeficiency virus (HIV) rates. Fifteen percent of adolescents/young adults with syphilis are co-infected with HIV. When you detect syphilis, screen for HIV. Congenital syphilis occurs in 1 in 10000 pregnancies. Symptoms of syphilis are listed in Table 44.7.1.

Syphilis is caused by *Treponema pallidum* and is highly contagious with skin-to-skin contact; one-third of exposed individuals contract infection. The asymptomatic incubation period ranges from 10 to 90 days, usually lasting around 3 weeks.

Diagnosis

Treponema pallidum cannot be cultured. Testing involves use of an indirect (nontreponemal) test, which screens antibodies directed against lipoidal antigens from damaged host cells or possibly from treponemes, looking at dilutions of reactive serum. This provides a sensitive, inexpensive, easy means of detection:
- RPR: rapid plasma regain test
- VDRL: Venereal Disease Research Laboratory test
- TRUST: toluidine red unheated serum test.

If the indirect test is positive, it is followed by a treponemal test, which screens directly for antibodies targeting treponemal proteins:
- FTA-ABS: fluorescent treponemal antibody absorbed test
- MHA-TP: microhemaglutination assay for antibody to *Treponema pallidum*
- TP-PA: *Treponema pallidum* particle agglutination test
- EIAs: enzyme immunoassays (e.g. Trep-Chek and Trep-Sure)
- CIAs: chemiluminescence immunoassays
- MBIA: Microbead immunoassays (e.g. BioPlex2200 Syphilis IgM and IgG).

Once positive, the indirect tests may stay positive, but adequate treatment results in a four-fold decrease in nontreponemal titers; thus, if the RPR starts at 1:32, it will decrease to 1:4 after treatment.

Risk for re-infection in the adolescent remains high; RPR or other indirect tests should be followed every 6–12 months to detect a rise, necessitating retreatment for the patient and partner.

Management

One dose of benzathine penicillin (PCN) G 2.4 million units IM should be given (this means Bicillin LA, *not* Bicillin CR). An alternative is azithromycin 2 g for treatment resistance.

Practical Pediatric and Adolescent Gynecology, First Edition. Edited by Paula J. Adams Hillard.
© 2013 John Wiley & Sons, Ltd. Published 2013 by John Wiley & Sons, Ltd.

Table 44.7.1 Symptoms of syphilis

Presentation	Symptoms
Primary	Nontender inguinal nodes
	Hard, painless chancre at site of inoculation (teaming with spirochetes)
	Lesion resolves within 6 weeks
Secondary	Fever, malaise, weight loss, headache, myalgia, rash not sparing palms and soles
	Occurs 2 weeks to 6 months after primary chancre
Tertiary	Progressive central nervous system destruction, cardiovascular destruction (thoracic aneurysms), skin lesions (gumma), bone destruction
Latent	Seroreactivity (initial positive or four-fold increase in nontreponemal test) but asymptomatic

---

✋ Caution

With any genital ulcer (Table 44.7.2), test for syphilis and HIV.

Table 44.7.2 Differentiation of ulcers with adenopathy

Disease	Ulcer tender?	Nodes tender?
Syphilis	Painless ulcer	Nontender nodes
Herpes simplex virus (HSV)	Tender blister/vesicles	Tender nodes
Chancroid	Ulcer crater-like and tender	Tender nodes, buboes
Granuloma inguinale	Painless ulcer	Nodes less prominent, pseudobuboes
Lymphogranuloma venereum	Painless ulcer	Tender, unilateral nodes

---

✋ Caution

- False positives for RPR or other indirect test occur in 1–2% of patients.
- Beware the prozone effect: false-negative results (especially in HIV patients and pregnant women) in the face of high titers of antibodies; serial dilutions will show a positive response. With a high index of suspicion and a negative test initially, ask the lab for serial dilutions.

✋ Caution

Jarisch–Herxheimer reaction

- If you treat a patient for syphilis and receive a call within hours that the patient *feels ill, faint or woozy*, they should be seen urgently. They may be experiencing the Jarisch–Herxheimer reaction, an acute febrile reaction as spirochetes are being lysed.
- Patients will present with fever, headache, myalgias, tachycardia, hypotension, and tachypnea, evolving into hypovolemic shock if they do not receive adequate supportive care.
- Patients should be warned to call you urgently if they do not feel right after their shot, or if they feel lightheaded with standing, see a new rash, or otherwise feel significantly unwell.
- The Jarisch–Herxheimer reaction occurs more frequently in patients with early syphilis, likely due to higher bacterial burdens in early stages of diseases.
- Treatment consists of supportive care, including antipyretics, intravenous fluids and further education about syphilis, STIs, and prevention.

Latent syphilis should be treated with benzathine PCN G 2.4 million units IM in a single dose. For late latent syphilis, the dose should be repeated weekly for 3 weeks.

⚛ Science revisited

Neurosyphilis
- Neurosyphilis is rare in adolescents. It is more common, but still rare, in HIV-infected individuals.
- This finding presents both diagnostic and therapeutic challenges, as both can have neurologic involvement. Consultation with an infectious disease expert is warranted.

If you need to retreat syphilis (due to re-infection from an untreated partner or a new infection), weekly injections of benzathine PCN G 2.4 million units IM should be given for 3 weeks.

⚛ Science revisited

- Azithromycin 2 g orally as a single dose is effective in the treatment of early syphilis.
- However, *Treponema pallidum* chromosomal mutations are associated with azithromycin; resistance and treatment failures have been reported. Benzathine PCN should be used if possible.
- An alternative for suspected resistance is doxycycline 100 mg PO BID for 14 days or tetracycline 500 mg PO QID for 14 days. The latter in teens can mean missed doses due to the dosing schedule and gastrointestinal distress.
- In the face of a penicillin allergy (pregnant patients included) where compliance cannot be guaranteed with either doxycycline or azithromycin, the patient should be desensitized and treated with benzathine PCN in a hospital or acute care setting.

Granuloma inguinale

Granuloma inguinale (GI), also called donovanosis, presents with a painless genital ulcer without adenopathy. You can also sometimes see subcutaneous

✋ Parent/patient advice

- A diagnosis of a sexually-transmitted disease (STD) provides a window of opportunity to help the adolescent understand that they are not invulnerable, that poor choices can result in significant hazards to their health, and that they can prevent future infections if they make safer choices.
- Parents may need coaching on how to talk to their teen about healthy sexuality.
- Parents can use the car as a vehicle of communication. On the way home from the doctor's office, discussion of healthy choices, keeping yourself safe, and other touchy subjects can occur. The teen may find it safer to answer questions while staring out the car window or avoiding eye contact.

granulomas (called pseudobuboes; real buboes go with chancroid). These highly vascular, beefy red lesions bleed easily with contact. The infection can also spread to the pelvis, intra-abdominally, to bones, or to the mouth (presumed transmission via oral sex).

Rare in the US, it is endemic in India, Papua New Guinea, the Caribbean, central Australia, and southern Africa. It is caused by an intracellular Gram-negative bacterium, *Klebsiella granulomatis*, formerly called *Calymmatobacterium granulomatis*.

Klebsiella granulomatis is hard to culture, and diagnosis relies on visualization of dark-staining Donovan bodies on biopsy.

Management

- For practical purposes, if you suspect GI, treat for GI. Anyone who has had sexual contact with the person within 60 days of diagnosed infection should be treated, despite little data on partner treatment success rates. The cheapest and most convenient treatment regimen should be used:Doxycycline 100 mg orally BID for 3 weeks (CDC STD 2010 Treatment Guidelines first choice; but *not* for pregnant patients)).
- Azithromycin 1 g orally a week for 3 weeks (unproven but likely to work well).

• Trimethoprim–sulfamethoxazole DS (160 mg/800 mg) orally BID for 3 weeks (but *not* for pregnant patients).
• Ciprofloxacin 750 mg orally BID for 3 weeks (but *not* for pregnant patients).
• Erythromycin 500 mg orally QID for 3 weeks (QID a day dosing is less convenient for the patient).

Treating should continue until all lesions have completely healed; they will heal from the inside out. Relapse can occur 6–18 months after therapy. If lesions recur, the patient should be treated again. If lesions do not seem to be getting better after the first few days of treatment, consider adding IV gentamycin 1 mg/kg every 8 hours (or other aminoglycoside).

> ### ✋ Caution
>
> Do not use doxycycline, ciprofloxacin, or trimethoprim–sulfamethoxazole in pregnant women.

Lymphogranuloma venereum

Lymphogranuloma venereum (LGV) causes tender inguinal and/or femoral lymphadenopathy, usually one-sided, with a genital ulcer or papule at the initial site of contact. The latter will go away on its own. For those having anal intercourse, symptoms can include proctocolitis, with anal mucus or bleeding, fever, anal pain, constipation, and tenesmus.

The primary lesion appears as an elevated, firm, raised papule, vesicle or pustule, 2–10 mm in size, round or oval in shape. An adolescent may not notice the initial ulcer, which is usually (but not always) nontender, while the unilateral nodes are usually quite tender.

LGV is caused by certain subtypes of *Chlamydia trachomatis*, specifically L1, L2, or L3. Unlike the more common asymptomatic chlamydial infections at the cervix or urethra, LGV strains create an invasive, systemic infection, which if untreated can create colorectal fistulas and strictures with chronic pain. These lesions can also become superinfected with other STDs/pathogens.

Diagnosis

LGV is diagnosed in a patient with a painless ulcer, unilateral tender adenopathy, a positive chlamydia test, and no other cause for proctocolitis or genital/perianal ulcers.

> ### ✋ Caution
>
> • Nucleic acid amplification tests (NAATs) are the most sensitive test to diagnose gonorrhea and chlamydia.
> • They are not yet FDA approved for rectal use, but many clinicians still use them for this.

Management

• The first-line antibiotic recommended by the Centers for Disease Control and Prevention (CDC) is doxycycline 100 mg orally BID for 3 weeks.
• Azithromycin 1 g a week for 3 weeks also should be effective but is untested to date.
• Erythromycin is effective, but the required regimen of 500 mg orally QID for 21 days make it harder to use.

Patients should be treated until all symptoms have resolved. HIV-positive individuals may require longer than 3 weeks of treatment.

All partners who have had sexual contact with the person within 60 days of infections should be treated with azithromycin 1 g orally as a single dose, or doxycycline 100 mg orally BID for 7 days.

Molluscum contagiosum

Molluscum contagiosum, caused by a poxvirus, appears as 2–5-mm small, pearly papules with a central depression (umbilication). Expressing the core of the papule can produce a white, cheesy discharge. The lesions are usually painless but can become inflamed, erythematous, and enlarged, especially if picked at or irritated via lotions. The incubation period is 2 weeks to 6 months.

Molluscum may be self-limited, spontaneously disappearing within 6–12 months, but they can also take up to 4 years to resolve. Parents and patients tend to want the lesions gone much faster.

Molluscum is considered a pediatric disease, as it is common in children, with atopic dermatitis serving as a risk factor due to immune cell dysfunction in atopic skin and local breaks in the skin barrier. Atopic children also itch and then scratch, allowing for autoinoculation.

Children, adolescents, and adults who are immunocompromised may develop "giant" lesions, over 15 mm in diameter, or they may have multiple lesions resistant to standard therapy. When an abundance of pearly papules present, screen for HIV.

Genital molluscum contagiosum can be acquired through skin-to-skin contact. It can mimic condyloma accuminata.

In patients with solid organ transplant, ongoing chemotherapy, or other form of immuncompromise, other opportunistic infections can mimic molluscum, such as histoplasmosis, cryptococcosis, keratoacanthoma, coccidiodomycosis, and verruca vulgaris.

Diagnosis

Diagnosis is usually based on visual appearance; the skin biopsy is typically reserved for those who are immunocompromised and have giant sized lesions.

✋ Patient/parent advice

- Adolescents and young adults should be warned to wear shorts that cover their inner thighs, long pants, or to sit on a towel when using equipment at the gym as molluscum may be acquired from work-out equipment seats used by an infected person.

  Transmission has been found in nonsexually active college age students whose only risk factor was use of "short shorts" while on the exercise bike at the gym.
- Shaving and electrolysis may be another form of autoinoculation.
- Children with molluscum can still go swimming.

Management

Some lesions may resolve with benign neglect, but this route is not the preference of most families and patients. Atopic children and adolescents, those with visible lesions, and immunocompromised patients should be treated. Options include curettage to remove the pearl, cryotherapy (freezing with liquid

nitrogen), and laser therapy, although the latter is far more expensive. Each of these methods may result in scarring.

★ Tips and tricks

- Use EMLA or other topical numbing medicine 25–30 minutes before curettage. With appropriate numbing, even very young children can tolerate depearling.
- For facial lesions, try azeleic acid topically twice a day for several months; this will avoid the scarring that may occur with curettage or cyrotherapy.
- Oral cimetidine has been used in children, and is safe, painless, and well tolerated. It does less well with facial lesions.
- Tretinoin has been reported as useful, as has imiquimod (a T-cell modifier) and cantharidin (a blistering agent applied in the office setting).
- In immunocompromised patients with widespread molluscum resistant to standard therapy, intralesional interferon has been used successfully. However, treatment comes with a high prevalence of influenza-like symptoms, site tenderness, depression, and lethargy.

Pubic lice (Pthirus pubis)

Pubic lice are parasitic insects that survive by feeding on human blood. Pubic lice are cousins of the common head louse, Pediculus humanus capitis, and the body louse, Pediculus humanus corporis. Pubic lice are usually spread by skin-to-skin sexual contact. Unlike body lice, pubic lice do not actually spread disease. If you diagnose pubic lice, you should screen for other STIs.

Adult lice are 1.1–1.8 mm in length, or the size of a pinhead. They are usually found in the pubic hair, but sometimes may gravitate to other course hairs such as beard, eyebrows, eyelashes, armpits, or other reachable areas (especially with oral sex or other positional opportunities). Nits or eggs take 6–10 days to hatch, at which time the immature louse is called a nymph. Nymphs take around 2–3 weeks to mature, feeding on human blood to grow. Adult lice are grayish–white to tan in color, have two pincer-like claws and four smaller other legs, with females bigger than males. If the louse falls or crawls off a person, it dies within 1–2 days.

🖐 Patient/parent advice

- You cannot get pubic lice from your dog, cat, or other pet.
- Lice prefer people, and they do not fly or hop like fleas; they move by crawling.
- You can see them with the naked eye; they are the size and shape of a pinhead.
- A diagnosis of any STD, including pubic lice, provides a perfect time for parents to "have that talk," specifically on healthy choices and values clarification.

🖐 Caution

- Pubic lice found on the eyelashes or eyebrows of a child may be a red flag for abuse, especially if there are no signs of head lice (which crawl more speedily than do pubic lice).
- Bed linen, towels, and close contact with an infected person can also result in transmission, assuming the contact occurs before the 1–2 days it takes the louse to die without feeding.
- You cannot get pubic lice from a toilet seat as their feet do not grasp porcelain easily.

Management

Over-the-counter 1% permethrin lotion or a mousse containing pyrethrins and piperonyl butoxide can be used simply and easily. Prescription medicines are also available.

🖐 Parent/patient advice

Application of treatment for pubic lice
- Wash the infested area, then towel dry.
- Douse the louse-infected area generously with the medication. Leave it on for the recommended time (usually 10 minutes).

- Wash the area with soap and water, then remove nits with a fine-toothed comb or fingernails.
- Wash all clothes/bedding with hot water/ detergent before sleeping in that bed/wearing those clothes again. For items that cannot be washed, put them in a sealed plastic bag for 72 hours (CDC recommends 2 weeks, but theoretically the nits should die within 1–2 days).
- Put on clean clothes and underwear immediately after treatment!
- Make sure any partner is treated before having skin-to-skin contact again (ditto for their clothes/ bedding).
- If live lice are still found, repeat in 9–10 days.
- For eyebrow lice in small numbers, remove nits/lice with fingernails or a nit comb.
- If further treatment for eyelash lice is needed, apply an ophthalmic-grade petrolatum ointment (available by prescription only) to the eyelid margins two to four times a day for 10 days. Do not use vaseline or regular petrolatum as it can be irritating to the eyes.

🖐 Caution

- Avoid lindane shampoo as first-line therapy, as it can result in neurotoxicity.
- Also avoid use of lindane shampoo in pregnant or breastfeeding patients, those with a seizure disorder, premature infants, and anyone under 110 lbs.
- Other prescription lotions are available but not yet FDA approved for treatment of lice, such as malathion lotion 0.5% (Ovide) and ivermectin.

♀ Pearls

- Consider testing for syphilis and herpes in all patients with ulcers.
- Whenever you diagnose chancroid, think co-infection with syphilis and HIV.
- With any rash, put on gloves *before* you touch.

Further reading

Rac MW, Greer LG, Wendel GD Jr. Jarisch-Herxheimer reaction triggered by group B streptococcus intrapartum antibiotic prophylaxis. *Obstet Gynecol* 2010;116 (Suppl 2):552–556.

Silverberg NB. Pediatric molluscum contagiosum: optimal treatment strategies. *Pediatr Drugs* 2003;5:505–512.

Workowski KA, Berman S; Centers for Disease Control and Prevention. Sexually transmitted diseases treatment guidelines, 2010. *MMWR Recomm Rep* 2010;59(RR-12):1–110.

45 Dysmenorrhea

Michelle Forcier and Zeev Harel

Division of Adolescent Medicine, Hasbro Children's Hospital and Department of Pediatrics, Warren Alpert Medical School of Brown University, Providence, RI, USA

Dysmenorrhea (severely painful menstruation) is one of the most common sources of cyclic abdominal pain and the leading cause of recurrent school and work absenteeism among young women. Most teens report painful periods, with 15% reporting severe dysmenorrhea symptoms that limit their activities of daily living and that do not improve with pain medications.

While dysmenorrhea is a common chronic problem, many adolescents do not seek medical attention for this disorder or are undertreated. Adolescent healthcare providers should screen for menstrual symptoms at every encounter with the adolescent female. Ascertaining the last menstrual period (LMP) should be considered an essential vital sign for adolescent females. Asking teens detailed questions about their menstrual experience may elicit common conditions that can be treated with reassurance or simple outpatient therapies. A detailed menstrual history is an important component of adolescent pelvic pain evaluation, and some teens may use this common complaint as a gateway symptom, opening the door to more confidential and in depth discussions of reproductive and sexual health.

Primary dysmenorrhea, monthly menstrual symptoms with no pelvic pathology, usually appears within a couple years after menarche as ovulatory cycles become established. Secondary dysmenorrhea, due to pelvic structural abnormalities, has a more severe clinical presentation, typically later in adolescence. Most symptoms are cyclic, occurring with menstruation, resulting from monthly reproductive system hormonal changes, and involving inflammatory mediators.

> ### ⚘ Science revisited
>
> **Proposed pathophysiology of dysmenorrhea**
> - With the drop in progesterone late in each menstrual cycle, arachidonic acid and other omega-6 fatty acids are released, triggering an inflammatory response cascade involving prostaglandins and leukotrienes.
> - Subsequent vasoconstriction of endometrial arteries and resultant myometrial contractions are the main source of uterine ischemia and ensuing pain.

Evaluation

A detailed menstrual and general medical history is the most important component of evaluating dysmenorrhea, especially as the physical exam may offer minimal diagnostic yield. Age of menarche, frequency,

---

> ### ★ Tips and tricks
>
> - The LMP should be considered a "vital sign" that is obtained for all adolescent encounters.
> - A menstrual history should be included as an important part of preventive health visits.
> - In addition to menstrual cramps, many adolescents experience other menstrual symptoms such as nausea/vomiting and headaches.
> - Most dysmenorrhea can be managed with proper use of NSAIDs or contraceptive hormones.

> ### ☝ Caution
>
> - Consider a diagnosis of endometriosis for difficult to manage dysmenorrhea.
> - Early diagnosis and treatment of endometriosis is important for future pain and fertility management.

duration, and volume of menses are important screening questions in any well woman's medical history.

The most common symptoms of dysmenorrhea include cyclic pelvic or lower back pain and/or abdominal cramping. In addition to assessing pain (location, scale of severity, radiation, aggravating/alleviating factors, interruption of daily living activities), the adolescent healthcare provider should assess other dysmenorrhea-associated symptoms such as gastrointestinal symptoms (nausea, vomiting, diarrhea, bloating, and appetite changes), psychologic symptoms (mood changes, irritability, energy), headaches, and acne exacerbation.

Symptoms of primary dysmenorrhea typically start several hours before or with the onset of menses and are most severe the first day or two of menstruation. Girls who have experienced early menarche and menorrhagia may have more severe complaints.

Secondary dysmenorrhea due to pelvic abnormalities should be considered in patients with dysmenorrhea that is particularly difficult to manage. Secondary dysmenorrhea usually occurs several years after menarche, and can present atypically in adolescents. Pain in youth may be acyclic or cyclic (perimenstrual) in timing, and is not usually accompanied by uterosacral nodularity, although posterior uterine tenderness may be present. The most common pelvic source of secondary dysmenorrhea is endometriosis, but adenomyosis, leiomyomas, endometrial polyps, and obstructing Müllerian abnormalities (imperforate hymen, transverse vaginal septum, cervical stenosis, bicornuate uterus with a noncommunicating rudimentary horn, uterine didelphys) may also be considered in the differential of cyclic abdominal pain.

Pelvic pain related to endometriosis is generally more continuous and progressive than primary dysmenorrhea, as cyclic hormonal and inflammatory changes in tissues outside the uterine cavity create recurrent swelling, stretching, scarring, and nerve damage within the endometriotic lesions. Even cyclic pain may begin more than 24 hours prior to menses, and may last throughout the days of menstrual flow, not just the first couple of days. The pathologic positive feedback loop in endometriosis consists of elevated local levels of estrogen that stimulate the enzyme cyclooxygenase-2 and synthesis of prostaglandin PGE2, which in turn increase aromatase activity, leading to a further increase in local estrogen levels. Endometriosis may also be associated with menstrual irregularities, dyspareunia, dysuria, dyschezia, irritable bowel and other gastrointestinal complaints, back and lower extremity pains, and a positive family history of the disease.

There are no imaging modalities that predictably and reliably pick up small lesions of endometriosis. Even laparoscopy may be difficult in the early and mid pubertal female who has small, difficult to image endometriosis lesions. Ultrasonography (US) of the pelvis, including transvaginal or transrectal US, can be an initial modality for investigating pelvic pain. US has high sensitivity (84–100%) and specificity (90–100%) for large ovarian endometriomas and is similar in diagnostic accuracy to magnetic resonance imaging (MRI) for deeply infiltrative lesions. MRI is better for imaging vaginal and bladder lesions, while there are no good imaging modalities for typically small peritoneal implants. Therefore, a diagnostic laparoscopy with resection/ablation of lesions is indicated in patients with dysmenorrhea refractory to treatments with NSAIDs and hormones.

Management

Treatment of primary dysmenorrhea typically targets this inflammatory response with prostaglandin

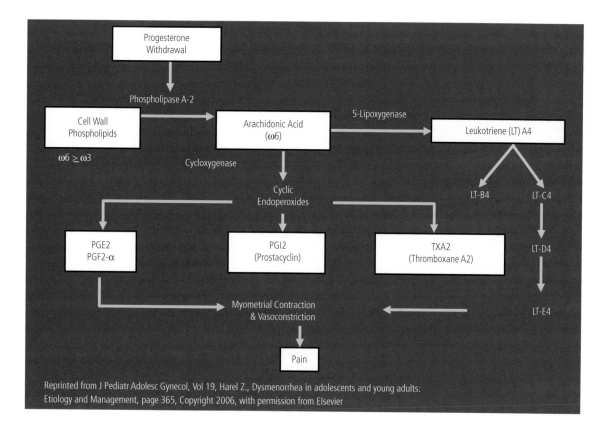

Reprinted from J Pediatr Adolesc Gynecol, Vol 19, Harel Z., Dysmenorrhea in adolescents and young adults: Etiology and Management, page 365, Copyright 2006, with permission from Elsevier

synthetase inhibitors/ nonsteroidal anti-inflammatory agents (NSAIDs) forming the basis of treatment. A variety of NSAIDs have been demonstrated to be most effective when given 1 day prior to or at the very start of menses (prophylactically), often with a loading dose, continuously with scheduled (i.e. around the clock) dosing for the first several days of menstruation to maintain consistent serum levels, and in weight-appropriate doses. While many teens may report having tried NSAIDs without success, providers who take a detailed history often elicit suboptimal self-management with significant room for improving therapy (Table 45.1). NSAIDs available over the counter and by prescription seem to have equivalent effectiveness. Administration based on principles of pharmacology is the key to maximal benefit.

Hormones are an additional treatment modality for dysmenorrhea and may be considered a first-line option for sexually-active teens. Many of today's contraceptive methods, including combined hormone therapy, offer significant relief, as well as providing contraceptive benefits for the sexually-active teen.

Hormone effectiveness for contraception and menstrual regulation is dependent on adherence and continuation of use. Longer-acting reversible hormonal contraceptives as well as extended cycling of hormonal contraceptives may offer more optimal control over time. Hormonal contraceptives typically prevent or improve dysmenorrhea by decreasing endometrial growth and amount of tissue, thus decreasing prostaglandin and leukotriene build up. Indirectly, hormonal contraceptives decrease progestin production, as they inhibit ovulation. Extended cycle regimens of oral contraceptive pills, the transdermal patch, or vaginal ring decrease the total number of annual menses, and thereby alleviate dysmenorrhea symptoms.

Progestin-only methods, such as the injectable medroxyprogesterone acetate, the etonorgestrel implant, and the levonorgestrel intrauterine system

Table 45.1 Summary of treatments for dysmenorrhea

NSAIDs	Best if used prior to onset of menses and with around the clock dosing for days 1–3 of menstruation
Ibuprofen	600–800 mg q 6–8 hours
Naproxen	500 mg q 12 hours
Mefenamic acid	500 mg initial loading dose, then 250 mg q 6 hours
Celecoxib	400 mg initial loading dose, then 200 mg q 12 hours (girls >17 years)
Off-label, additional treatments	
Combined estrogen and progestin hormonal contraceptives	Includes daily combined oral contraceptive pills of any formulation, Ortho-Evra transdermal patch, and the vaginal ring NuvaRing. Consider extended cycle dosing to provide fewer episodes of withdrawal bleeding
Depot medroxyprogesterone injection	IM 150 mg, SC 104 mg
Levonorgestrel intrauterine system (Mirena)	20 μg daily slow release up to 5 years after insertion
Etonorgestrel (Implanon or Nexplanon)	68-mg device, releasing 25–70 μg daily up to 3 years
Omega-3 fatty acids	In diet or nutritional supplements may decrease potency of inflammatory mediators
Exercise	Improves blood flow to pelvis and produces natural pain relievers (due to release of endorphins)
Vitamin and herbal remedies	Vitamin B1 and magnesium supplement have been shown to be effective. There is insufficient evidence to recommend the use of any of the other herbal and dietary supplements
Acupuncture	Acupuncture has been associated with significant reductions in pain compared with baseline, medication, or herbal treatments
Transcutaneous nerve stimulation (TENS)	High-frequency TENS has been shown to be effective in a number of small trials. There is insufficient evidence to determine the effectiveness of low-frequency TENS

(LNG-IUS), also limit growth of the uterine lining, inhibiting ovulation and monthly hormonal changes. Medroxyprogesterone often leads to cessation of monthly menses, decreasing uterine bleeding and relief of other perimenstrual symptomatology. The implant has been linked to improvements in dysmenorrhea but has the side effect of unpredictable uterine bleeding. The LNG-IUS also limits endometrial growth and has the predictable side effect of amenorrhea in 50% of users within the first year. This IUS is FDA approved for menometrorrhagia and has been shown to alleviate dysmenorrhea symptoms in adolescents.

It is important to remember that pain secondary to Müllerian anomalies can be related to both outflow

✋ **Patient/parent advice**

- Start taking NSAIDs the day before menstruation begins or with the first signs of menstrual pain, take an appropriate dose, and continue them around the clock for the first 1–3 days
- Hormonal therapy has many uses in addition to contraception, including treatment of menstrual pain and associated symptoms, treatment of heavy bleeding, and treatment of irregular bleeding.
- There is no evidence that taking hormone therapy leads to earlier initiation of sexual activity.

obstruction and resultant endometriosis. Repairing the anomalous tract relieves obstruction and may relieve endometriosis.

Early diagnosis and treatment of suspected endometriosis may minimize progression and severity over time, and may protect future fertility. Conservative treatment in adolescent populations includes medical management with NSAIDs and contraceptive hormones. While there is a paucity of strong evidence, extended cycle regimens of combined estrogen and progestin oral contraceptive pills have long been used for young women who have severe dysmenorrhea and/or are suspected to have endometriosis. Progestin-only hormones also provide excellent pain relief. The progestin norethindrone is FDA approved for endometriosis, and both subcutaneous and intramuscular medroxyprogesterone also have excellent long-term benefits.

Short-term treatment with gonadotropin-releasing hormone (GnRH) analogs is an additional option for medical management of endometriosis. GnRH analogs create a hypogonadal, hypoestrogenic state. Because of its side effects profile and potential for the development of low bone mineral density over time, it is not FDA approved for prolonged use (see Chapter 49).

Summary

Dysmenorrhea is a common reproductive health concern for many adolescents. Early diagnosis and long-term medical management are important for severe cases associated with possible endometriosis. NSAIDs and contraceptive hormones are the mainstay of therapy and when used prophylactically can lead to significant improvement of symptoms and less impairment of activities of daily living.

Further reading

Falcone T, Lebovic DI. Clinical management of endometriosis. *Obstet Gynecol* 2011;118(3):691–705.

Harel Z. Dysmenorrhea in adolescent and young adults: etiology and management. *J Pediatr Adolesc Gynecol* 2006;19:365.

Harel Z. Dysmenorrhea in adolescents and young adults: from pathophysiology to pharmacological treatments and management strategies. *Expert Opin Pharmacother* 2008; 9(15):1–12.

Harel Z. Dysmenorrhea in adolescents and young adults: an update on pharmacological treatments and management strategies. *Expert Opin Pharmacother* 2012;13(15):2157–2170.

46 Congenital anomalies

Amy M. Vallerie[1] and Lesley L. Breech[2]

[1]Department of Pediatrics, Division of Adolescent Medicine, New York Medical College, Valhalla, NY, USA
[2]Department of Surgery, Division of Pediatric and Adolescent Gynecology, University of Cincinnati College of Medicine, Cincinnati, OH, USA

The uterus, cervix, Fallopian tubes, and upper vagina are derived from the Müllerian ducts. Differentiation of the female reproductive tract begins during the fifth week of gestation, with development, descent, canalization, and fusion of the paramesonephric ducts into a single midline uterus with communicating cervix and bilateral Fallopian tubes (Figure 46.1). The female reproductive tract is anomalous in 0.5–10%, depending on the study population. These anomalies present as menstrual dysfunction, pelvic pain, infertility, or obstetric complications in adolescence and early adulthood. Patients with obstructive anomalies present during middle to late puberty, following normal adrenarche and thelarche. Müllerian anomalies are associated with renal anomalies and anorectal malformations. Three classifications systems have been proposed:

- American Society of Reproductive Medicine, formerly American Fertility Society (AFS), classification system, which is the most widely used (Table 46.1)
- Vaginal–Cervical–Uterine–Adnexal-associated Malformation (VCUAM) system
- Acien's embryologic–clinical classification.

This chapter will review combined and isolated anomalies of the uterus, vagina, and Fallopian tubes.

Uterine anomalies

The uterus is comprised of a fundus, body, and cervix. The prepubertal uterus is tubular in shape with a 1:1

> ### Science revisited
>
> - Müllerian system development was originally hypothesized as a default pathway when the *SRY* gene failed to stimulate differentiation of the Wolffian, or male reproductive, system.
> - In 1999, discovery of the critical role of the *Wnt-4* gene in female mouse uterine and vaginal differentiation debunked this hypothesis.
> - Several reports exist in the literature of adult women with congenital Müllerian tract agenesis and *Wnt-4* mutations.
> - Additional genes actively expressed during Müllerian system differentiation include *SHOX*, *PAX*, *Cftr*, and *AMH*.
> - Studies evaluating these gene signaling pathways have failed to demonstrate a consistent role in female reproductive tract development, but point to a heterogeneous, multifactorial etiology.

ratio of uterine body to cervix. During puberty, the uterine body develops further, taking on a balloon shape, increasing in size relative to the cervix. Given the size and structure of the prepubertal uterus, and an asymptomatic state, anomalies are rarely detected in preadolescence. Anomalies of the uterus can affect the fundus, body, and/or cervix. There is a strong

---

Practical Pediatric and Adolescent Gynecology, First Edition. Edited by Paula J. Adams Hillard.
© 2013 John Wiley & Sons, Ltd. Published 2013 by John Wiley & Sons, Ltd.

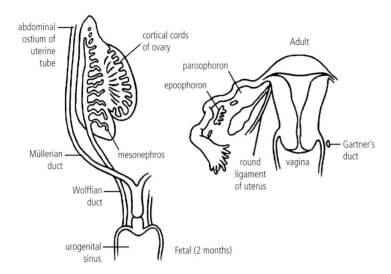

abdominal
ostium of
uterine
tube

cortical cords
of ovary

paroophoron

Adult

epoophoron

Müllerian
duct

mesonephros

round
ligament
of uterus

vagina

Gartner's
duct

Wolffian
duct

urogenital
sinus

Fetal (2 months)

Figure 46.1 Diagram of the genital ducts at 2 months and their mature female remnants. Mesonephros or Wolffian duct development is suppressed. The paramesonephric or Müllerian duct system differentiates into the uterine, Fallopian tube, and upper vaginal structures. The kidneys are derived from the adjacent metanephric ducts (not pictured). Reproduced with permission from Lin PC, Bhatnagar KP, Nettleton GS, Nakajima ST. Female genital anomalies affecting reproduction. *Fertil Steril* 2002;78(5):899–915. Elsevier.

association between uterine, renal, and anorectal malformations.

Uterine anomalies can be classified as symmetric and asymmetric.

Symmetric uterine anomalies

Symmetric uterine anomalies include arcuate, septate, bicornuate, and didelphys configurations. These variations result from incomplete fusion of the bilateral uterine horns.

Arcuate, septate, and bicornuate uteri have one uterine body and a single, but variable, uterine cavity and fundus. Both bicornuate and arcuate uteri have a midline fundal muscular indentation, resulting in a heart-shaped uterine cavity (Figure 46.2). An arcuate uterus has a normal, convex fundus. Bicornuate uteri exhibit a midline depression in both the cavity and fundus. A uterine septum is an avascular membranous division of the uterine cavity and may extend the entire length of the uterine cavity. Patients with a complete uterine septum may have cervical duplication.

Patients typically present with infertility and pregnancy complications during adulthood. As adolescents, patients may present with imaging suggestive of an anomaly on evaluation for unrelated complaints or related anomalies, menorrhagia or dysmenorrhea. Diagnosis can be made through imaging with 3D ultrasound or MRI, and is best performed during the luteal phase when a thickened endometrial lining allows improved delineation of the uterine cavity. These studies may soon replace diagnostic laparoscopy and hysteroscopy as the gold standard for evaluation.

Uterine didelphys is comprised of two equal, well-developed hemiuteri, each with a cervix and unilateral Fallopian tube. Seventy-five percent of patients with uterocervical duplication have a longitudinal vaginal septum dividing the vaginal cavity into two hemivaginas. Hence, these patients may present complaining of difficulty with tampon insertion, leaking of menstrual fluid with a tampon in place, or dyspareunia. Patients with uterine didelphys have mildly impaired fertility and increased rates of preterm labor, miscarriage, and fetal malpresentation. There is no surgical intervention for uterine didelphys. Pregnancy should be managed by a maternal–fetal medicine (MFM) specialist.

Asymmetric uterine anomalies

Asymmetric uterine anomalies, or unicornuate hemiuterus with an incompletely developed or absent contralateral uterine horn, account for approximately 5% of all uterine anomalies. The uterine horn may be functional or nonfunctional (74%), as defined by the presence of hormonally responsive endometrial tissue, and may or may not communicate (92%) with the dominate unicornuate uterus (Figures 46.3 and

Table 46.1 Classification of Müllerian anomalies according to the ASRM classification system

Type I	"Müllerian" agenesis or hypoplasia
	A. Vaginal (uterus may be normal or exhibit a variety of malformations)
	B. Cervical
	C. Fundal
	D. Tubal
	E. Combined
Type II	Unicornuate uterus
	A. Communicating (endometrial cavity present)
	B. Noncommunicating (endometrial cavity present)
	C. Horn without endometrial cavity
	D. No rudimentary horn
Type III	Uterus didelphys
Type IV	Uterus bicornuate
	A. Complete (division down to internal os)
	B. Partial
Type V	Septate uterus
	A. Complete (septum to internal os)
	B. Partial
Type VI	Arcuate
Type VII	*DES-related anomalies
	A. T-shaped uterus
	B. T-shaped with dilated horns
	C. T-shaped

*DES, diethylstilbestrol

Adapted from Buttram VC, Jr. Müllerian anomalies and their management. *Fertil Steril* 1983;40:159; Buttram VC Jr, Gibbons WE. Müllerian anomalies: a proposed classification (an analysis of 144 cases). *Fertil Steril* 1979;32:40; The American Fertility Society. The American Fertility Society classifications of adnexal adhesions, distal tubal occlusion, tubal occlusion secondary to tubal ligation, tubal pregnancies, Müllerian anomalies, and intrauterine adhesions. *Fertil Steril* 1988;49:944. Elsevier.

46.4). Patients with a nonfunctional uterine horn may present with dysmenorrhea or pelvic pain secondary to rudimentary horn adenomyosis, hydrosalpinx, or endometriosis. The classic presentation of a noncommunicating, functional uterine horn is progressive dysmenorrhea and a palpable pelvic mass. Unfortunately, only half of these patients present with these symptoms, delaying diagnosis and putting them at risk for ectopic pregnancy in the rudimentary horn. Such pregnancies have been reported in patients with communicating and noncommunicating uterine horns and have high morbidity. Therefore, patients with a unicornuate uterus require surgical intervention by an experienced gynecologic surgeon to remove the functional horn prior to reproduction.

⭐ **Tips and tricks**

Uterine and renal anomalies
- The literature consistently demonstrates a strong association between uterine and renal anomalies.
- Approximately one-third of patients with uterine didelphys, unicornuate uteri, and uterovaginal agenesis have a solitary functioning kidney.
- Additionally, in patients with a uterine anomaly, unilateral renal agenesis was predictive of an obstructive Müllerian anomaly in 55–70% of cases.
- Therefore, while evaluation of the renal system is part of the standard work-up in patients with uterine anomalies, all females with a solitary functioning kidney should undergo evaluation of the reproductive tract with ultrasound during early puberty.

✋ **Patient/parent education**

- Reproductive tract anomalies are extremely concerning to both patients and their families.
- Patients have concerns regarding optimal treatment as well as the impact on fertility potential.
- In patients with anomalies that require surgical management, it is not always necessary to intervene immediately.
- Gonadotropin-releasing hormone (GnRH) agonists, continuous oral contraceptives or continuous progesterone therapy can be administered as a temporizing measure, preventing further accumulation of hematometrocolpos until the optimal time for surgery is reached.

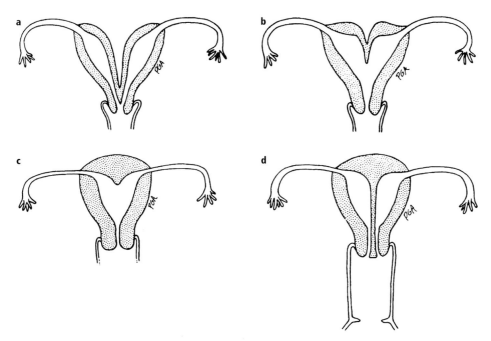

Figure 46.2 The AFS classifications of anomalies. (A) Complete uterus bicornuate, (B) Partial uterus bicornuate, (C) Arcuate uterus, (D) Complete septate uterus.
Reproduced with permission from Reichman DE, Laufer MR. Congenital uterine anomalies affecting reproduction. *Best Pract Res Clin Obstet Gynaecol* 2010;24(2):193–208. Elsevier.

• Alternatively, the hematometrocolpos can be drained percutaneously or laparoscopically.
• Such delay allows the patient to mature and become an active participant in the decision for surgery.
• Additionally, advances continue in high-risk obstetric and neonatal care, as well as reproductive technology.
• Patients may benefit from a counseling session with an appropriate specialist prior to surgery.

Isolated anomalies of the uterine cervix

Isolated anomalies of the uterine cervix are extremely rare and can be divided into two groups: cervical agenesis and cervical dysgenesis (Figure 46.5). Patients present with amenorrhea, pain, and a palpable mass secondary to hematometra. Retrograde menstruation can result in endometriosis and hematosalpinx. The vaginal cavity is variable in length and development, but the uterine cavity is typically singular. A preliminary diagnosis can be made by MRI, but the extent of dysgenesis is not fully appreciated until the time of surgery. Referral to an experienced gynecologic surgeon is imperative, as surgical correction has historically been associated with significant morbidity, a high risk of multiple procedures, and rarely, mortality. Recent case reports suggest that surgical repair techniques are improving and specific candidates can be successfully repaired. Patients and parents should be counseled extensively prior to any surgical intervention.

Vaginal agenesis

Congenital absence of the uterus and vagina (CAUV), known as Mayer–Rokitansky–Küster–Hauser (MRKH) syndrome, affects approximately 1

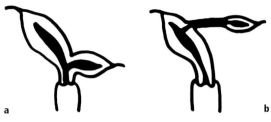

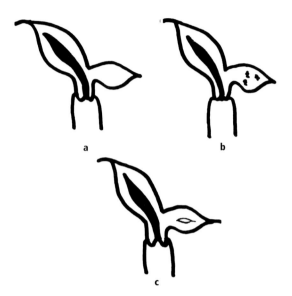

Figure 46.3 Communicating rudimentary horn.
(A) Nonseparated and (B) separated. Patients have normal menstruation. All types of unicornuate uterus with a functional rudimentary horn are at risk for ectopic pregnancy.
Reproduced with permission from Jayasinghe Y, Rane A, Stalewski H, Grover S. The presentation and early diagnosis of the rudimentary uterine horn. *Obstet Gynecol* 2005;105:1460. Lippincott Williams & Wilkins.

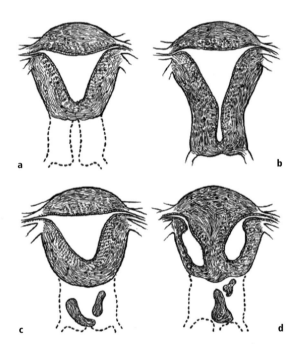

Figure 46.4 Noncommunicating rudimentary horn. (A) Nonseparated and (B) separated. If endometrium is present within the horn (C), patients will have menstrual obstruction.
Reproduced with permission from Jayasinghe Y, Rane A, Stalewski H, Grover S. The presentation and early diagnosis of the rudimentary uterine horn. *Obstet Gynecol* 2005;105(6):1460. Lippincott Williams & Wilkins.

Figure 46.5 Four types of cervical dysgenesis. (A) The fundus of the uterus is without a cervix. (B) The cervical body is intact with obstruction of the cervical os. (C, D) Fragmentation of the cervix in which portions of the cervix have no connection to the uterine body.
Reproduced with permission from Rock JA, Roberts CP, Jones HWJ. Congenital anomalies of the uterine cervix: lessons from 30 cases managed clinically by a common protocol. *Fertil Steril* 2010;94(5):1858–1863. Elsevier.

in 5000 newborn females. Müllerian agenesis presents during adolescence as painless primary amenorrhea. Patients undergo otherwise normal pubertal development with mature secondary sexual characteristics. On physical exam, there is blind ending pouch of distal vaginal tissue. The size of the vaginal dimple is variable; therefore, visual inspection is not sufficient. The uterine structures are typically bilateral rudimentary hemiuteri (Figure 46.6). Five percent of cases have a functional uterine lining, which results in secondary hematometra, endometriosis, and cyclic lateralized abdominal, pelvic or flank pain.

Renal, skeletal, auditory, and cardiac anomalies are associated with MRKH. Additionally, patient siblings have an increased prevalence of congenital anomalies. The majority of cases are sporadic, but familial cases have been reported. The diagnosis is made by physical exam, and ultrasound or MRI. Karyotyping and testosterone levels are necessary to exclude complete androgen insensitivity syndrome (CAIS).

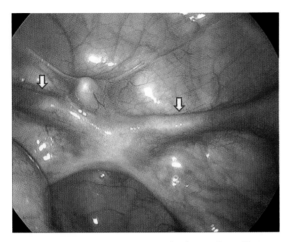

Figure 46.6 Laparoscopic image of pelvis with Müllerian agenesis with bilateral nonfunctional uterine horns (arrows).

response to circulating androgens, is 10 times more common than partial AIS. In CAIS, the presence of Müllerian inhibiting substance (MIS) suppresses the development of the internal female reproductive tract. Additionally, the male system fails to develop as the signals cannot be received secondary to nonfunctioning receptors. During puberty, when testosterone surges, but fails to evoke the appropriate response, excess testosterone is produced by the functioning gonads and peripherally converted to estrogen. Therefore, phenotypic females present during mid-puberty with primary amenorrhea, complete breast development, minimal acne, and scant pubic and axillary hair. The genitalia are consistent with an estrogenized female perineum with a blind ending vaginal pouch. Patients with partial AIS will present with varying degrees of ambiguous genitalia. Gonads may be palpable in the labia or inguinal canal. Laboratory evaluation will show an XY karyotype and elevated luteinizing hormone and testosterone levels. Diagnosis can be confirmed by human chorionic gonadotropin (hCG) stimulation test or androgen receptor studies. Ultrasound and/or MRI demonstrate abdominal, pelvic, or inguinal gonads and absent uterine tissue.

★ Tips and tricks

- A transabdominal pelvic ultrasound is a satisfactory method of evaluation for the presence or absence of a uterus.
- While transvaginal ultrasound is the preferred modality to evaluate the ovaries, transperineal, transrectal, or transvaginal ultrasound is not required as this can be both physically and emotionally uncomfortable for the patient.
- Additionally, the ovaries may not be seen on pelvic ultrasound, as one or both fail to completely descend into the ovarian fossa in 16% of patients; however, the presence of ovarian function is obvious on exam, as normal breast development is present, and patients can be reassured that the ovaries are present. Thus, transabdominal pelvic and abdominal ultrasound is needed to completely define the reproductive and renal anatomy.

✋ Caution

Complete androgen insensitivity syndrome
- CAIS accounts for 1–2% of cases of female children with inguinal herniation of the gonads and should be considered in the differential diagnosis of all female children with inguinal hernia or mass.
- Diagnosis can be made by ultrasound imaging combined with laboratory testing, biopsy of the gonadal tissue at the time of surgical repair, or a laparoscopic approach to hernia repair with diagnostic evaluation of the pelvic organs.

Androgen insensitivity syndrome (AIS) is a rare X-linked congenital defect, affecting 1–5 in 100 000 newborns, in which the androgen receptors function abnormally. CAIS, in which the receptor has no

Management of vaginal agenesis is a multidisciplinary endeavor. Patients should be referred to a specialist with experience in the management of Müllerian anomalies, such as a pediatric gynecologist or reproductive endocrinologist. Ideally, patients with CAIS should be cared for at a center for disorders of sexual development (see Chapter 2) with a core team consisting of endocrinology, genetics, urology, and gynecology. Psychology and patient and family support groups are important and valuable throughout diagnosis and treatment. There is no urgency to creating a vaginal space. Management is patient directed and driven. The American College of Obstetricians and Gynecologists (ACOG) recommends progressive perineal dilation as the primary method of vaginal construction. Patients who are unable to achieve an adequate vaginal space can be managed surgically. Patients with MRKH can achieve fertility via IVF and a gestational carrier. However, patients with CAIS are infertile and the gonads should be surgically removed secondary to a 2–5% risk of malignancy. These patients will require lifetime hormone replacement and are at an increased risk for osteoporosis and heart disease.

Transverse vaginal septum

The prevalence of transverse vaginal septum is unknown, but has been estimated to be from 1 in 2100 to 1 in 70 000 women. This defect is thought to result from failure of the urogenital sinus to fuse

with the upper Müllerian-derived vagina, resulting in a segment of fibrotic tissue obstructing menstruation (Figure 46.7 and Table 46.2). A small perforation in the septum is not uncommon. A septum can occur anywhere along the length of the vaginal canal, but has a slight preponderance for the upper vagina. Transverse septa greater than 1 cm in thickness are referred to as segmental vaginal atresia, and are

Table 46.2 Classification of vaginal septa

Classification	Features
Class I	Transverse
	A. Obstructing
	B. Nonobstructing
Class II	Longitudinal
	A. Obstructing
	B. Nonobstructing
Class III	Stenosis/iatrogenic

Reproduced with permission from Attaran M, Gidwani G. Management of emergencies associated with congenital malformations of the female genital tract, In: Gidwani G, Falcone T (eds). *Congenital Malformations of the Female Genital Tract, Diagnosis and Management*. 1999. Lippincott Williams & Wilkins.

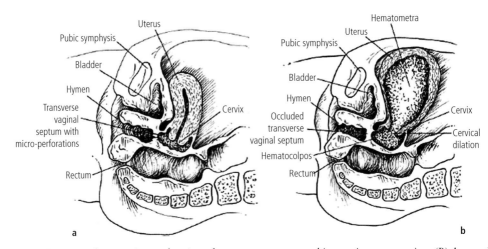

a

b

Figure 46.7 (A) An incomplete or microperforation of a transverse septum; this permits menstruation. (B) A complete transverse septum or secondary scarring of a perforated septum will result in accumulation of hematometrocolpos. Reproduced with permission from Nichols JL, Bieber EJ, Gell JS. Secondary amenorrhea attributed to occlusion of microperforate transverse vaginal septum. *Fertil Steril* 2010;94(1):351.e5 – 351.e10. Elsevier.

surgically more difficult to repair. The uterus, cervix, and Fallopian tubes are anatomically and functionally normal. There does not appear to be an increased incidence of renal anomalies. Patients present in mid-puberty with hematometrocolpos and cyclic pelvic pain if the septum is imperforate. Patients with large hematometrocolpos may have a palpable mass and compression symptoms, such as urinary retention and constipation. Patients can be managed medically to prevent further accumulation of hematometrocolpos, pending evaluation and surgical repair. MRI will define the level of obstruction, thickness of the septum, and involvement of the upper genital tract. Patients should also be evaluated for possible hydrone-phrosis, as this would necessitate immediate interven-tion. Percutaneous or laparoscopic drainage are temporizing measures for patients in acute pain prior to surgical correction by a qualified gynecologist, although there is a risk of introducing infection into the upper vaginal segment.

> ### ☝ Caution
>
> • A low transverse septum can be misdiagnosed as an imperforate hymen. Transverse septa are composed of tough fibrous tissue, while an imperforate hymen is a thin compliant membrane.
> • With a transverse septum, there is no blue bulge at the perineum as would be seen with hematocolpos behind a thin hymenal membrane.
> • MRI should be used if the diagnosis is unclear.
> • Surgical management of a transverse vaginal septum as an imperforate hymen can result in complications and scarring, with high morbidity.

Obstructed hemivagina, ipsilateral renal agenesis syndrome

Obstructed hemivagina, ipsilateral renal agenesis (OHV-IRA) syndrome is a unique entity in which an oblique vaginal septum obstructs one side of a septated vagina and uterine didelphys (Figure 46.8). The resulting unilateral obstruction results in signifi-cant delay in diagnosis, as patients are menstruating

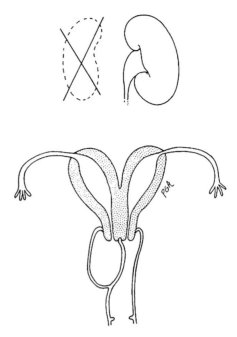

Figure 46.8 Obstructed hemivagina, ipsilateral renal agenesis (OHV-IRA). Oblique vaginal septum occluding unilateral uterus didelphys and hemivagina, associated with renal agenesis. Reproduced with permission from Reichman DE, Laufer MR. Congenital uterine anomalies affecting reproduction. *Best Pract Res Clin Obstet Gynaecol* 2010;24(2):193–208. Lippincott Williams & Wilkins.

regularly. Hence patients are often diagnosed in an emergency room setting with uncontrolled pain. There may be a palpable mass and lateral bulge in the vagina on bimanual exam. The communicating cervix is difficult to palpate because it is superiorly displaced by the contralateral hematometra. Diagnosis is confirmed by ultrasound or MRI of a single normal hemiuterus and cervix and a pelvic mass of hematomet-rocolpos. Patients undergo urgent correction with transvaginal resection of the septum. If detected in the outpatient setting, patients with OHV-IRA should be referred to a gynecologist with expertise in this condi-tion for surgical treatment.

Longitudinal vaginal septum

As previously mentioned, longitudinal vaginal septum is most commonly noted in the setting of a duplicated uterine anomaly, but can be an isolated anomaly as well. Patients present in adolescence with difficult tampon insertion, vaginal bleeding with a tampon in place, dyspareunia, or significant vaginal bleeding following intercourse. Adult women may present with obstetric symptoms related to the associated uterine anomaly. MRI is recommended to define the uterine cavity. Patients should be referred to a gynecologist for appropriate counseling and elective septum excision.

★ Tips and tricks

- Duplication of the vagina is not always obvious, as one side may be dominant.
- A speculum may be inserted into one side without discomfort or complication, occluding the other without the practitioner's knowledge.
- Careful inspection of the vaginal introitus and bimanual exam may improve detection.
- Ninety-five percent of patients with a vaginal septum will have a uterine anomaly, while 75% of patients with uterocervical duplication have a longitudinal vaginal septum.
- If a vaginal septum is noted on exam, evaluation of the upper genital tract is indicated.
- When performing a Pap smear for cervical cancer screening, it is necessary to collect a sample from each cervix separately and label them accordingly for appropriate follow-up.

Fallopian tube anomalies

Congenital anomalies of the Fallopian tube are rare. These anomalies include accessory or duplicated Fallopian tubes, accessory ostia, and complete or segmental atresia. Congenital tubal atresia places patients at risk for adnexal torsion and hydrosalpinx. Adolescents may present with acute symptoms of adnexal torsion or pelvic infection, such as acute, severe unilateral pain with associated nausea, vomiting, and/or fever. At the time of surgery, a Fallopian tube anomaly is noted. Adult women with bilateral tubal atresia will present with infertility. Surgical cor-

rection of tubal atresia is limited to those patients with infertility. A reproductive endocrinology and infertility specialist (REI) can excise the atretic area and re-approximate the fimbria to the proximal Fallopian tube.

Conclusion

Müllerian anomalies are a heterogeneous group of isolated and combined defects of female reproductive tract development. These anomalies are relatively common, making it likely that a general practitioner will encounter an adolescent with a Müllerian anomaly. Diagnosis most often occurs during adolescence, a pivotal period of physical and emotional development, creating unique challenges in counseling and management. Patients present with subtle or progressive symptoms, delaying diagnosis. Incomplete Müllerian fusion can best be explained on the basis of polygenic/multifactorial inheritance. There is a strong association between uterine, vaginal, renal, and anorectal anomalies. Patients with an anomaly of the urogenital system should undergo evaluation to rule out other associated anomalies. The key elements of evaluation are physical exam and imaging. A high index of suspicion, knowledge of associated anomalies, and awareness of diagnostic tools allow appropriate evaluation, early detection, and referral to an experienced pediatric/adolescent gynecologist, REI, or multidisciplinary center.

Further reading

Brucker SY, Rall K, Campo R, Oppelt P, Isaacson K. Treatment of congenital malformations. *Semin Reprod Med* 2011;29:101–112.

Damario MA, Rock JA. Uterovaginal anomalies. In: Koehler Carpenter SE, Rock JA (eds). *Pediatric and Adolescent Gynecology*, 2nd edn. Philadelphia: Lippincott Williams & Wilkins, 2000, pp. 332–353.

Rackow BW, Arici A. Reproductive performance of women with Müllerian anomalies. *Curr Opin Obstet Gynecol* 2007;19:229–337.

Simpson JL. Genetics of the female reproductive ducts. *Am J Med Genet* 1999;89:224–239.

47 Ectopic pregnancy

Michelle Vichnin

Merck Vaccines, West Point, PA, USA

Ectopic pregnancy (EP) is defined as a pregnancy that occurs outside of the uterus, most commonly in the ampullary section of the Fallopian tube. Ruptured EP is a leading cause of morbidity and mortality in women in the first trimester of pregnancy. It is important to make a timely diagnosis and implement treatment to ensure the best clinical outcomes.

Evidence at a glance

- The risk factors for EP have been well studied. Any damage to the Fallopian tube increases the risk for development of an EP. Common risk factors include prior tubal surgery, prior pelvic inflammatory disease (PID), previous EP, *in utero* exposure to diethylstilbestrol, and intrauterine device (IUD) *in situ*. Cigarette smoking is an independent risk factor.
- A history of a diagnosed chlamydial infection is associated with a two-fold increased EP risk.
- Contraceptives decrease the number of intrauterine pregnancies as well as EPs.

It is difficult to ascertain the true incidence of EP because many patients are treated in an outpatient setting. While it is true that EP is more likely to occur in adults, one study at a large institution showed that 12% of ectopic pregnancies occurred in adolescents.

✋ Caution

- It is critical to rule out EP in any adolescent (or any woman of child-bearing age) who presents with amenorrhea, pelvic pain, and/or irregular vaginal bleeding.
- Other conditions that may present in a similar fashion are appendicitis, spontaneous abortion (miscarriage), ovarian torsion, PID, ruptured corpus luteum cyst, tubo-ovarian abscess, and urinary calculi.

Evaluation

Patients with an EP may present in one of two ways: ruptured (hemodynamically unstable/surgical emergency) and unruptured EP.

A patient presenting with pelvic pain, hypotension, and a positive pregnancy test has a surgical emergency, and most likely, a diagnosis of an EP, although a ruptured corpus luteum cyst with hemoperitoneum is also a diagnostic possibility. She may be dizzy and she may have shoulder pain due to referred pain from diaphragmatic irritation by the hemoperitoneum. *Immediate* surgery is the only treatment option in these cases, and if performed quickly enough, transfusion may be avoided. A large bore IV line should be placed and fluid resuscitation started. A complete

Practical Pediatric and Adolescent Gynecology, First Edition. Edited by Paula J. Adams Hillard.
© 2013 John Wiley & Sons, Ltd. Published 2013 by John Wiley & Sons, Ltd.

blood count (CBC), type-and-screen, and β-human chorionic gonadotropin (β-hCG) should be requested and the operating room called. Experienced surgeons may perform laparoscopy, but laparotomy is acceptable. In the case of a ruptured EP, the Fallopian tube may need to be removed partially (partial salpingectomy) or completely (complete salpingectomy).

A patient with an unruptured EP may be managed conservatively (see later).

The patient with a positive urine pregnancy test should undergo a transvaginal ultrasound (TVUS). If an intrauterine pregnancy (IUP) or EP is clearly visualized on TVUS (sometimes a beating fetal heart may be seen in the adnexa), the diagnosis is made. Unfortunately, half of the time the ultrasound is nondiagnostic (no definitive gestation seen inside or outside of the uterus). The patient with a nondiagnostic ultrasound needs further evaluation with serum β-hCG levels.

★ Tips and tricks

- It is often timesaving/convenient to order bloodwork when the ultrasound is ordered.
- Send off a β-hCG, CBC, and type-and-screen, and include liver function tests (LFTs), blood urea and nitrogen (BUN), and creatinine, since these tests are required prior to starting methotrexate.
- In this way, the patient will avoid a "second stick" if she is diagnosed with an EP and methotrexate is chosen as the treatment option.

A β-hCG level of ~1500 mIU/mL is associated with the ability to visualize a normal singleton IUP with TVUS (the so-called "discriminatory zone" of β-hCG). If the β-hCG level is less than 1500 mIU/mL, *the level should be repeated in 48 hours.* In a normal IUP, the β-hCG level increases by at least 53%. Once the level reaches the 1500 mIU/mL threshold, a TVUS should be repeated to confirm the presence if an IUP.

In an abnormal IUP or an EP, the levels of β-hCG may plateau, rise inappropriately (i.e. not increase by at least 53%) or decline. If levels of β-hCG follow these patterns, dilation and curettage (D&C) or in-office Manual Vacuum Aspiration (MVA) is performed to determine the presence of chorionic villi in

the uterus. Suction curettage is felt to be more accurate by some specialists than sharp curettage. If chorionic villi are absent, EP is likely.

✋ Patient/parent advice

- Patients must understand the need for close follow-up when being followed for a possible EP, which is a potentially life-threatening condition.
- Most patients, even teens, can be followed as outpatients, with instructions to go to the emergency room immediately with increased pain or vaginal bleeding, dizziness, or fainting ("ectopic precautions").
- If there is uncertainty that the patient will be compliant, she may be admitted for observation.

Management

Immediate surgery is the only treatment option for a ruptured EP. Many gynecologists were taught that "the sun never sets on an ectopic," meaning that any patient with an EP should be taken to the operating room immediately. However, with very accurate assays for β-hCG and proven effectiveness of methotrexate for medical treatment, that mantra no longer holds true. Appropriate treatment options for the patient with an unruptured EP include expectant, medical, or surgical management.

Expectant management

Expectant management is appropriate only when the β-hCG levels are low and declining. A good candidate for expectant management has a β-hCG level of less than 1000 mIU/mL and declining on repeat levels, an ectopic mass less than 3 cm, no fetal heart beat, and is compliant.

Medical management

Medical management with methotrexate (a folic acid antagonist which inactivates the enzyme dihydrofolate reductase) has been well studied. There are case reports of its successful use in adolescents.

When selecting patients for medical therapy, keep the following in mind:
• The lower the β-hCG levels at the time of treatment, the higher the success rate.
• A gestational adnexal mass of greater than 4 cm or adnexal fetal cardiac activity are predictors of treatment failure.
• Compliance is very important, especially with adolescents, and daily follow-up may be necessary.
• Contraindications include kidney disease, liver disease, blood dyscrasias and active pulmonary disease (need to confirm normal CBC, creatinine, and LFTs, which should be sent with the initial β-hCG, and type-and-screen when the patient presents).
• Side effects include nausea, vomiting, and stomatitis.

There are three published protocols for methotrexate administration to treat EP:
• Single dose ($50\,mg/m^2$): simple, effective
• Two doses
• Fixed multidose: may be more effective than single dose, but needs folinic acid rescue to minimize side effects.

The time to resolution of the EP is 3–7 weeks after methotrexate therapy. Failure of therapy occurs when:
• β-hCG levels do not decrease by at least 15% from day 4 to day 7 after administration.
• A patient develops severe pain, hypotension, or other signs of rupture and needs surgical intervention.

Surgical management

Surgical management is still an important treatment option, especially in patients who are anxious about medical treatment side effects or their ability to follow-up so frequently. Also, some patients desire definitive management. Laparoscopy with salpingostomy (preservation of Fallopian tube) is the preferred method of treatment, but treatment failure occurs 5–20% of the time. Follow-up patients with serial serum β-hCG levels postoperatively until the levels are less than 5 mIU/mL. Methotrexate may be used if the β-hCG levels plateau postoperatively.

✋ **Caution**

Contraception should be emphasized after treatment, since a new pregnancy can cause confusion when following β-hCG levels.

⚲ **Pearls**

• Screening adolescents for chlamydia is very important to decrease the risk of EP.
• In young women who present with amenorrhea, pelvic pain, and/or abnormal vaginal bleeding, EP must be ruled out.
• Ruptured EP is a surgical emergency.
• Compliant patients with unruptured EP may be treated conservatively.

Further reading

American College of Obstetricians and Gynecologists. ACOG Practice Bulletin. *Medical Management of Ectopic Pregnancy*, Number 94. ACOG, 2008.

Barnhart KT, Sammel MD, Gracia CR, *et al*. Rick factors for ectopic pregnancy in women with symptomatic first-trimester pregnancies. *Fertil Steril* 2006;20:36.

Menon S, Sammel MD, Vichnin M, *et al*. Risk factors for ectopic pregnancy: A comparison between adults and adolescent women. *J Pediatr Adolesc Gynecol* 2007;20: 181–185.

48.1 Ovarian cysts

Paula J. Adams Hillard

Department of Obstetrics and Gynecology, Stanford University School of Medicine, Stanford, CA, USA

An ovarian cyst is a very common diagnosis in patients who have pelvic pain, particularly those who have been to an emergency medical facility. While ovarian cysts can certainly cause pelvic pain, many "cysts" that are diagnosed on the basis of ultrasound findings may be "red herring" diagnoses. In thinking about ovarian cysts, it is helpful to consider the algorithm in Figure 48.1.1 that aids in reaching a logical diagnosis.

The clinician may find it helpful to ask themselves a series of dichotomous questions about the clinical situation. The first consideration should be a focus on symptoms. Other factors include the characteristics of the mass (cystic, mixed echogenicity including hemorrhagic, solid), child's age (prepubertal vs pubertal/adolescent in whom ovarian functional cysts may be present), and the size of the mass. A "functional" cyst will be either a follicular cyst (an exaggeration of the physiologic process in which a single follicle becomes the dominant follicle in the first half of the cycle prior to ovulation) or a cystic corpus luteum (an exaggeration of the development of a normal corpus luteum, which typically involves hemorrhage into the cystic cavity of the corpus luteum). The development of a normal dominant ovarian follicle in the follicular phase of the menstrual cycle can be confused with the development of a pathologic cyst; the normal follicle can reach a size of 2–3 cm, which should *not* be described as a cyst, but rather as a cystic follicle. Similarly, small follicles within the ovary are a normal finding; the pathologic condition of polycystic ovaries, in which 12 or more sub-centimeter follicles are present in each ovary, while associated with metabolic changes (see Chapter 50), does not cause pain.

👆 Patient/parent information

- Most ovarian cysts of less than 3 cm in size in adolescents are "functional" cysts that simply reflect normal functioning of the ovary, occurring each month on a regular basis.
- A hormone imbalance called polycystic ovary syndrome often includes the presence of multiple small (<1 cm) ovarian cysts. These cysts and this condition do not cause pain, and are different from other ovarian cysts (see Chapter 50).
- Functional cysts are rarely the cause of pain, typically resolve with time, and do not need to be treated.
- Persistent pelvic pain should be evaluated, and management options discussed.
- Because hormonal contraceptives prevent ovulation, they typically prevent cyclic pelvic pain, and may be helpful for managing mid-cycle pain or pain with menstruation.

Practical Pediatric and Adolescent Gynecology, First Edition. Edited by Paula J. Adams Hillard.
© 2013 John Wiley & Sons, Ltd. Published 2013 by John Wiley & Sons, Ltd.

★ Tips and tricks

Categorizing ovarian masses
- Symptoms:
  - ○ Asymptomatic: incidental finding
  - ○ Acute-onset symptoms. Mechanisms of pain:
    - – Hemorrhage into cystic cavity (hemorrhagic corpus luteum)
    - – Torsion
    - – Cyst rupture (typically corpus luteum)
    - – Versus nongynecologic causes (appendicitis)
  - ○ Chronic symptoms of pelvic pain:
    - – Consider pelvic endometriosis
    - – Slow growing neoplasm
- Age:
  - ○ Prepubertal
  - ○ Adolescent with cyclic ovarian function
- Size:
  - ○ <10 cm: likely functional or benign neoplasm
  - ○ >10 cm: likely neoplasm
- Neoplasm:
  - ○ Benign
  - ○ Malignant
- Functional:
  - ○ Follicular cyst
  - ○ Corpus luteum cyst

Asymptomatic mass

The presence of a mass, detected on imaging (e.g. renal or bladder ultrasound, or an abdominal CT scan), in the absence of pelvic symptoms, allows time for a measured approach to the mass. While a transvaginal pelvic ultrasound offers the most information about a pelvic mass, it may not be feasible in a young adolescent. In this case, a transabdominal ultrasound with a focus on the *pelvis*, not the abdomen, will have to suffice. Ultrasound provides more information about the mass than a CT scan, allowing the determination not only of accurate size, but also of characteristics of the mass: a unilocular cyst, a cyst with septations, a mass of mixed solid and cystic components, the presence of characteristics indicating hemorrhage or clot, or the presence of a predominantly solid mass.

☟ Caution

A *solid* ovarian mass is a likely neoplasm, which can be *benign or malignant*.
- The most common solid ovarian mass in the pediatric age group is a germ cell tumor (see Chapter 48.2).
- Referral to a specialist (pediatric gynecology, gynecologic oncology, or pediatric surgery) is warranted.

An asymptomatic unilocular cyst ("simple" with no internal septations or vascularity) of less than 10 cm in size is almost certainly benign, but could be a benign neoplasm (such as a mucinous cystadenoma) or a follicular cyst. Table 48.1.1 lists the differential diagnosis for a unilocular ovarian cyst in the pediatric/adolescent age group (see also Table 5.1). While a simple ovarian cyst is likely functional or benign, the

Evidence at a glance

Torsion in adolescents
- Data from adults indicates that ovarian torsion accounts for 3% of acute abdominal pain in females.
- Annual incidence of torsion is 4.9 in 100 000 females aged 1–20 years, similar to the rate of testicular torsion.
- In a national inpatient database, adolescents aged older than 12 years accounted for 83% of all torsions for girls younger than 20 years.
- In the same national sample, malignancy was seen in only 0.4% of cases of torsion for ages 1–20 years.
- Thromboembolic events were not seen in this large sample.
- Ovarian torsion is much less common than appendicitis.
- Detorsion and ovarian preservation is successful in more than 90% of cases, with follicular development or normal ovarian morphology, in spite of a "necrotic" appearance.
- The association between successful detorsion and duration of symptoms is not clear.

Table 48.1.1 Differential diagnosis of a unilocular cyst in the pediatric age group

- Follicular cyst
- Cystadenoma:
  - Mucinous: can get very large
  - Serous
- Paratubal (para-ovarian) cyst
- Hydrosalpinx, salpingitis, pelvic inflammatory disease
- Mesenteric cyst
- Urachal cyst
- Appendiceal abscess
- Obstructed genital lesions (imperforate hymen, noncommunicating uterine horn)

presence of a cystic mass can lead to adnexal torsion (see Chapters 5 and 39.1).

In the absence of symptoms, observation of ovarian cysts is typically warranted, with a repeat ultrasound to assess for growth (indicating neoplasm) or a decrease in size/resolution. Benign follicular cysts can be seen on prenatal ultrasound, in the pediatric age group (most commonly in the first year of life), or in adolescents during the first half of the menstrual cycle as an exaggeration of the normal process of selection of a primary ovarian follicle prior to ovulation. In the neonatal age group, an incidentally noted small (<4 cm) cyst will likely resolve, and can be managed with serial ultrasound to assess resolution by 6 months. Complex cysts, those that persist beyond 6 months, symptomatic cysts, and enlarging cysts warrant surgical intervention. In the prepubertal age group, observation with periodic ultrasound assessment is warranted for simple cysts without symptoms (see Chapter 5). In an adolescent, follicular cysts are typically asymptomatic, and cysts of less than 10 cm in size are likely to resolve over 6–8 weeks. The persistence or enlargement of a cystic mass over this time period suggest the presence of a neoplasm, and warrants consideration of surgical intervention, in which normal ovarian tissue should be conserved. Figure 48.1.1 shows an algorithm for the management of asymptomatic ovarian cyst.

Similar to the presence of a solid mass, in the prepubertal age group, a mass with mixed echogenicity suggests a neoplasm, and requires referral, even if asymptomatic. In the adolescent age group, a mass with mixed echogenicity may be a functional ovarian cyst, most commonly a corpus luteum cyst with evi-

dence of hemorrhage. An endometrioma is another diagnosis to consider, although rare in adolescents. Germ cell tumors must also be considered (see Chapter 48.1). The differential for ovarian masses of mixed echogenicity is listed in Table 48.1.2.

Evidence at a glance

- Combined hormonal contraceptives, while suppressing ovarian activity, do not hasten the resolution of a functional ovarian cyst.
- Time alone is as likely to result in resolution as is treatment with combined hormonal contraceptives.
- Combined hormonal contraceptives, by suppressing ovulation and thus the development of ovarian follicles as well as a corpus luteum, can minimize the development of *subsequent* ovarian cysts. They should not be prescribed as *treatment* for the presence of an ovarian cyst.

Acute onset of pelvic pain

Corpus luteum cysts are common, and a menstrual history will typically reveal a last menstrual period around 3 weeks earlier. They are more likely to be symptomatic than are follicular cysts, and can be associated with acute pain, due to bleeding into the enclosed cystic cavity or to intraperitoneal hemorrhage. While these mechanisms may account for acute pain, corpus luteum cysts can also cause torsion, and thus the distinction between a symptomatic corpus luteum cyst and torsion of a corpus luteum cyst is challenging. A corpus luteum cyst without torsion will resolve over time, even in the presence of a small hemoperitoneum, and surgery is rarely required. Ovarian torsion is a surgical emergency and requires detorsion, which can be performed laparoscopically; even hemorrhagic cysts that appear nonviable can usually be detorsed and observed with ovarian preservation. Persistent cysts should usually be managed with cyst removal (cystectomy) rather than oophorectomy, as even large cysts typically have some normal ovarian tissues present. Figure 48.1.2 illustrates the management of cysts with acute pain.

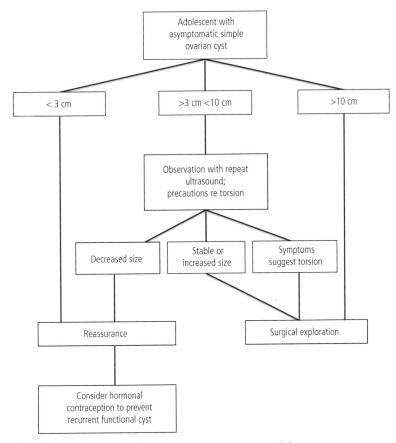

Figure 48.1.1 Algorithm for the management of a simple ovarian cyst in an adolescent.

Table 48.1.2 Differential diagnosis of mixed echogenic adnexal masses in the adolescent age group

- Corpus luteum cyst
- Germ cell neoplasms:
  - Benign cystic teratoma: –most common (see Chapter 48.2)
  - Serous cystadenoma
  - Mucinous cysadenoma
  - Malignant ovarian germ cell tumors (see Chapter 48.2)
- Endometrioma
- Ectopic pregnancy
- Pelvic inflammatory disease:
  - Tubo-ovarian abscess
  - Tubo-ovarian complex
  - Pyosalpinx

Management of acute pain in an adolescent requires that an ectopic pregnancy be considered in the differential diagnosis (see Chapter 47). A positive urine or serum qualitative human chorionic gonadotropin (hCG) with evidence on ultrasound of a hemoperitoneum requires surgical management.

If the hCG is negative and a hemoperitoneum is present, management is dependent on the clinical presentation. A ruptured corpus luteum cyst is the most likely diagnosis, although other types of cysts can occasionally rupture and cause intra-abdominal hemorrhage. If the vital signs are unstable or the hematocrit is low or falling, surgical intervention is indicated. A diagnostic laparoscopy will isolate the site of bleeding and allow for therapeutic management with a cystectomy or cauterization of the bleeding site. If the vital signs are stable and the hematocrit

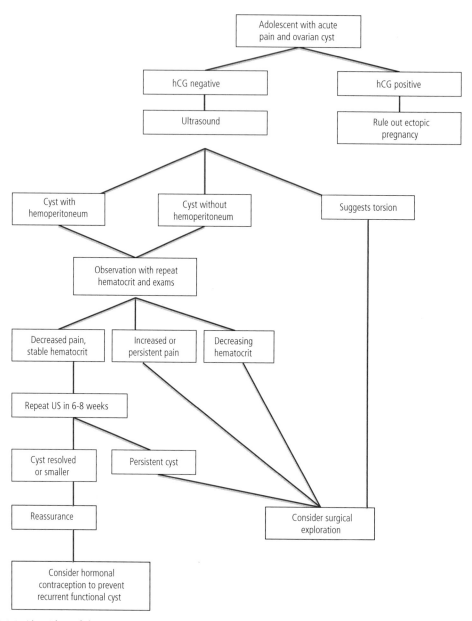

Figure 48.1.2 Algorithm of the management of the adolescent with acute pain and an ovarian cyst.

also stabilizes, management can be expectant with close observation for 24 hours. If stable, a repeat ultrasound in 6–8 weeks will typically demonstrate resolution of a functional cyst, or at least a decrease in size. Oral contraceptive pills, by preventing ovulation, will markedly decrease the risk of recurrence of a ruptured corpus luteum cyst, and can be offered as preventive treatment. Persistent masses may be neoplastic, and consideration should be given to surgical exploration, typically via laparoscopy (Figure 48.1.2).

Further reading

Grimes DA, Jones LB, Lopez LM, *et al.* Oral contraceptives for functional ovarian cysts. *Cochrane Database Syst Rev* 2011;9:CD006134.

Levine D, Brown DL, Andreotti RF, *et al.* Management of asymptomatic ovarian and adnexal cysts imaged at US; Society of Radiologists in Ultrasound Consensus Conference. *Ultrasound Q* 2010;26:121–131.

Strickland JL. Ovarian cysts in neonates, children and adolescents. *Curr Opin Obstet Gynecol* 2002;14:459–465.

48.2 Ovarian germ cell tumors

Claire Templeman

Department of Obstetrics and Gynecology, University of Southern California, Los Angeles, CA, USA

Pediatric germ cell ovarian tumors are a rare, heterogeneous group that are thought to occur as a result of *in utero* events, but whose etiology is largely unknown. They are grouped together based upon a presumed common cell of origin, the primordial germ cell. During normal development these cells migrate to the gonads from their site of origin in the embryonic yolk sac. They are classified into two broad groups: dysgerminomas of the ovary (seminomas in the testis of boys) and nondygerminomatous tumors of the ovary, which comprise yolk sac tumors, teratomas, embryonal carcinomas, and choriocarcinomas (Table 48.2.1). Teratomas are the most common germ cell tumors of the ovary and comprise tissue from all three germ cell layers (ectoderm, mesoderm and endoderm).

Germ cell tumors may be benign or malignant. The most commonly encountered benign tumors are mature cystic teratomas, also known as dermoid cysts. These tumors comprise 70% of benign ovarian neoplasms in women younger than 30 years of age. Malignant ovarian germ cell tumors (MOGCTs) may occur in girls and young women with a peak incidence in the teenage years. A reported 25% of germ cell tumors in patients younger than 15 years of age are malignant.

The most common presenting symptoms are abdominal pain and a palpable pelvic/abdominal mass (approximately 85% of patients). A further 10% of patients will present with acute abdominal pain, which may be associated with ovarian torsion. Vague symptoms such as abdominal distension and pressure may also occur. Rapid onset of abdominal distension or mass is indicative of a MOGCT.

In prepubertal patients, vaginal bleeding associated with isosexual precocious puberty may be the presenting symptom of an estrogen-secreting germ cell tumor, typically a granulosa cell tumor.

> ### ✋ Caution
>
> - In young girls and adolescents (≤18 years) presenting with ovarian torsion, the reported malignancy rate is 1.8%.
> - 40–50% of patients undergoing oophorectomy for ovarian torsion do not have any ovarian pathology.
> - Therefore, conservative management involving detorsion of the ovary with preservation of ovarian tissue should be strongly considered.

Diagnosis

A thorough history and physical exam will enable appropriate investigations to be ordered.

Based upon the clinical suspicion of a MOGCT, a pelvic ultrasound, abdominal computerized axial

Table 48.2.1 Classification of ovarian germ cell tumors

I. Primitive germ cell tumors
   A. Dysgerminoma
   B. Yolk sac tumor
   C. Embryonal carcinoma
   D. Polyembryoma
   E. Nongestational choriocarcinoma
   F. Mixed germ cell tumor
II. Biphasic or triphasic teratoma
   A. Immature teratoma
   B. Mature teratoma
III. Monodermal teratoma and somatic-type tumors associated with biphasic or triphasic teratoma

Table 48.2.2 Germ cell tumor markers and their associated tumors

Possible elevated tumor marker	Tumor
Alpha-fetoprotein (AFP)	Endodermal sinus tumor
	Embryonal cell carcinoma
	Mixed germ cell tumor
	Some immature teratomas
Lactate dehydrogenase (LDH)	Dysgerminoma
Human chorionic gonadotropin (hCG)	Embryonal cell carcinomas
	Choriocarcinoma
	Mixed germ cell tumors
	Some dysgerminomas

Science revisited

- Patients with dysgenetic gonads (the presence of a Y chromosome in the karyotype) are at increased risk for gonadoblastoma, a rare ovarian tumor in which 90% of cases occur in patients with dysgenetic gonads.
- 50–60% of gonadoblastomas are associated with MOGCTs, the majority of which are dysgerminomas.
- In these patients, both gonads should be removed even if there is only evidence of a tumor in one ovary.

---

tomography (CAT) scan and chest X-ray should be performed to evaluate for metastatic spread.

Tumor markers (tumor products that can be measured in the serum) may be elevated in certain types of malignant tumors. These are important not only in the initial diagnosis, but also in monitoring treatment, and post-treatment surveillance. The most likely markers to be elevated and their associated pathologies are listed in Table 48.2.2.

If there is a history of primary amenorrhea, Turner syndrome with mosaic karyotype or intersex condition, and dysgenetic gonads are suspected, and karyotyping should be performed.

Management

Surgery is the primary therapy for both mature cystic teratomas (MCTs) and MOGCTs. Once the diagnosis of an adenxal mass is made, the approach may be either via laparoscopy or laparotomy. If after imaging and evaluation of tumor markers, the suspicion for malignancy is low, laparoscopic management of the mass may be undertaken. A laparotomy may be appropriate if the mass is very large, there is a high suspicion for a MOGCT, or the surgeon judges this to be the best approach. In patients with a MCT, an ovarian cystectomy, with careful avoidance of cyst spillage to minimize the risk of a chemical peritonitis, is the treatment of choice. This will allow the preservation of as much ovarian tissue as possible.

Tips and tricks

A frozen section is important in determining the appropriate surgical procedure: cystectomy versus salpingo-oophorectomy with staging.

With the exception of 10–15% of pure dysgerminomas, the majority of MOGCTs are unilateral and 60% are confined to the ovary at diagnosis. Even in the setting of bilateral ovarian tumors, MCT may occur in one ovary despite malignancy in the other. These MOGCT tumor characteristics make fertility-sparing surgery the treatment of choice for the majority of patients. Hence unilateral salpingo-oophorectomy with surgical staging has become the standard of care for patients in the absence of dysgenetic gonads.

There is some debate in the literature about what constitutes adequate surgical staging in the context of MOGCT tumors, since the guiding principle has been extrapolated from epithelial ovarian tumors. Standard staging involves the collection of peritoneal washings for cytology, biopsies from pelvic and abdominal peritoneum, and omentectomy. The issue of whether routine lymphadenectomy should be performed is contested. It has been demonstrated that survival is not affected by deviation from standard surgical staging guidelines, so it has been proposed that palpation of pelvic and paraortic lymph nodes with sampling of any suspicious or enlarged nodes may be appropriate pending further research.

Currently patients with stage 1A dysgerminoma and stage 1A grade 1 immature teratomas are managed with surgery alone. Recurrence risk is relatively low in this group of patients, and recurrence can be effectively salvaged with chemotherapy. The combination of bleomycin, etoposide, and cisplatin (BEP) is the standard treatment for patients with MOGCT. Currently there is a trend for following surgery with close surveillance rather than chemotherapy for all stage 1 MOGCTs; however, this is the subject of current trials.

Follow-up

Close post-treatment surveillance is required after treatment for all stages of MOGCT. The optimal strategy is unknown, but recommendations include history and physical exam, along with a CT scan of the chest, abdomen and pelvis, and serum tumor markers every 3 months for the first 2 years and then every 6 months for a further 3 years. Nondysgerminomatous tumors require follow-up for 5 years. Dysgerminomas , due to the risk of late recurrence, require follow-up for 10 years.

Prognosis

Tumor stage, histologic subtype, residual disease, and elevation of the preoperative tumor markers human chorionic gonadotropin (hCG) and alpha-fetoprotein (AFP) appear to be prognostic parameters for patients with MOGCTs. Patients treated appropriately with surgery and postoperative BEP chemotherapy have an excellent chance for remission without recurrence.

For patients with early-stage disease, the likelihood of cure after adjuvant chemotherapy is near 100%. In patients with advanced disease, cure rates are about 75%. Recurrences in patients generally occur within 24 months of diagnosis. In patients who have had surgery for MCTs and followed for up to 10 years, the ipsilateral recurrence rate is reported to be 2–4%.

Evidence at a glance

Late effects if treatment

• The majority of studies suggest there is no adverse effect on fertility or teratogenicity after fertility-preserving surgery and chemotherapy for MOGCT.

• Following fertility preservation surgery, a Gynecological Oncology Group (GOG) study found that 87% of patients reported normal post-treatment menstrual function, and a number have reported healthy live births.

• There is no evidence to suggest treatment predisposes to early pregnancy loss or congenital malformation of the fetus; however, it has been recommended that young women avoid pregnancy for at least a year after treatment.

Summary

In general, the treatment principles for all types of MOGCT are similar, and include surgery for diagnosis and complete surgical staging, cytoreductive surgery if advanced disease is present, and adjuvant chemotherapy in most cases.

Further reading

Gershenson DM. Management of ovarian germ cell tumors. *J Clin Oncol* 2007;25:2938–2943.

Gershenson DM. Ovarian germ cell tumors: Pathology, clinical manifestations, and diagnosis. *UpToDate* Oct 2011. www.uptodate.com

Templeman C, Fallat ME, Lam AM, *et al.* Managing mature cystic teratomas of ovary. *Obstet Gynecol Surv* 2000;55 (12):738–745.

49 Endometriosis

Mary Anne Jamieson

Queen's University, Kingston, ON, Canada

Endometriosis, the presence of endometrial glands and stroma outside of the uterus, definitely occurs in adolescents. Adults who have been diagnosed with endometriosis will often retrospectively report symptoms beginning during their teen years. Clinicians who do not acknowledge endometriosis as a possible cause of chronic pelvic pain and intractable dysmenorrhea in a teen may unintentionally delay diagnosis, which can have devastating physical, emotional, and psychosocial consequences.

Adolescents who are ultimately diagnosed with endometriosis have often originally presented with common gynecologic complaints: dysmenorrhea, acute and/or chronic pelvic pain, and dyspareunia. For each of these complaints, the differential diagnosis is quite broad (see Chapters 39.1 and 45), but the index of suspicion for endometriosis should increase if the teen presents with more than one of these symptoms, or if dysmenorrhea has been unresponsive to traditional therapies, and particularly if there is a family history of endometriosis. While endometriosis symptoms may respond to therapies recommended for primary dysmenorrhea, such as nonsteroidal anti-inflammatory drugs (NSAIDs) and combined hormonal contraceptives (CHCs), endometriosis should be considered if these therapies are either ineffective from the outset or become ineffective after an initial response. Recognizing that dyspareunia in teens can be complex and multifactorial, endometriosis-related dyspareunia is usually related to deep penetration.

While adolescents can present with other endometriosis symptoms such as pain with defecation, it is this author's opinion that they can also present with abnormal uterine bleeding (which is often painful or accompanied by cramps). On the other hand, teens with an inherited bleeding disorder are more likely to develop endometriosis, presumably from increased retrograde flow.

★ Tips and tricks

- If an adolescent with dysmenorrhea fails to respond to traditional therapies, think endometriosis.
- Make private time part of your routine gynecologic visit with an adolescent (see Chapter 17). You need to ask about dyspareunia; plus it is important to know if the teen also requires contraception when deciding on treatment options for possible or confirmed endometriosis. (See Chapters 18 and 19)

⚛ Science at a glance

If an individual has a first-degree relative with confirmed endometriosis, there is a 7% chance that she will develop endometriosis.

Practical Pediatric and Adolescent Gynecology, First Edition. Edited by Paula J. Adams Hillard.
© 2013 John Wiley & Sons, Ltd. Published 2013 by John Wiley & Sons, Ltd.

> ### ✋ Caution
>
> - If a teen presents with severe pain *at menarche*, or if the dysmenorrhea is *consistently one-sided*, consider an obstructed hemiuterus or hemivagina (see Chapter 46). These can cause/coexist with endometriosis.
> - Be suspicious of the teen with advanced endometriosis. Think Müllerian anomaly, immunocompromise or inherited bleeding disorder.

> ### ★ Tips and tricks
>
> - Individualize the need for a gynecologic exam.
> - In a teen, the physical exam is often not a reliable way of making the diagnosis of endometriosis.
> - The goal is to rule out other possible diagnoses.
> - Have a low threshold for performing a transabdominal pelvic ultrasound.

Diagnosis

The physical exam may or may not point directly to endometriosis. It is often used more to rule in/out other etiologies in the differential diagnosis, such as abdominal mass or abdominal wall trigger points (see Chapter 39.2). While musculosketelal causes of pelvic pain are prevalent as primary etiologies, teens with endometriosis may secondarily develop a myofascial pain syndrome. In endometriosis, the lower abdomen may be tender to deep palpation in multiple spots but there is seldom a presentation of peritonitis. Teens do not tend to present with advanced disease or a ruptured endometrioma (unless they have an obstructing Müllerian anomaly). The need for a speculum exam, cervical sexually-transmitted disease (STD) testing, Pap smear, and bimanual/rectovaginal exam must be individualized, especially if the patient is credibly precoital and has never used tampons. The bimanual or rectovaginal exam *may* identify tender uterosacral ligaments and occasionally nodules typical of endometriosis, but often the findings are nonspecific, noncontributory, and/or difficult to interpret. Many adolescent gynecologists have a low threshold for requesting a transabdominal pelvic ultrasound to document normal pelvic anatomy and rule out adnexal masses, because of the limitations of the pelvic exam in young women.

While taking a good history, being attentive to the teen's complaints and having a high index of suspicion for the possibility of endometriosis is paramount; endometriosis in adolescents can only be definitively diagnosed by laparoscopy (+ biopsy). Teens seldom get endometriomas, making ultrasound unreliable for diagnosis; and they seldom have deep infiltrating lesions making MRI unreliable. However, imaging is recommended in an effort to rule in/out other etiologies in the differential diagnosis. Anyone performing a diagnostic laparoscopy to rule out endometriosis in an adolescent should not only appreciate that the lesions can look different in this age group (clear vesicle, petechial, flame-like), but also be prepared to treat the lesions surgically where/when appropriate. On the other hand, repeated laparoscopies should be avoided not only in the context of a negative first-look laparoscopy, but also when the patient is known to have endometriosis.

> ### ✋ Caution
>
> - Teens usually present with minimal/mild endometriosis.
> - Their lesions can look atypical: clear vesicles, and small petechial-like or flame-like lesions.
> - Powder-burn lesions, when present, can be subtle.

Management

While many algorithms exist for the investigation and management of endometriosis, they are seldom specific to teens. Some teens and their families feel that they really need to know whether or not they have endometriosis, even if they have not explored or exhausted medical therapies, while others are content to know that they could have endometriosis and want to try medical therapies on speculation first. With the latter group, it is crucial to have been thorough in ruling out worrisome or sinister etiologies for the presenting complaints. When the problem has been narrowed to primary dysmenorrhea versus endometriosis, it is reasonable to move through some of the recommended medical treatment strategies before surgery. Preserving fertility in teens is most certainly a goal of treatment, but there is no clear evidence that surgical ablation of endometriosis in a teen is any more advantageous than medical therapies to delay progression and protect future fertility. Successful treatments for pelvic endometriosis may be as much about reducing menstrual flow (and thus retrograde flow) with or without endometrial atrophy as they are about creating a hypoestrogenic environment.

Treatments include:
- **Medical therapies:**
  - NSAIDs + acetaminophen
  - Combined hormonal contraceptives (CHCs): pill, transdermal patch or vaginal ring
  - Extended cycle combined hormonal contraceptives
  - Long-acting systemic progestins: implant or injection
  - Levonorgestrel intrauterine system (LNG-IUS)
  - Gonadotropin-releasing hormone (GnRH) analogs with add-back hormone therapy consisting of 5 mg of norethindrone acetate (NA) daily or 0.625 mg of conjugated estrogen plus 5 mg of NA daily.
  - Future? Dienogest oral progestin, a daily tablet that contains both 19-nortestosterone and progesterone derivatives. It is not androgenic. It is a relatively new endometriosis therapy and currently is not labeled as a contraceptive, although it reduces the likelihood of conceiving during the course of therapy. Its role in the treatment of adolescents with endometriosis is yet to be clarified.
- **Surgical therapies** usually involve laparoscopic ablation with electrocautery or laser or resection, depending on the surgeon's skill, equipment available, and location/extent of implants/adhesions.
- **Alternative therapies:**
  - Heating pad/hot water bottle or chemical heat wrap patches
  - Yoga
  - Acupuncture
  - Regular exercise
  - Biofeedback
  - Relaxation.

Multidisciplinary care and pain management teams that include a psychologist are important resources for those patients who prove challenging.

★ Tips andtricks

The LNG-IUS can be challenging to insert in an adolescent. Consider whether it would be appropriate to insert it at the time of laparoscopy.

✋ Caution

- While there are concerns about the impact of GnRH analogs or long-acting systemic progestins on bone density in adolescents, even when calcium and vitamin D are adequate and when there is hormone therapy add-back, usually the benefits outweigh the risks, especially with short courses of less than 8 months.
- The impact of these medications on bone density appears to be reversible after discontinuation.

When trying to decide on a treatment strategy, it is useful to ask the following questions:
- Psychologically, does she need to know whether she has endometriosis or not?
- What has she tried already, and did she try it properly and for long enough to consider that method a failure? For example, she only tried one pack of birth control pills and abandoned them because of breakthroughbleeding or she tried NSAIDs but did not take an appropriate dose at an appropriate frequency.
- Is her pain predominantly cyclic, and are her menses relatively predictable? NSAIDs in combination with acetaminophen are only likely to be satisfactory if her primary complaint is dysmenorrhea and other symptoms are infrequent. Even then, she must be prepared with medications on hand at all times so she can medicate prophylactically.
- Does she need reliable contraception?
- Are there other noncontraceptive benefits to be exploited by using a particular method? For example,

CHCs can improve acne, regulate cycles and reduce heavy flow; long-acting progestins and the LNG-IUS can reduce heavy flow.

• Are there any restrictions secondary to drug costs or health benefit subsidy programs? For example, can the patient afford the LNG-IUS?

• Would the patient comply with the proper mode of administration? For example, would she take a daily pill, would she be able to tolerate an IUD insertion or is she willing to accept an injection?

• Are there any contraindications to a particular method? For example, does she have complex migraines with neurologic features that under most circumstances preclude the use of a CHC, or has she had recent/recurrent/active STIs that would under most circumstances preclude the insertion of an IUS in the near future?

★ Tips and tricks

• It is very important to correct misinformation about endometriosis and the treatment options. Teens and their families will often have unfounded fears and concerns, e.g. safety of CHCs or infertility as a result of endometriosis.

• Stress prophylactic NSAIDs + acetaminophen for endometriosis symptoms. These meds should always be readily available. (Schools may require a written note from a physician authorizing medication use.)

• Forewarn and reassure about anticipated treatment-related side effects so that the teen and her family will give the treatment an adequate trial.

✋ Patient/parent advice

• www.youngwomenshealth.org
• www.EndometriosisAssn.org
• Endometriosis does not necessarily mean infertility. Many women with endometriosis are fertile.
• Take NSAIDs (in combination with acetaminophen if necessary) prophylactically for endometriosis-related dysmenorrhea or pelvic pain. It is not harmful to do so unless treatment is required for several consecutive weeks.
• CHCs are safe and effective in all but the most rare circumstances, and have not been shown to lead to the initiation of sexual activity in a teen who would otherwise have abstained.
• Calcium (1500 mg/day) and vitamin D (800 U/day), are important through diet or supplements in all teens, but especially in those on depomedroxyprogesterone acetate or a GnRH analog; ask your healthcare provider if you are unsure about the need for supplements.

Further reading

American College of Obstetricians and Gynecologists. ACOG Committee Opinion. Number 310, April 2005. Endometriosis in adolescents. *Obstet Gynecol* 2005;105: 921.

Ballweg ML, Laufer MR. Adolescent endometriosis: Improving the comfort level of health care providers treating adolescents with endometriosis. *J Pediatr Adolesc Gynecol* 2011;24:(5 Suppl):S1.

Endometriosis: diagnosis and management. *J Obstet Gynaecol Can* 2010;32(7; Suppl 2). Entire supplement, but especially Endometriosis in adolescents, S25–S27.

Laufer MD. Diagnosis and treatment of endometriosis in adolescents. UpToDate. www.uptodate.com

50 Polycystic ovary syndrome

Samantha M. Pfeifer

Perelman School of Medicine at University of Pennsylvania, Philadelphia, PA, USA

Polycystic ovary syndrome (PCOS) is one of the most common disorders in reproductive age women occurring in approximately 5–10%. PCOS is currently thought of as a heterogeneous disorder caused by overproduction of androgens primarily by the ovary, and is associated with insulin resistance. The syndrome is characterized by oligomenorrhea and signs of hyperandrogenism, and is frequently seen in association with obesity. For many women symptom onset is during adolescence, and therefore it is important to recognize and understand this disorder in this age group, and to facilitate the initiation of therapy to treat symptoms and decrease the risk of long-term sequelae.

> ### ⚗ Science revisited
>
> • PCOS is considered to be a genetic disorder, as it has been demonstrated to occur in 25–30% of first-degree female relatives.
> • However, the gene or genes responsible for PCOS have yet to be characterized.

The causes of PCOS are unknown and remain an active area of investigation. However, PCOS has been associated with an increase in production of luteinizing hormone (LH) as well as insulin resistance, both leading to overproduction of androgens from the ovary. Insulin resistance has been demonstrated in 20–60% of women with PCOS, although it is believed that all women with PCOS have some degree of insulin resistance. In addition, insulin resistance is seen in lean as well as obese individuals with PCOS.

> ### ⚗ Science revisited
>
> There are several proposed mechanisms for the stimulation of ovarian androgen production in women with PCOS:
> • Decreasing sex hormone-binding globulin, thereby increasing available and active androgens.
> • Directly increasing production of LH.
> • Increasing production of androgens from the ovary and adrenal gland by directly binding insulin and insulin-like growth factor (IGF)-I receptors, by upregulating IGF-I receptors, and decreasing insulin-like growth factor binding protein (IGFBP)-I.

Health consequences

It is important to diagnose and treat PCOS in adolescence in order to decrease the risk of associated

---

Practical Pediatric and Adolescent Gynecology, First Edition. Edited by Paula J. Adams Hillard.
© 2013 John Wiley & Sons, Ltd. Published 2013 by John Wiley & Sons, Ltd.

adverse health sequelae. Long-term health consequences of PCOS relate to both the insulin resistance and the hyperandrogenism seen with this disorder, and include:

- Obesity
- Diabetes
- Metabolic syndrome
- Endometrial hyperplasia
- Anovulatory infertility
- Depression.

Obesity is seen in 50–75% of women with PCOS. In the adolescent, this may present around the time of or just after puberty. The weight accumulation is predominantly abdominal, and is reflected in an increased waist-to-hip ratio. Obesity in adolescents is correlated with obstructive sleep apnea, orthopedic disorders, fatty liver, and decreased quality of life.

Diabetes and impaired glucose tolerance are seen more frequently in adolescents with PCOS. The incidence increases with obesity. An abnormal 2-hour glucose tolerance test (GTT) has been observed in approximately 33% of adolescents with PCOS. The incidence in normal-weight individuals is lower.

Metabolic syndrome is defined as cardiovascular disease risk factors associated with insulin resistance, including glucose intolerance, dyslipidemia, hypertension, and central obesity. Metabolic syndrome is seen more frequently in adolescents with PCOS compared to the general population (37% vs 5%). The frequency of metabolic syndrome in adolescents is directly proportional to the body mass index (BMI), with the incidence in normal weight, overweight, and obese PCOS girls being 0%, 11%, and 63%, respectively. In girls with PCOS, hyperandrogenism is also correlated with an increased risk for development of metabolic syndrome, independent of obesity.

Endometrial hyperplasia is a potential result of unopposed estrogen stimulation to the endometrium. Adolescents are at risk due to chronic anovulation associated with PCOS. The prevalence of endometrial hyperplasia in the adolescent PCOS population is unknown, but is probably very low.

Infertility in women with PCOS appears to be related to oligo- or anovulation. This condition is treatable. It is important to reassure the adolescent that pregnancy is possible with current treatments, as many are left with the impression that they will never be able to conceive; this impression may even result in unprotected sexual activity and unintended pregnan-cies. Clomiphene citrate is the first-line drug to treat anovulation associated with PCOS when pregnancy is desired if anovulation results in infertility. Other treatment options include letrozole, metformin, gonadotropins, ovarian drilling, and *in vitro* fertilization.

Depression and perceived decreased quality of life have been reported in women with PCOS. In adolescents with PCOS, quality of life scores have been inversely correlated with BMI, highlighting the fact that obesity is the most significant factor.

Diagnosis

PCOS is most commonly defined by the Rotterdam Criteria, which require two of the following three elements:

- Oligomenorrhea defined as menses occurring at greater than intervals of 40 days
- Evidence of hyperandrogenism either by clinical criteria (acne, hirsutism) *or* biochemical measurements (elevated total testosterone)
- Evidence of polycystic ovary morphology on ultrasound.

To make the diagnosis of PCOS, all other causes of the presenting symptoms must be excluded, such as hyper- or hypo-thyroidism, hyperprolactinemia, nonclassical adrenal hyperplasia (NCAH), Cushing syndrome, and androgen-producing tumor (either adrenal or ovarian).

> ### ☝ Caution
>
> - Diagnosing PCOS in the adolescent may be difficult, as some of the symptoms, such as acne and menstrual irregularity, are often seen transiently as part of the normal progression through puberty.
> - In addition, the most sensitive method of assessing ovarian morphology, a transvaginal ultrasound, may not be feasible or appropriate in young adolescents.
> - Assigning a diagnosis of PCOS incorrectly may lead to unnecessary therapies and impose psychological distress.

Diagnostic factors in the history include irregular menstruation, usually dating to menarche with cycles occurring irregularly and at greater than 40-day intervals. However, more frequent menses may reflect anovulatory bleeding as well. This may be difficult to assess in the adolescent, as menses can be irregular following menarche. Persistent irregular menses for more than 2 years post menarche are suggestive of a hormonal condition. Cycles of longer than 90 days are above the 95% centile, even in the first gynecologic year.

Clinical signs of PCOS include signs of hyperandrogenemia and insulin resistance. In the adolescent, hyperandrogenism is more likely to initially present as persistent and severe acne rather than excess hair growth. However, transient acne is not uncommon in the teenage years. Since acne may not represent hyperandrogenism, some believe that hirsutism is a more specific sign of hyperandrogenism in the adolescent. These symptoms may predate menarche. Premature adrenarche is associated with the development of PCOS. A history of rapid development (several months) of hair growth, acne or virilizing symptoms is more suggestive of an androgen-producing tumor. Acanthosis nigricans, a velvety darkening of the skin typically on the dorsal surface of the neck and intertrigenous areas such as the upper thigh and axilla, is a marker of insulin resistance (Figure 50.1). Onset of obesity following menarche is also associated with PCOS.

Lab studies to diagnose PCOS are aimed at diagnosing other causes of oligo or amenorrhea and assessing biochemical evidence of hyperandrogenism.

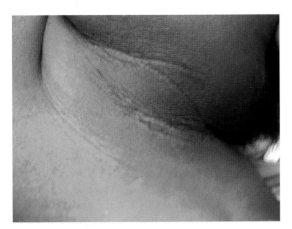

Figure 50.1 Acanthosis nigricans of the neck in African-American woman.

Serum follicle-stimulating hormone (FSH), estradiol, thyroid-stimulating hormone (TSH), and prolactin should be performed to evaluate for evidence of ovarian insufficiency (failure), thyroid dysfunction, and hyperprolactinemia, all causes of irregular menses. In addition, thyroid dysfunction can be associated with hair loss, and hyperprolactinemia can be associated with hirsutism. An LH:FSH ratio of greater than 2 is often seen in nonobese adolescents with PCOS, but is not a diagnostic criterion.

Given the difficulties of interpreting clinical signs of hyperandrogenism in the adolescent, biochemical assessment is considered to be more specific. Total testosterone is frequently used to assess androgen excess in PCOS (see Chapter 35). However, levels may be in the upper normal range or only slightly elevated. Most commercially available assays for free testosterone have poor validity in females, and therefore this test is of questionable significance. Dehydroepiandrosterone (DHEAS) is elevated in about 25–50% of women with PCOS, and thus this test is nondiagnostic for PCOS. There is no need to measure androstenedione or sex hormone-binding globulin levels. If there is clinical suspicion of an androgen-producing tumor, then obtaining total testosterone or DHEAS is warranted, and high values (testosterone >200 ng/dL or DHEAS >8000 ng/mL) require further evaluation with imaging studies.

It is important to exclude the diagnosis of NCAH, especially in those of Eastern European Jewish or Hispanic descent. A fasting morning serum 17-hydroxyprogesterone level obtained in the follicular phase of the menstrual cycle should be obtained, as adrenal function is highest in the morning, and ovarian production of 17-hydroxyprogesterone in the luteal phase may confuse the results. If the value is greater than 200 ng/dL, then an adrenocorticotropic hormone (ACTH) stimulation test should be obtained to exclude NCAH. If there is suspicion of Cushing syndrome, a 24-hour urinary free cortisol, overnight dexamethasone suppression test, or midnight salivary cortisol test is warranted.

Ultrasound is necessary to diagnose PCOS. In the adolescent this is usually done by the transabdominal approach. A transvaginal ultrasound is more specific and may be appropriate for some adolescents. The criteria for diagnosing polycystic ovary morphology is the presence of 12 or more follicles of 2–9 mm in diameter on the ovary. Increased ovarian volume of greater than 10 mL is also suggestive, and is easier to determine using a transabdominal approach than a follicle count. Only one ovary demonstrating this morphology is sufficient for diagnosis.

Once the diagnosis of PCOS has been determined, then additional testing for associated health sequelae is recommended. Assessment of BMI and blood pressure should be performed. Testing for impaired glucose tolerance or diabetes is advised, especially in the overweight or obese individual. In an adolescent with PCOS this is best accomplished by performing a 75-g 2-hour GTT. Fasting glucose and hemoglobin A1c may be obtained. There is no accurate outpatient test for insulin resistance. Fasting insulin levels are nondiagnostic and are therefore not recommended. A fasting lipid profile and assessment of liver function is also recommended.

Management

Treatment options for PCOS in the adolescent include weight loss for obese individuals, symptom-directed therapy for irregular menstruation and hyperandrogenism, and metabolic correction of the underlying insulin resistance using insulin-sensitizing medications.

Weight loss should be the first-line therapy in overweight or obese adolescents with PCOS. A weight reduction of 5–10% has been shown to result in decreased testosterone levels, increased sex hormone-binding globulin, resumption of menses, and improved reproductive outcomes in those with PCOS. Weight loss is best accomplished by lifestyle/behavioral changes incorporating dietary modification combined with increase in exercise. This approach has been shown to be more effective than dietary restriction alone. Dietary intervention should focus on calorie restriction. A low calorie diet is considered to be 1000–1200 kcal/day, which should reduce total body weight by 10% over 6 months. Low glycemic diets have been shown to be more effective in restoring menstruation and improving response to GTT compared to a low calorie diet. Regular physical exercise is essential for weight loss and long-term weight management. A minimum of 30 minutes of moderately intense exercise at least 3 days per week is recommended. Unfortunately, like all chronic conditions, lifestyle modifications must be maintained to avoid

regaining weight. This is particularly difficult for the adolescent who may not be offered healthy food choices at home or school, and who also may have difficulty maintaining a strict diet in front of peers.

For those adolescents who are morbidly obese, bariatric surgery may be an option. More data are needed in adolescents to evaluate the short- and long-term risks and benefits, and to determine who would most benefit from this approach.

Symptom-directed therapy

This approach involves utilizing techniques and medications directed at treating the acne, hirsutism, and irregular menstrual bleeding seen with PCOS. Adolescents in general have self-esteem issues. For a young adolescent female with PCOS, severe acne or hirsutism can compound those issues; therefore, optimizing treatment is important. A multidisciplinary approach is favored utilizing hair removal techniques and consultation with a dermatologist in conjunction with other medical therapies (see Chapter 35). The earlier the treatment is instituted, the better the long-term results. It is important to stress this concept, as many parents are reluctant to use medical therapy in an adolescent for fear of side effects.

Hair removal techniques include waxing, shaving, plucking, threading, use of depilatories, electrolysis, and laser therapy; bleaching may also be helpful in girls with dark hair.

✋ Patient/parent advice

Early treatment of acne and hirsutism improves long-term results by preventing scarring from acne, and minimizing the impact of hirsutism and acne on self-esteem.

First-line medical therapy to control acne, hirsutism and irregular menses is combined hormonal contraceptive therapy. Although only a few combined contraceptives have FDA approval for control of hirsutism, all are equally effective. If hormonal contraceptives fail to control hyperandrogenic symptoms effectively, then therapy with an antiandrogen such as spironolactone, flutamide, or finasteride can be added. In the US, spironolactone is the preferred antiandrogen, whereas in Europe, flutamide is more commonly used.

Insulin-sensitizing medications

Insulin-sensitizing medications have been proposed for treatment for PCOS due to the strong association with insulin resistance and hyperandrogenism in PCOS. The most commonly studied medication is metformin, a biguanide that increases insulin sensitivity in the liver and peripheral glucose uptake. Thiazolidenediones, another class of insulin-sensitizing medication, have not been adequately studied in adolescents.

In adult women with PCOS, metformin has been shown to decrease serum androgens, decrease insulin, improve ovulatory rates, and lead to resumption of menstrual cyclicity. However, studies in the adolescent are few, involve small numbers of subjects, and are of short duration; most are observational not randomized controlled trials, and are predominantly focused on a population of relatively lean girls with history of precocious puberty, hyperinsulinemic hyperandrogenism, and PCOS, and therefore may not be generalizable to a more heterogeneous population.

Dosing of metformin in adolescents is similar to adults: 1000–2000 mg daily in divided doses. Available data in the adolescent show metformin to be associated with a decrease in androgens, improved glucose tolerance, and improvement in menstrual cyclicity. Metformin alone does not result in weight loss, and there are few studies evaluating the effect of metformin on hirsutism. Metformin is not a weight-loss drug; however, when metformin is combined with a low calorie diet, decreases in weight and BMI have resulted. In a small study of thin adolescent girls with hyperinsulinemic hyperandrogenism, low-dose metformin has been associated with an improvement in ovarian hyperandrogenism, hyperinsulinemia, hirsutism, and menstrual cyclicity.

Metformin has been used in combination with combined oral contraceptives (COCs). In obese adolescent girls, the addition of metformin to COC and lifestyle modification offered no benefit over COC and lifestyle modification with respect to weight loss, reduction in free androgen index, and improved hirsutism. In contrast, studies in lean adolescent girls with hyperinsulinemic hyperandrogenism suggest that the addition of metformin and flutamide to COC is beneficial. Further studies are needed to evaluate the short- and long-term effects of metformin used alone or in combination therapy in the adolescent, and to determine which PCOS phenotype would most benefit from this therapy.

★ Tips and tricks

- Metformin is associated with significant nausea and gastrointestinal side effects.
- Start medication with a 500-mg pill daily, and increase the dose by one pill weekly to the desired dose.
- If side effects persist, start with half a pill and increase in half-pill increments.

♀ Pearls

- PCOS is characterized by hyperandrogenism and insulin resistance.
- Diagnosis in the adolescent can be difficult.
- Early diagnosis facilitates treatment of symptoms such as acne, hirsutism, and irregular menses, which can be disturbing to an adolescent.
- Diagnosis of PCOS can identify treatment options that can decrease the risk of long-term sequelae.
- Combined hormonal contraceptives and antiandrogens have been shown to treat symptoms of hyperandrogenism and menstrual irregularity.
- Insulin-sensitizing medications have been shown to be beneficial in reducing androgens, and improving glucose tolerance and menstrual regularity in adolescents with PCOS, but further studies are needed to determine long-term benefits and which PCOS phenotypes would most benefit from this therapy.

Further reading

Carmina E, Oberfield SE, Lobo RA. The diagnosis of polycystic ovary syndrome in adolescents. *Am J Obstet Gynecol* 2010;203:201.e1–5.

Geller DH, Pacaus D, Gordon CM, Misra M. State of the art review: Emerging therapies: The use of insulin sensitizers in the treatment of adolescents with polycystic ovary syndrome (PCOS). *Int J Pediatr Endocrinol* 2011; 2011:9.

Rotterdam ESHRE/ASRM-Sponsored PCOS Consensus Workshop Group. Revised 2003 consensus on diagnostic criteria and long-term health risks related to polycystic ovary syndrome (PCOS). *Hum Reprod* 2004;19:41–47.

51 Pelvic inflammatory disease

Colleen McNicholas and Jeffrey F. Peipert

Division of Clinical Research, Department of Obstetrics and Gynecology, Washington University School of Medicine in St. Louis, St. Louis, MO, USA

Pelvic inflammatory disease (PID), as defined by the Centers for Disease Control and Prevention (CDC), covers a spectrum of female upper genital infections, including endometritis, salpingitis, pyosalpinx, tubo-ovarian abscess (TOA), and pelvic peritonitis. In the US, PID accounted for nearly 45 000 hospitalizations and 100 000 initial office visits for women aged 15–45 years in 2009. Acute episodes of PID have immediate and long-term sequelae, including psychologic, economic, and public health implications, as well as infertility, ectopic pregnancy, and chronic pain.

Risk factors for PID include both modifiable and nonmodifiable factors. Young age is a major risk factor for sexually-transmitted diseases (STDs), including PID. Although 15–24-year olds represent only one-quarter of the sexually-active population, they account for nearly half of new cases of STDs each year. Adolescent are at higher risk of developing PID than their adult counterparts because of both behavioral and anatomic differences. High-risk behaviors include unprotected sex, multiple sex partners, and short duration serial monogamous relationships. Forty-six percent of high school students surveyed reported being sexually active, with nearly 40% of them not using condoms. Adolescence is a time of concrete thinking, with less ability to think abstractly, conceptually, or to foresee long-term consequences of actions. Thus, adolescents are not as likely to plan ahead for condom use or consider the long-term consequences of unprotected intercourse.

Eliciting risk factors at the annual adolescent health maintenance visit can help clinicians to better identify high-risk adolescents.

> ### ✋ Parent/patient advice
>
> **Minimize your risk! Risk factors for PID**
> - Young age
> - Early age of intercourse
> - Smoking or other substance abuse
> - Prior or current sexually-transmitted infection
> - Multiple sexual partners
> - Number of lifetime partners
> - New recent partner (within 1 month)
> - Sex with menses
> - Lack of barrier contraception (condoms)

PID is a polymicrobial infection. Most cases are caused by ascending sexually-transmitted infections (STI) from the lower genital tract, mainly *Chlamydia trachomatis* and *Neissseria gonorrhoeae*, with smaller contributions from endogenous vaginal flora, genital mycoplasmas, and mycobacterium tuberculosis. In 2007, the CDC reported 1.1 million cases of chlamydia and 356,000 cases of gonorrhea in young women

---

Practical Pediatric and Adolescent Gynecology, First Edition. Edited by Paula J. Adams Hillard.
© 2013 John Wiley & Sons, Ltd. Published 2013 by John Wiley & Sons, Ltd.

aged 15–24 years. It is estimated that roughly 10–40% of untreated chlamydia cases will lead to PID, and that as many as 20% of women with PID will develop infertility. Bacterial vaginosis is a common cause of vaginal discharge; however, its relationship to PID remains controversial. There are limited data investigating an association between trichomoniasis and PID, and no data that specifically address the question in adolescents.

While most cases of PID are caused by STD pathogens, sexual activity is not a requisite. Instrumentation or ascending abnormal vaginal flora may contribute a small proportion of cases. Although clinicians are concerned about intrauterine device (IUD)-associated infections in young women, the true incidence of PID after insertion is low, and an increased risk is limited to the first 21 days after insertion. PID has been found in prepubertal and sexually naïve girls; however, this mechanism is rare.

♨ Science revisited

- Anatomically, the cervix of an adolescent is immature, with a larger proportion of columnar epithelium on the ectocervix, offering a larger surface area for potential infection.
- The adolescent cervix may have alterations in cervical mucus and/or endocervical defense mechanisms which predispose them to PID.
- The persistent high-estrogen state associated with adolescent anovulation has been hypothesized to allow easier penetration of the cervical mucus by microorganisms and subsequent upper genital tract ascension.

Diagnosis

PID can present with a variety of signs and symptoms, which are often mild in severity, making diagnosis imprecise and difficult in any age group. However, PID is a significant source of reproductive morbidity. Thus, a low threshold for diagnosis and treatment should be maintained. Although the signs and symptoms of PID do not differ in adolescents when compared to adult women, making the diagnosis in

adolescents may be more challenging. Adolescents may have concerns about confidentiality, limiting their disclosure of risky sexual behavior. Additionally, many adolescents are naïve to pelvic exams, resulting in difficult and inadequate exams.

The current CDC diagnostic criteria support the use of minimum criteria and additional supportive criteria. Evaluation for the presence of *N. gonorrhoeae* and *C. trachomatis* should be performed in all sexually-active adolescents, and certainly if PID is suspected. More specific diagnostic tools such as transvaginal ultrasonography, MRI, laparoscopy, or endometrial biopsy are available, but are invasive and costly. A transvaginal ultrasound or other testing should be considered when clinical diagnosis is difficult or the patient is not responding to conservative management.

★ Tips and tricks

Minimum and supportive criteria for diagnosing PID

- Minimal criteria for women with abdominal or pelvic pain:
  - Cervical motion tenderness, or
  - Uterine tenderness, or
  - Adnexal tenderness
- Supportive criteria:
  - Oral temperature >101 °F
  - Cervical or vaginal mucopurulent discharge
  - Presence of abundant white blood cells on saline microscopy
  - Elevated erythrocyte sedimentation rate
  - Elevated C-reactive protein
  - Documentation of *C. trachomatis* or *N. gonorrhoeae*

In general, PID should be suspected in all sexually-active adolescents with adnexal, cervical motion, or uterine tenderness. The differential diagnosis for PID should be thoroughly evaluated (Table 51.1).

Management

The 2010 CDC STD treatment guidelines recommend initiating empiric treatment for PID in women at risk

Table 51.1 Differential diagnosis of pelvic inflammatory disease

- Gastrointestinal disorders:
  - Appendicitis
  - Cholecystitis
  - Gastroenteritis
- Gynecologic disorders:
  - Dysmenorrhea
  - Endometriosis
  - Ovarian cysts/tumors/torsion
  - Ectopic pregnancy
- Urologic disorders:
  - Urinary tract infection
  - Pyelonephritis
  - Nephrolithiasis

Table 51.2 Parenteral treatment regimens for pelvic inflammatory disease (2010 CDC guidelines: http://www.cdc.gov/std/treatment/2010/pid.htm Accessed 21-12-12)

Regimen A
Cefotetan 2 g IV every 12 hours
or
Cefoxitin 2 g IV every 6 hours
plus
Doxycycline 100 mg orally (or IV) every 12 hours

Regimen B
Clindamycin 900 mg IV every 8 hours
plus
Gentamicin loading dose IV or IM (2 mg/kg of body weight), followed by a maintenance dose (1.5 mg/kg) every 8 hours. Single daily dosing (3–5 mg/kg) can be substituted

Alternative regimen
Ampicillin/sulbactam 3 g IV every 6 hours
plus
Doxycycline 100 mg orally (or IV) every 12 hours

for STDs, who are experiencing pelvic or lower abdominal pain, meet the minimum criteria, and do not have another clear etiology for their signs and symptoms. Treatment regimens must provide broad-spectrum coverage for the most likely pathogens, including *N. gonorrhoeae*, *C. trachomatis*, anaerobes, Gram-negative facultative bacteria, and streptococci.

Routine hospitalization of adolescents for PID is not recommended. No difference in long-term outcomes (pregnancy, recurrent PID, chronic pelvic pain, ectopic pregnancy) has been shown for inpatient therapy for mild-to-moderate PID, even in the subgroup of adolescents. There is also no evidence to suggest that adolescents do not have the ability to comply with outpatient therapy.

Indications for hospitalization do not differ for young adolescents. If the adolescent meets hospital admission criteria (e.g. severe illness, surgical emergencies, pregnancy, failed outpatient treatment, TOA), parenteral therapy is indicated (Table 51.2).

> ✋ **Caution**
>
> Intravenous doxycycline is painful and should be avoided even in hospitalized patients when possible.

If the patient has been diagnosed with a TOA, inpatient observation is suggested for at least 24–48 hours. Transition to an oral regimen for theses cases should include broadening anaerobic coverage with clindamycin (450 mg QID) or metronidazole (500 mg BID), to be taken with doxycycline (100 mg BID) to complete a 14-day course. For uncomplicated PID (without TOA), patients should transition to an oral antibiotic regimen of doxycycline or clindamycin to complete a 14-day course.

Outpatient management guidelines (Table 51.3) should be followed for all patients with mild-to-moderate PID.

Follow-up

Women treated for PID should be re-evaluated for clinical response in 48–72 hours. Patients should show significant clinical improvement within 72 hours of initiating therapy, and parenteral therapy should be instituted if there is no response to the ambulatory regimen. In addition, diagnostic imaging should be considered. In cases of uncertain diagnosis or severe illness, diagnostic laparoscopy may be performed. Repeat testing for *N. gonorrhoeae* and *C. trachomatis* 3–6 months following treatment, regardless of the treatment status of the patient's partner, should be performed.

Table 51.3 Outpatient treatment regimens for pelvic inflammatory disease (2010 CDC guidelines: http://www.cdc.gov/std/treatment/2010/pid.htm Accessed 21-12-12)

Regimen A

Ceftriaxone 250 mg IM in a single dose

plus

Doxycycline 100 mg orally twice a day for 14 days

with or without

Metronidazole 500 mg orally twice a day for 14 days

Regimen B

Cefoxitin 2 g IM in a single dose and probenecid 1 g orally, administered concurrently in a single dose

plus

Doxycycline 100 mg orally twice a day for 14 days

with or without

Metronidazole 500 mg orally twice a day for 14 days

Regimen C

Other third-generation cephalosporin (ceftizoxime or cefotaxime)

plus

Doxycycline 100 mg orally twice a day for 14 days

with or without

Metronidazole 500 mg orally twice a day for 14 days

The risk of developing sequelae from PID depends on the severity and number of episodes. After a single episode, one in four women will develop a serious long-term complication. Among these long-term complications are ectopic pregnancy, infertility, recurrent PID, and chronic pelvic pain. Risk of ectopic pregnancy following a single episode of PID is six times that of controls, and further increases to 17-fold following two episodes.

PID has a strong association with tubal factor infertility (TFI). Reported rates of TFI range from 10% to 21% for mild PID, 35–45% for moderate PID, and 40–67% for severe PID. The single most important predictor of TFI is the number of episodes of PID, with each new episode approximately doubling the rate. This emphasizes the importance of prevention and education, especially when an adolescent with many reproductive years ahead is diagnosed with PID.

TOAs are estimated to occur in 3–16% of women with acute salpingitis, and can cause considerable morbidity and even mortality. Women with TOAs may present with fever, leukocytosis, abdominal pain, and pelvic mass. Broad-spectrum antibiotic therapy should be the initial treatment of these abscesses. However, if the patient is not responding, percutaneous drainage or surgical exploration must be considered. It is estimated that 20% of patients that present with TOAs require surgical intervention during hospital admission, with an additional 31% requiring surgical intervention in the follow-up period. Size of TOA is strongly associated with increased hospital stay and complication rates. Ruptured TOAs are a surgical emergency and patients often present with diffuse peritonitis and the possibility of progressing to sepsis. Although total hysterectomy with bilateral salpingo-oophorectomy was once the preferred surgical treatment of choice, fertility-sparing procedures such as laparoscopic drainage or unilateral adnexectomy are preferred in adolescents.

Chronic pelvic pain is another important sequela of PID. Pelvic pain has been noted in 36% of patients just 36 months following the diagnosis of mild or moderate PID. Consistent use of condoms after the diagnosis of acute PID has been shown to reduce the risk of chronic pain by 40%.

Prevention

With adolescents acquiring nearly half of all reported new STDs, efforts should focus on screening and education. There is good evidence that screening for and treating C. trachomatis reduces the incidence and sequelae from PID. The US Preventive Services Task Force recommends screening for all sexually-active females aged 25 years and younger at routine healthcare visits. Adolescents generally prefer to be screened with first-void urine or self-collected swabs rather than swabs collected at the time of pelvic exams. Home-based screening may increase testing rates, as compared to clinic-based screening. In 2006, 66% of high schools taught students about condom efficacy, but only 39% were taught proper use. Among teens aged 18–19 years, 41% reported knowing little or nothing about condoms. Educational efforts including the use of barrier contraception, assessing high-risk behaviors, performing regular STD screening, and intervening with early treatment are the most important prevention measures to reduce rates of PID and resulting sequelae among adolescents.

Further reading

Center for Disease Control and Prevention. *Pelvic Inflammatory Disease. 2010 Sexually Transmitted Disease Treatment Guidelines.* Atlanta: CDC, 2010.

Ness RB, Soper DE, Holley RL, *et al*. Effectiveness of inpatient and outpatient treatment strategies for women with pelvic inflammatory disease: results from the Pelvic Inflammatory Disease Evaluation and Clinical Health (PEACH) Randomized Trial. *Am J Obstet Gynecol* 2002; 186(5):929–937.

Westrom L, Joesoef R, Reynolds G, Hagdu A, Thompson SE. Pelvic inflammatory disease and fertility. A cohort study of 1,844 women with laparoscopically verified disease and 657 control women with normal laparoscopic results. *Sex Transm Dis* 1992;19(4):185–192.

Acknowledgement

This work was supported in part by an anonymous foundation, by a Clinical and Translational Science Award (UL1RR024992), and by Grant Number KL2RR024994 from the National Center for Research Resources (NCRR), a component of the National Institutes of Health (NIH) and NIH Roadmap for Medical Research. Its contents are solely the responsibility of the authors and do not necessarily represent the official view of NCRR or NIH. Information on NCRR is available at http://www.ncrr.nih.gov/. Information on Re-engineering the Clinical Research Enterprise can be obtained from http://nihroadmap.nih.gov/clinicalresearch/overview-translational.asp.

52

Gonadal dysgenesis

Courtney A. Marsh and Yolanda R. Smith

University of Michigan Health System, Ann Arbor, MI, USA

Gonadal dysgenesis refers to a variety of conditions within the spectrum of disorders of sex development characterized by abnormal gonadal development. As organogenesis of gonads is complex and highly regulated by multiple genes, understanding normal gonadal differentiation is helpful in better understanding gonadal dysgenesis.

⬡ Science revisited

Sex determination and differentiation

- At 8 weeks' gestation, bipotential gonads begin to differentiate.
- In normal male development, the sex determining region (*SRY*) on the Y chromosome activates genes downstream to promote testis organogenesis.
- A variety of genes including *SOX9* (*SRY* related box 9), SF1 (steroidogenic factor 1), *DAX-1* (dosage-sensitive sex reversal, adrenal hypoplasia critical region, on chromosome X, gene 1), and *DHH* (desert hedgehog) play key roles in Sertoli and Leydig cell proliferation, and formation of tubular cords.
- Sertoli cells secrete anti-Müllerian hormone (AMH) causing Müllerian duct regression and Leydig cells secrete testosterone and insulin-like peptide 3, causing Wolffian duct development.

- Although less understood, ovarian organogenesis is no longer thought to be the "default" pathway.
- Several autosomal genes are involved with ovarian development including: *WNT4/FST* (wingless type mouse mammary tumor virus integration site family, member 4/follicostatin), *RSPONDIN-1*, *FOXL2* (forkhead transcription factor 2), and *FST* (follicostatin). In particular, *RSPONDIN-1* acts synergistically with *WNT4/FST* to maintain oocyte viability and stabilize β-catenin; involved with follicle cell development. *FOXL2* represses *SOX9*, promoting ovarian differentiation and granulosa cell formation.
- Although there may be a factor responsible for suppressing the testes-determining pathway in XX individuals, this pathway remains an active area of research.

Historically, many terms were used to describe variants within gonadal dysgenesis. With recent advances in molecular genetics, a new classification system was developed in 2006 which emphasized chromosomal status. Within the spectrum of gonadal dysgenesis there are many variants including pure, partial, or mixed gonadal dysgenesis. Diagnosis is based on appearance and histologic features of both

Practical Pediatric and Adolescent Gynecology, First Edition. Edited by Paula J. Adams Hillard.
© 2013 John Wiley & Sons, Ltd. Published 2013 by John Wiley & Sons, Ltd.

gonads. Types of pure gonadal dysgenesis include Turner syndrome (45, XO), pure gonadal dysgenesis XX, and pure gonadal dysgenesis XY (Swyer syndrome). With pure gonadal dysgenesis, individuals have characteristic "streak gonads" which, although difficult to visualize radiographically, can be diagnosed with surgical visualization. Distinguishing partial (bilateral dysgenetic gonads) from mixed (one streak, one dysgenetic gonad) gonadal dysgenesis is difficult and requires biopsy (or removal) of both gonads for definitive diagnosis.

Turner syndrome

Turner syndrome, a form of pure gonadal dysgenesis, occurs in approximately 1 in 2000–4000 female births and is caused by partial to complete deletion of one of the X chromosomes. Diagnosis is made through standard 30-cell karyotype, although if suspicion is high and initial karyotype is normal, fluorescent *in-situ* hybridization (FISH) or comparative genomic hybridization (CGH) can be performed to find microdeletions on the X chromosome. Although a karyotype of 45, XO is most common, up to 30% of females diagnosed will have some degree of mosaicism and a minority will have Y chromosomal material identified on karyotype.

⚕ Caution

- Presence of Y chromosomal material confers risk of tumor.
- Individuals with gonadal dysgenesis and Y chromosomal material have increased risk of gonadoblastoma and germ cell tumors.
- By age 30 years, up to 30% of individuals with gonadal dysgenesis and Y chromosomal material will have a gonadal tumor, typically a gonadoblastoma. Up to 60% of those with gonadal tumors will have malignant transformation to a germ cell tumor.
- Gonadal biopsy with or without gonadectomy may be indicated, although risk of malignancy and recommended treatment varies with diagnosis, presence of Y chromosomal material and location of gonads.

Timing of diagnosis may vary depending on degree of mosaicism and phenotype. Some females with Turner syndrome are diagnosed prenatally after ultrasound reveals characteristic findings, such as cystic hygroma, webbed neck, shortened femur, cardiac anomalies, and lymphedema, and amniocentesis reveals XO karyotype. Diagnosis can also be made in infancy or childhood as growth disorders with short stature in the majority will prompt evaluation. Some may be diagnosed in adolescence during evaluation for primary or secondary amenorrhea with high follicle-stimulating hormone (FSH), prompting chromosomal analysis with karyotype. Finally, women may be diagnosed with Turner syndrome during a fertility evaluation. A later timing of diagnosis may be associated with a milder phenotype or greater degree of mosaicism.

Many features and conditions are associated with Turner syndrome (Table 52.1).Screening for associated conditions is important as some conditions can be life-threatening.

Management of females with Turner syndrome should involve a team of specialists individualized to the patient's associated conditions. Growth hormone (GH) therapy is initiated when growth failure is diagnosed and continued until projected adult height is attained or growth is less than 2 cm/year. While on GH therapy, patients are often followed with insulin-like growth factor (IGF) 1 and IGF binding protein 3 to titrate the dose. An increase in height of 7.2 cm in females taking GH for an average of 5.7 years as compared to those who did not take GH has been demonstrated.

⚕ Caution

Growth hormone
- When discussing initiation of GH therapy, risks and benefits associated with GH should be discussed.
- Although adverse effects associated with GH therapy are rare (<0.4%), an increase in scoliosis, diabetes, serious cardiovascular events, intracranial hypertension, slipped capital femoral epiphysis, pancreatitis, and new malignancies is seen in patients with Turner syndrome taking GH as compared to controls.

Table 52.1 Screening for features and conditions associated with Turner syndrome

Screening tool	Associated feature/condition	Approximate timing; frequency
Physical exam	Low posterior hairline, unfavorable body composition, prominent ears, lymphedema, nail dysplasia	At time of diagnosis
Growth chart	Short stature	Throughout childhood
Orthodontic exam	Narrow palate, retrognathia	At age 7 years
Follicle-stimulating hormone	Gonadal failure/infertility	At age 10–12 years
Neuropsychological, developmental, and/or educational exam	Learning disabilities: visuospatial, mathematic, and memory	At time of diagnosis, then variable
Tanner staging	Delayed puberty	Throughout adolescence
Dual emission X-ray absorptiometry (DEXA)	Low bone mineral density	At age 18 years
Formal audiology exam	Sensorineural hearing loss*	At time of diagnosis; q 1–3 years
Thyroid-stimulating hormone	Hypothyroidism*	At age 4
Electrocardiogram with echocardiogram and/or cardiac magnetic resonance imaging	Cardiac anomaly*	At time of diagnosis; q 5–10 years
Renal ultrasound	Renal anomaly*	At time of diagnosis
Fasting blood glucose or 2-hour oral glucose tolerance test	Diabetes mellitus*	At age 15 years (earlier if risk factors)
Serum immunoglobulin A (IgA) and tissue transglutaminase IgA antibody	Celiac disease*	At age 4 years; q 2–5 years
Complete metabolic profile	Renal and/or hepatic dysfunction*	At age 15 years
Fasting lipid profile	Metabolic dysfunction*	At age 15 years (earlier if risk factors)

*Associated conditions found in ≤50% of females with Turner syndrome; all other associated conditions found in >50% of females with Turner syndrome.

Pure gonadal dysgenesis XX

Pure gonadal dysgenesis with 46, XX karyotype is a rare disorder typically diagnosed during a work-up for delayed puberty or primary amenorrhea. Patients will be phenotypically female but upon lab evaluation will have elevated FSH and luteinizing hormone (LH) with undetectable anti-Müllerian hormone, consistent with hypergonadotropic hypogonadism. Stimulation with human chorionic gonadotropin (hCG) will not induce a normal rise in FSH and LH. FSH receptor mutations, sporadic or recessive, are a rare cause of pure gonadal dysgenesis with XX karyotype. Females with this condition should be screened for sensorineural hearing loss as they may have a recessive disorder; Perrault syndrome. Familial ovarian dysgenesis has been reported in an autosomal recessive fashion associated with consanguinity with mutation of the FSH receptor gene at 2p16 or translocation at Xq13.3–q26.

Pure gonadal dysgenesis XY

Individuals with pure gonadal dysgenesis with 46, XY karyotype (Swyer syndrome) are phenotypically female with unambiguous female genitalia and normal Müllerian structures. The etiology is linked to *SRY* mutations, mostly found within the high mobility box (HMG) domain, with over 60 mutations characterized. Similar to other females with pure gonadal dysgenesis, those with pure gonadal dysgenesis with XY karyotype have streak gonads and an intact uterus, necessitating estrogen therapy to induce puberty. Although they have XY karyotype, spermatogenesis is absent. Presence of Y chromosomal material increases the risk of gonadal tumors and malignancy and gonadectomy is recommended.

Partial or mixed gonadal dysgenesis

Individuals with partial (bilateral dysgenetic gonads) or mixed (one streak, one dysgenetic gonad) gonadal dysgenesis have a urogenital sinus and ambiguous external and internal genitalia. As previously mentioned, diagnosis may be suggested by radiographic findings but requires pathologic confirmation for definitive diagnosis. Management of patients with partial or mixed gonadal dysgenesis is complex and should be done in coordination with a multidisciplinary care team to ensure comprehensive care of the patient.

In partial and mixed gonadal dysgenesis, initial gender assignment is a frequent concern of the family and should be handled with open communication in a respectful manner (see Chapter 2). Factors that may help guide decision-making include: karyotype, future fertility, degree of virilization, and endocrine status.

✷ Tips and tricks

Multidisciplinary care team
• When managing patients with gonadal dysgenesis, it is important to provide comprehensive care for the patient through a team of specialists.
• The care team may include, but is not limited to, providers from the following specialties: urology and/or surgery, neonatology, genetics, social work, psychology, psychiatry, endocrinology (medical and/or reproductive), gynecology, nursing, ethics, and primary care provider.
• Females with Turner syndrome may also need care providers in orthodontia, gasteroenterology, education, audiology, ophthalmology, cardiology, and otolaryngology, depending on the associated conditions.
• Although there are little data regarding long-term outcomes of individuals with gonadal dysgenesis, a holistic approach is recommended to optimize patient care.

✋ Patient/parent advice

Gender assignment
• Assigning gender in individuals with ambiguous genitalia is a complex, individual decision made by consensus.
• The decision should be made by the patient's family and the multidisciplinary care team early in life.
• Surgical reconstruction is a separate decision which may be delayed unless function is compromised.

Adolescence and gonadal dysgenesis

Females with gonadal dysgenesis often have specific needs during adolescence. Adolescence is a time of transition which can be difficult for those with gonadal dysgenesis. Concerns may include developing sexual identity, gender assignment, and genital anatomy. Specialized care with therapists trained in disorders of sex development can help address anxiety regarding intimacy and relationships. Approximately a quarter of individuals with a history of ambiguous genitalia experience gender dysphoria regardless of the initial gender assignment. If gender reassignment is considered, it should be initiated by the patient only and in coordination with care from a trained psychiatric care provider. Anatomic concerns should be addressed on an individual basis. In adolescent females, a vaginal assessment is typically performed and, if appropriate, an individualized care plan is discussed.

Additionally, as gonadal failure is common in gonadal dysgenesis, estrogen replacement is needed for pubertal development and to prevent adverse effects associated with hypoestrogenism, including lack of secondary sexual characteristics, osteoporosis, endothelial dysfunction, dyslipidemia, and early death. Although many routes for estrogen therapy exist, transdermal administration of estradiol bypasses the first-pass metabolism in the liver and may reduce thrombotic risk as compared to oral administration. While on estrogen therapy, serum estradiol may be monitored to titrate the dose. When breast development is adequate or breakthrough bleeding occurs, progesterone should be added to counteract effects of unopposed estrogen and prevent endometrial hyperplasia. In those without a uterus, progesterone is not necessary.

Summary

Gonadal dysgenesis is a heterogeneous group of conditions within disorders of sex development resulting from abnormal development of the gonads. Although gonadal differentiation is a complex process, advances in molecular genetics have improved our understanding of gonadal dysgenesis. In adolescence, issues that may arise include: medical conditions specific to the diagnosis, reassessment of anatomy, gender dysphoria, development of secondary sexual characteristics, and psychosocial development. Optimal management of gonadal dysgenesis includes a multidisciplinary care team providing individualized care with open communication and respect.

♀ Pearls

- Sex steroid therapy is often needed to induce puberty and maintain bone and cardiac health.
- Spontaneous puberty may occur in females with Turner syndrome and a mosaic karyotype.
- The presence of intra-abdominal gonads in individuals with Y chromosomal material confers increased risk of gonadal tumors.
- A multidisciplinary care team is best suited to address specific needs in adolescence.

Further reading

Davenport ML. Approach to the patient with Turner's syndrome. *J Clin Endocrinol Metab* 2010;95:1487–1495.

Hughes IA, Houk C, Ahmed SF, *et al.* LWPES Consensus Group; ESPE Consensus Group. Consensus statement on management of intersex disorders. *Arch Dis Child* 2006; 91:554–563.

Strauss JF, Barbieri RL (eds). *Yen and Jaffe's Reproductive Endocrinology, Physiology, Pathophysiology and Clinical Management*. Philadelphia: Saunders Elsevier, 2009.

53 Sexual assault and date rape

Beth L. Emerson and Kirsten Bechtel

Yale School of Medicine, Department of Pediatrics, Section of Pediatric Emergency Medicine, Yale New-Haven Children's Hospital, New Haven, CT, USA

Sexual assault, defined as any forced or unwanted sexual activity, is unfortunately, a common problem during adolescence. In the US, over half of reported sexual assault victims are between the ages of 12 and 24 years. The prevalence of sexual assault may be as high as 18% for females in middle and high school.

The immediate care of the adolescent sexual assault victim requires the coordination of medical, legal, and psychosocial disciplines. Social work and victim support services should be involved as soon as possible to evaluate mental health needs and coordinate outpatient medical services and psychological support.

☆ Tips and tricks

• The patient should be informed as to what the medical and forensic examination will entail and given as much control over the examination as possible.
• The medical provider should use open-ended questions when obtaining the history, such as "Why did you come to the Emergency Department?" and "Can you tell me what happened?"
• When documenting the history, the use of the patient's own words in direct quotes can be helpful to fully convey the patient's experience of the assault.

• In situations where a physical exam is paramount, such as a history of severe genital pain or bleeding, inability to urinate or defecate, utilize the services of the child life therapists if available.
• A careful medical exam should first exclude any significant, life-threatening injury.
• If there is a history of abdominal or genital pain, vaginal bleeding or difficulty with urination or defecation, a speculum exam should be considered.
• Adolescents' comfort with and consent to the exam should be ensured prior to proceeding.
• Sedation or examination under anesthesia may be necessary in rare circumstances.

The history of the assault should be obtained in a confidential, safe setting. Having all the necessary members of the team present, including a support person as a victim advocate, may avoid repetitive, unnecessary questioning of the patient. Information about the circumstances of the assault, the identification of the perpetrator (if known), and any other injuries can guide the evaluation. Clear, concise documentation of the history is essential.

Practical Pediatric and Adolescent Gynecology, First Edition. Edited by Paula J. Adams Hillard.
© 2013 John Wiley & Sons, Ltd. Published 2013 by John Wiley & Sons, Ltd.

If the alleged sexual contact was within 72 hours, the patient should be given the option of evidence collection for a forensic (rape) kit. There may be regional variation in the contents of the kit, but the kit often includes the patient's clothing, scalp and pubic hair samples, blood samples for DNA typing, fingernail scrapings, swabs of any bodily fluids seen under ultraviolet light, and swabs of the genitalia. A sexual assault nurse examiner (SANE), available in some regional centers, should perform evidentiary

---

🔬 Science revisited

- Use of the BlueMaxx BM 500 lamp (SIrchie Laboratories, Raleigh, NC, USA) may be better than a Wood's lamp to detect biologic fluids such as seminal fluids.
- If the patient presents more than 72 hours after the assault, or if obtaining body swabs for forensic evidence collection would be traumatic for the patient, obtain clothing worn at the time of the assault if possible, as it may yield evidence that could potentially identify the perpetrator.

---

collection if available. An experienced clinician should perform the exam to minimize further trauma.

If the patient presents with altered mental status, amnesia or impaired motor skills, an evaluation for concomitant alcohol or drug use (voluntarily or otherwise) should be considered. Blood and urine samples for toxicology, as well as specialized laboratory testing for the "date rape" drugs, gamma-hydroxybutyrate (GHB) and flunitrazepam (Rohypnol), should be obtained with the patient's consent if the alleged assault occurred within the preceding 72 hours.

Testing for sexually-transmitted infection (STI) should be offered (Table 53.1) Appropriate follow-up of results within 1 week should be arranged prior to discharge, as well as serial testing for HIV at 6 weeks, 3 months, and 6 months. Depending on regional prevalence in the adolescent/adult population, STI prophylaxis can be offered (http://www.cdc.gov/std/treatment/2010/sexual-assault.htm).

Table 53.1 STI testing

Neisseria gonorrhoeae and *Chlamydia trachomatis*	Nucleic acid amplification tests (NAATs)
Trichomonas vaginalis	Wet mount and culture
HIV, syphilis, hepatitis B	Serum testing

While the overall risk of human immunodeficiency virus (HIV) transmission following sexual assault is low, it should be considered after higher risk exposures. Appropriate screening includes HIV enzyme immunoassay (EIA) and if performed, HIV post-exposure prophylaxis (PEP) should be considered. The Centers for Disease Control and Prevention (CDC) recommends consultation with an HIV treatment specialist if PEP is considered.

Prophylaxis with hepatitis B vaccine can be considered for incompletely vaccinated patients. Tetanus toxoid should be provided for patients with any cutaneous injury without a tetanus toxoid booster in the last 5 years.

After a negative urine pregnancy test, pregnancy prophylaxis can be administered up to 120 hours after the assault. Two levonorgestrel 0.75-mg tablets

---

✋ Caution

- When documenting the physical exam, refrain from using the term "intact" to describe the anatomy of the hymen. Instead use terms such as "no interruptions in the edge of the hymen" or "V-shaped interruption of the hymen at 6:00."
- Offer emergency contraception, with a repeat pregnancy test if no menses within 3 weeks.
- In rare cases where sedation is required to facilitate the examination, the type of sedation and time of administration should be clearly documented in the medical record. Any sedation should be done after a history has been obtained from the patient.

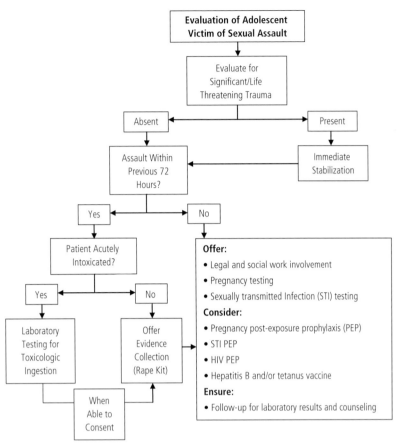

Figure 53.1 Management algorithm.

given immediately help ensure completion of therapy. Co-administration with an antiemetic may be helpful.

Following the completion of the sexual assault evaluation, the local police department should be contacted to maintain the appropriate chain of custody for the evidence collected. If the patient has any significant traumatic injury or the inability to arrange a safe discharge plan, hospital admission should be considered. Upon discharge, coordination with the patient's primary care provider is also essential to ensure follow-up of laboratory testing and supportive psychological care.

An algorithm for the management of the sexual assault victim is shown in Figure 53.1.

✋ Patient/parent advice

• Sexual violence (SV) refers to sexual activity where consent is not obtained or freely given. Anyone can experience SV, but most victims are female. The person responsible for the violence is typically male and is usually someone known to the victim. The person can be a friend, co-worker, neighbor, or family member.
• Psychological disturbances are the most common sequelae from sexual assault. A wide range of reactions can interfere with daily

(Continued)

functioning, such as: guilt/shame/
embarrassment; fear/distrust/sadness;
nightmares/flashbacks/posttraumatic stress
disorder (PTSD); depression/anxiety/phobias. It is
important to respect a victim's choice and style
of coping and to support the victim as much as
possible. It is also important to arrange for
professional mental health support/counseling if
the victim so desires. This can include advocacy-
based counseling in an individual, family or
group setting and 24-hour crisis intervention
assistance.

• It is important to follow-up with a primary
care provider for the results of any STI testing,
such as HIV, and to take all antibiotic and
antiretroviral medications as prescribed.

• Pregnancy is the most common medical
sequela after sexual assault. After emergency
contraception, the next menstrual cycle will
come at an earlier time and will have heavier
flow. If the next menstrual cycle is delayed, it is
important to get another urine pregnancy test,
as emergency contraception is not 100%
effective. It is important that contraception
(either hormonal or barrier based) be used with
any future consensual sexual activity.

Further reading

Kaufman M. Care of the adolescent sexual assault victim. *Pediatrics* 2008;122(2):462–470.

Santucci KA, Hsiao AL. Advances in Clinical Forensic Medicine. *Curr Opin Pediatr* 2003;15:304–308.

Thackeray JD, Hornor G, Benzinger EA, Scribano PV. Forensic evidence collection and DNA identification in acute child sexual assault. *Pediatrics* 2011;128(2):227–232.

Appendix 1 Essential information

Practical Pediatric and Adolescent Gynecology, First Edition. Edited by Paula J. Adams Hillard.
© 2013 John Wiley & Sons, Ltd. Published 2013 by John Wiley & Sons, Ltd.

Appendix 1.1.2 History of vulvovaginal symptoms in prepubertal girls

- Duration of symptoms
- Time of day when symptoms are worse
- Presence of discharge:
  - Color
  - Presence of foul odor
- Vaginal bleeding
- Itching
- Dysuria
- Burning and/or vulvar pain
- Irritant exposure including:
  - Bubble baths
  - Harsh detergent
  - Poor wiping techniques
- Prior home or prescribed regimens:
  - Recent antibiotics
  - Recent steroid use (inhaled or topical)
- Voiding habits
- Bowel habits

Appendix 1.1.3 Review of systems for prepubertal girls with vulvovaginal symptoms

- History of trauma
- Topical allergies
- Atopy
- Skin conditions:
  - Eczema
  - Psoriasis
- Potential risk of sexual abuse
- Signs of early puberty
- History of previous or current urinary tract infections,
- Recent gastroenteritis
- Enuresis
- Encopresis
- Recent respiratory infection

Appendix 1.1.4 Differential diagnosis of vulvovaginitis in prepubertal girls

- Nonspecific vulvovaginitis
- Specific vulvovaginitis
- Dermatologic skin disorders, e.g. lichen sclerosus
- Vaginal foreign bodies
- Sexually-transmitted infections
- Urinary tract infection
- Ectopic ureter
- Sexual abuse
- Pinworms
- Systemic disorders, e.g. Kawasaki disease
- Vulvodynia – rare
- Congenital enteric fistula

Appendix 1.2 Vulvar conditions that may present in girls of any age

- Lichen sclerosus
- Condyloma
- Contact irritant
- Epidermoid cysts (also termed sebaceous cysts)
- Molluscum contagiosum
- Pigmented nevus
- Psoriasis
- Vulvar abscess
- Vulvar vestibulitis
- Vulvar ulcers

Appendix 1.3 Causes of anogenital signs and symptoms in children: differential diagnosis

Sign or symptom	Trauma	Infection	Inflammation	Other
Genital or anal bleeding	Abusive trauma Accidental trauma, e.g. straddle injury	Shigella Group A beta-hemolytic strep Candidiasis	Intravaginal foreign body Excoriation due to irritants, hygiene, diaper dermatitis	Anal fissures Dehisced labial adhesions Urethral prolapse
Genital or anal bruising	Abusive blunt trauma Accidental blunt trauma, e.g. straddle injury		Lichen sclerosus et atrophicus	Hemangiomas Urethral prolapse Bruise mimics (nevi, Mongolian spots)
Genital or anal erythema	Abusive abrasive trauma	N. gonorrhoeae C. trachomatis Candidiasis Streptococcus or staphylococcus infections	Irritants, including soaps, fecal material, diaper dermatitis Folliculitis Psoriasis Lichen sclerosus et atrophicus	Normal prepubertal mucosa
Scarring of the hymen, vestibule or anus	Healed abusive blunt force or penetrative trauma			Labial adhesion Linea vestibularis Anatomic variants (usually midline), e.g. linea vestibularis, diastasis ani, failure of midline fusion
Dilatation of hymenal or anal openings	Uncommon, nonspecific finding for abuse			Obesity in females Decreased sphincter tone due to neurologic condition or sedation Presence of stool in rectal vault Encopresis Prolonged exam or change in exam position
Genital discharge	Healing genital trauma	N. gonorrhoeae C. trachomatis T. vaginalis Streptococcal infection Bacterial vaginosis Candidiasis	Intravaginal foreign body Overgrowth of normal vaginal flora	Semen Physiologic leukorrhea Smegma
Vesicles		Herpes simplex virus 1 or 2 Varicella zoster virus Epstein-Barr virus Impetigo	Behçet disease Pyoderma gangrenosum	
Papules and nodules		Condylomata acuminata Molluscum contagiosum Condylomata lata	Crohn disease Perianal pseudo-verrucous papules and nodules	Anal skin tags Urethral/peri-urethral cysts

Appendix 1.4 Assessment of vulvovaginal conditions in an adolescent

History
- Symptoms:
  - Vaginal discharge
  - Pruritus
  - Dyspareunia
  - External dysuria
  - Vaginal pain
  - Vulvar rash
- Duration of symptoms
- Relationship to menses
- Previous sexual activity
- Contraceptive use
- Pregnancy
- Recent course of antibiotics or steroid medications

Review of systems
- Symptoms of diabetes mellitus: polyuria, polydipsia, and polyphagia
- Immunologic deficiency: fevers, rashes, infections, hospital admissions for evaluation, and treatment of infections
- HIV: high-risk sexual behaviors, prior testing, and results

Physical exam
- There are rarely systemic signs of infection unless the patient is immunocompromised
- External genital examination:
  - Vulvar edema
  - Erythema
  - Fissures
  - Excoriations
  - Thick white curdy vaginal discharge
  - Pustulopapular peripheral skin lesions

Appendix 1.5 Goals of gynecologic care of an adolescent

- Establishing a relationship of trust with a clinician
- Facilitating patient/parent communication
- Screening for risks:
  - Unprotected sexual activity (risks for unintended pregnancy, STIs)
  - Substance use and abuse (comorbidities associated with unprotected sexual activity)
  - Depression and suicidal ideation
- Screening for adolescent antecedents of adult diseases (osteoporosis, polycystic ovary syndrome, diabetes mellitus, cardiovascular disease)
- Preventing menstrual morbidities (quality of life)
- Facilitating healthy psychosexual development
- Modeling appropriate health-seeking behaviors and development of self-efficacy
- Facilitating empowerment to learn about and care for her own body (first pelvic exam)
- Providing preventive guidance to patient and parent

Appendix 1.6.2 Reasons for a primary clinician to refer an adolescent to a gynecologist

- Vulvar, vaginal, or cervical lesion of unclear etiology or unresponsive to previous management
- Abnormal bleeding (heavy menstrual bleeding, amenorrhea, frequent bleeding) of unclear etiology or bleeding unresponsive to medical therapy or with anemia
- Dysmenorrhea unresponsive to NSAIDs and/or hormonal therapy
- Acute pelvic pain (concern about adnexal mass, ectopic pregnancy, pelvic infection)
- Chronic pelvic pain
- Adnexal mass
- Genital anomaly (duplication, imperforate hymen, vaginal septum, vaginal agenesis)
- Pregnancy
- Pelvic infection (if suspicion of tubo-ovarian complex or abscess or if clinician is not comfortable with management)
- Contraception in young women with chronic medical conditions
- Desire for contraceptive implant or IUD
- Genital trauma
- History of past gynecologic surgery with concerns about anatomy, risk of recurrence, genital anomalies, fertility

Appendix 1.6.3 Reasons to refer an adolescent to a gynecologist or specialist with greater experience in uncommon genital problems

- Genital anomaly:
  - Uterine duplication
  - Vaginal septum (transverse or longitudinal)
  - Vaginal agenesis
  - Obstructing anomaly:
    - Imperforate hymen,
    - Obstructing longitudinal or transverse vaginal septum with hematocolpos and/or hematometra
    - Cervical agenesis
    - Obstructed uterine horn
- History of specific gynecologic diagnoses:
  - Endometriosis
  - Germ cell tumor
  - Ovarian torsion
  - Lichen sclerosus
  - Vulvar aphthosis
  - Accidental vulvar trauma
  - Primary ovarian insufficiency
- Disorders of sex development (DSD): best managed with a team approach with genetics, endocrinology, urology, gynecology, social services, advocates for individuals with DSD
  - History of unknown diagnosis with genital surgery in infancy or childhood
  - History of virilization and subsequent surgery:
    - Congenital adrenal hyperplasia
    - Partial androgen insensitivity syndrome
  - Complete androgen insensitivity syndrome
  - Sex chromosome anomalies:
    - Turner syndrome/gonadal dysgenesis
  - Disorders of gonadal development
- Menstrual suppression for medical indications:
  - Developmental delay or autism
  - Bleeding disorders such as von Willebrand disease
  - Menstrual molimina
- Contraception for adolescents with complex medical problems
- Vulvar masses or lesions

Appendix 1.7 Indications for a pelvic exam in an adolescent

- Persistent vaginal discharge
- Dysuria or urinary tract symptoms in a sexually-active female
- Dysmenorrhea unresponsive to nonsteroidal anti-inflammatory drugs
- Amenorrhea
- Abnormal vaginal bleeding
- Lower abdominal pain
- Contraceptive counseling for an intrauterine device or diaphragm
- Perform Pap test
- Suspected/reported rape or sexual abuse
- Pregnancy

Appendix 1.8 Family history relevant to gynecologic conditions in adolescents

- Mother's age of menarche
- Family history of "early menopause"
- Family history of irregular menses during adolescent or young adult years
- Gynecologic diagnoses in the family:
  - Irregular menses
  - Heavy menses
  - Dysmenorrhea
  - Polycystic ovary syndrome:
    - Irregular menses
    - Hirsutism
    - Obesity
    - Infertility (specifically anovulatory)
  - Uterine fibroids
  - Endometriosis
- Family history of malignancies:
  - Breast cancer
  - Ovarian cancer
  - Uterine cancer
  - Colon cancer
  - Cervical cancer
- Family history of venous thromboembolism:
  - Deep vein thrombosis, pulmonary embolism
  - Recurrent miscarriages
  - Specific thrombophilias (Factor V Leiden, protein S, C, antithrombin III deficiency)
- Cardiovascular disease:
  - Diabetes
  - Hypertension
  - Hyperlipidemia
  - Sudden death
  - Stroke

Appendix 1.9.2 Adolescent developmental changes

	Body image	Cognitive	Family	Peer group	Sexuality
Early adolescent (11–14 years)	Onset of puberty Preoccupation with pubertal changes Self-conscious	Concrete thinking Daydreaming Mood swings Idealistic vocational goals	Less interest in family activities Anti-adult: appear to prefer friends to family Parents are a source of embarrassment	Same sex friendships Best friend Opposite sex interactions in school and large group activities Difficulty negotiating peer relationships, loneliness common	Physical attractiveness of partner most important; date in groups or non face-to-face "dating" (text, internet) Masturbation begins Gay/lesbian/bisexual/ transgender/questioning (GLBTQ): realize aroused by same gender, identity confusion in a heterosexist world
Middle adolescent (15–17 years)	General acceptance of body Concerns over making herself more attractive	Some abstract thinking; fall back to concrete thinking in times of stress Creativity Risk taking behavior and feelings of omnipotence, invulnerability, and immortality	Begin to question family rules/ values Parental concern and conflict peaks More time away from family	Mixed gender peer group, more time with peers Conformity with peer values	Intense, short-term romantic relationships. More concerned with herself in a relationship than she is about her partner Partner usually 2 years older Looking for image of ideal romantic partner Increased sexual activity and experimentation GLBTQ: Begins to think of herself as lesbian/ transgender and aligns with others
Late adolescent (18 years and older)	Acceptance of body	Adult reasoning skills Realistic vocational goals	Move toward adult relationship with parents	Peer group values less important Friendships based on similar interests/ activities	Long-term committed relationships Reciprocity in the relationship GLBTQ: Integration of homosexual identity into life

Appendix 1.9.3 Stages of adolescence

Early adolescence (11–14 years)	Middle adolescence (15–17 years)	Late adolescence (18–21 years)
Transition to middle school (e.g. multiple teachers, harder course work, higher expectations)	School and associated activities become central focus of life	May be entering college, starting first job, becoming a parent, or serving in the military
Increased logical, abstract, and idealistic thinking	May receive driving permit/license	Cognitive development still ongoing
Desire to belong to a peer group	Peers' importance as sources of information	May live in a variety of settings
Increased time without adult supervision	Increased interest in interpersonal relationships (e.g. dating, sexual activity)	Legally allowed to vote, smoke, or drink
Changes to family relationships (adolescent striving for greater independence)	Developmental period with highest risk for mental health disorders	Self-identity, rational and realistic conscience developed
		Moral, religious, and sexual values refined
		Decreased participation in health supervision visits

Appendix 1.9.4 Tanner staging of breast development

1 Preadolescent stage; nipple elevation only
2 Breast bud stage; elevation of breast and nipple as small mound, with enlargement of areola diameter
3 Further enlargement of breast and areola; increased pigmentation of areola
4 Further areola enlargement and pigmentation; nipple and areola form secondary mound above level of breast
5 Mature stage; smooth contour; projection of nipple only with recession of areola to level of breast

Appendix 1.10 Menstrual parameters in adolescents

Clinical description		Normal limits
Frequency (days)	Frequent	<21
	Normal	**21–45**
	Infrequent	>45
Regularity	Absent	
	Regular	**Approximately monthly**
	Irregular	Cycles <21 or >45 days
Duration of flow (days)	Prolonged	>8
	Normal	**3–7**
	Shortened	<3
Volume (mL)	Heavy	>80
	Normal	**5–80 (3–6 pads/day)**
	Light	<5

Appendix 1.11.2 Confidential sexual history

Ask about:
- All types of sexual behaviors including oral, vaginal, and anal intercourse
- Gender of sex partners
- Number of sex partners in the past 2 and 12 months
- New partners in the past 2 months
- Contraception use
- Condom use
- Difficulty with condom use (e.g. breakage, slippage)
- Negotiating condom use with partners
- Quality of relationships with partners (e.g. safety)
- Pregnancy history
- Past STI testing or infections

Appendix 1.11.3 The 5 Ps of sexual history taking

- Partners:
  - "Do you have sex with men, women, or both?"
  - "In the past 2 months, how many partners have you had sex with?"
  - "In the past 12 months, how many partners have you had sex with?"
  - "Is it possible that any of your sex partners in the past 12 months had sex with someone else while they were still in a sexual relationship with you?"
- Prevention of pregnancy:
  - "What are you doing to prevent pregnancy?"
- Protection from STDs:
  - "What do you do to protect yourself from STDs and HIV?"
- Practices:
  - To understand your risks for STDs. I need to understand the kind of sex you have had recently."
  - "Have you had vaginal sex, meaning 'penis in the vagina sex'?" If yes, "Do you use condoms never, sometimes or always?"
  - "Have you had anal sex, meaning 'penis in the rectum/anus sex'?" If yes, "Do you use condoms never, sometimes or always?"
  - "Have you had oral sex, meaning 'mouth on the penis or vagina'?"
- Past history of STDs:
  - "Have you ever had an STD?"
  - "Have any of your partners had an STD?"

Appendix 1.11.4 Review of systems if concerns about sexually-transmitted infections

Ask about:
- Change in vaginal discharge including:
  - Amount
  - Character
  - Color
  - Odor
- Vulvar discomfort, irritation, and pruritus
- Genital sores or lesions
- Dysuria
- Intermenstrual bleeding
- Bleeding with sexual intercourse
- Pain or discomfort with sexual intercourse
- Abdominal or pelvic pain

Appendix 1.11.5 Physical exam if concerns about sexually-transmitted infections

External genital exam
- Check for findings suggestive of an STI, such as:
  - Inguinal lymphadenopathy
  - Presence of vaginal discharge
  - Vulvar irritation
  - Vulvar lesions

Speculum exam
Allows for visualization of the cervix to assess for diagnostic signs of cervicitis including:
- Mucopurulent endocervical exudate and
- Endocervical friability
- (Both of these may be observed through use of endocervical cotton swab specimen to identify mucopurulent or bloody discharge respectively on the swab)

Bimanual exam
- Adnexal tenderness
- Uterine tenderness
- Cervical motion tenderness
- The presence of any one of these is clinically diagnostic for PID in the absence of other abdominal or pelvic pathology

Appendix 1.12.2 Percentage of women experiencing an unintended pregnancy during the first year of typical use and the first year of perfect use of contraception, and the percentage continuing use at the end of the first year: United States of America

Method (1)	% of Women Experiencing an Unintended Pregnancy within the First Year of Use		% of Women Continuing Use at One Year[3]
	Typical Use[1] (2)	Perfect Use[2] (3)	(4)
No method[4]	85	85	
Spermicides[5]	28	18	42
Fertility awareness-based methods	24		47
Standard Days method[6]		5	
TwoDay method[6]		4	
Ovulation method[6]		3	
Symptothermal method[6]		0.4	
Withdrawal	22	4	46
Sponge			36
Parous women	24	20	
Nulliparous women	12	9	
Condom[7]			
Female (fc)	21	5	41
Male	18	2	43
Diaphragm[8]	12	6	57
Combined pill and progestin-only pill	9	0.3	67
Evra patch	9	0.3	67
NuvaRing	9	0.3	67
Depo-Provera	6	0.2	56
Intrauterine contraceptives			
ParaGard (copper T)	0.8	0.6	78
Mirena (LNg)	0.2	0.2	80
Implanon	0.05	0.05	84
Female sterilization	0.5	0.5	100
Male sterilization	0.15	0.10	100

Emergency Contraception: Emergency contraceptive pills or insertion of a copper intrauterine contraceptive after unprotected intercourse substantially reduces the risk of pregnancy.[9] (See Chapter 6.).

Lactational Amenorrhea Method: LAM is a highly effective, *temporary* method of contraception.[10] (See Chapter 18.)

(Continued)

Appendix 1.12.2 (*Continued*)

Reproduced from Trussell J. Contraceptive Efficacy. In Hatcher RA, Trussell J, Nelson AL, Cates W, Stewart FH, Kowal D (eds) *Contraceptive Techology: 19th Revised Edition*. New York, NY: Ardent Media, 2007.

Notes:

[1]Among *typical* couples who initiate use of a method (not necessarily for the first time), the percentage who experience an accidental pregnancy during the first year if they do not stop use for any other reason. Estimates of the probability of pregnancy during the first year of typical use for spermicides, withdrawal, fertility awareness-based methods, the diaphragm, the male condom, the oral contraceptive pill, and Depo-Provera are taken from the 1995 National Survey of Family Growth corrected for underreporting of abortion; see the text for the derivation of estimates for the other methods.

[2]Among couples who initiate use of a method (not necessarily for the first time) and who use it *perfectly* (both consistently and correctly), the percentage who experience an accidental pregnancy during the first year if they do not stop use for any other reason. See the text for the derivation of the estimate for each method.

[3]Among couples attempting to avoid pregnancy, the percentage who continue to use a method for 1 year.

[4]The percentages becoming pregnant in columns (2) and (3) are based on data from populations where contraception is not used and from women who cease using contraception in order to become pregnant. Among such populations, about 89% become pregnant within 1 year. This estimate was lowered slightly (to 85%) to represent the percentage who would become pregnant within 1 year among women now relying on reversible methods of contraception if they abandoned contraception altogether.

[5]Foams, creams, gels, vaginal suppositories, and vaginal film.

[6]The Ovulation and TwoDay methods are based on evaluation of cervical mucus. The Standard Days method avoids intercourse on cycle days 8 through 19. The Symptothermal method is a double-check method based on evaluation of cervical mucus to determine the first fertile day and evaluation of cervical mucus and temperature to determine the last fertile day.

[7]Without spermicides.

[8]With spermicidal cream or jelly.

[9]ella, Plan B One-Step and Next Choice are the only dedicated products specifically marketed for emergency contraception. The label for Plan B One-Step (one dose is 1 white pill) says to take the pill within 72 hours after unprotected intercourse. Research has shown that all of the brands listed here are effective when used within 120 hours after unprotected sex. The label for Next Choice (one dose is 1 peach pill) says to take 1 pill within 72 hours after unprotected intercourse and another pill 12 hours later. Research has shown that both pills can be taken at the same time with no decrease in efficacy or increase in side effects and that they are effective when used within 120 hours after unprotected sex. The Food and Drug Administration has in addition declared the following 19 brands of oral contraceptives to be safe and effective for emergency contraception: Ogestrel (1 dose is 2 white pills), Nordette (1 dose is 4 light-orange pills), Cryselle, Levora, Low-Ogestrel, Lo/Ovral, or Quasence (1 dose is 4 white pills), Jolessa, Portia, Seasonale or Trivora (1 dose is 4 pink pills), Seasonique (1 dose is 4 light-blue-green pills), Enpresse (one dose is 4 orange pills), Lessina (1 dose is 5 pink pills), Aviane or LoSeasonique (one dose is 5 orange pills), Lutera or Sronyx (one dose is 5 white pills), and Lybrel (one dose is 6 yellow pills).

[10]However, to maintain effective protection against pregnancy, another method of contraception must be used as soon as menstruation resumes, the frequency or duration of breastfeeds is reduced, bottle feeds are introduced, or the baby reaches 6 months of age.

Appendix 1.12.3 Conditions that occur frequently in adolescents for which combined oral contraception can have a beneficial effect

- Dysmenorrhea
- Premenstrual syndrome
- Benign breast disease
- Iron-deficiency anemia
- Acne
- Menstrual irregularities

Appendix 1.12.4 Bleeding patterns after 1 year of continuous hormone use

- Combined oral contraceptives: amenorrhea rate – 50–70%
- DMPA: amenorrhea rate – 45–70%
- Levenorgestrel IUD: amenorrhea rate – 50%
- Transdermal patch*: amenorrhea rate at 3 months – 10%
- Vaginal ring: median number or bleeding or spotting days – 14 days in months 9 through 12 of use
- Subdermal etonorgestrel implant: mean number of bleeding or spotting days – 19 days in months 9 through 12 of use

*Information only available for 3 months of continuous patch use.

Appendix 1.12.5 Contraception method switching: how to switch to or from combined oral contraceptives (COCs)

Switching from	Switching *to*						
	COCs	Patch	Ring	Progestin shot ("Depo")	Progestin implant	Hormone IUD	Copper IUD (nonhormone)
COCs	*No gap:* take first pill of new pack the day after taking any pill in the old pack	Start patch *one day before* stopping pill	*No gap:* insert ring the day after taking any pill in the pack	First shot *7 days before* stopping pill	Insert implant *4 days before* stopping pill	Insert hormone IUD *7 days before* stopping pill	Can insert copper IUD *up to 5 days after* stopping pill
Patch	Start pill *1 day before* stopping patch						
Ring	Start pill *1 day before* stopping ring						
Progestin shot ("Depo")	Can take first pill up to *15 weeks after* the last shot						
Progestin implant	Start pill *7 days before* implant is removed						
Hormone IUD	Start pill *1 day before* IUD is removed						
Copper IUD	Start pill *7 days before* IUD is removed						

Adapted from Reproductive Health Access Project @ http://www.reproductiveaccess.org/fact_sheets/switching_bc.htm

Appendix 1.13 Psychological screening with sample questions

	Category	Sample questions
H	Home	Who do you live with at home?
		How do you get along with people at home?
		Do you feel safe at home?
E	Education/	What school do you go to? What grade are you in?
	employment	What types of grades do you usually make?
		What do you want to do after you finish school?
		Do you work? What type of work do you do, and how many hours a week do you work?
E	Eating	How do you feel about your body?
		What changes would you want to make to your weight or body?
		What do you usually eat?
		What are you doing to change your weight?
A	Activities	What do you like to do for fun?
		What do you do with your friends?
D	Drugs	Have you ever tried smoking cigarettes or marijuana or drinking alcohol?
		How often are you using?
		What do you think about quitting?
		What problems have you had because of using?
S	Sexuality	Are you attracted to males, females, or both?
		Are you in a relationship now?
		Have you ever had sex? How old were you when you first had sex?
		How often are you using condoms?
		Are you on any type of contraception or interested in it?
		Have you ever had a sexually-transmitted illness?
		Have you ever been pregnant?
S	Suicidality/depression	How would you describe your mood?
		Do you have trouble sleeping?
		Have you ever had any thoughts of or tried anything to hurt or kill yourself?
S	Safety	Has anyone been hurting you physically, emotionally, or sexually?
		Have you been bullied?
(S)	Spirituality	What do you consider to be your religion or spiritual background?
		How do your religious beliefs impact how you make decisions for your health?

Appendix 1.14 Etiologies of chronic pelvic pain

- Gynecologic causes:
  - Endometriosis
  - Pelvic inflammatory disease
  - Congenital anomalies
  - Pelvic adhesive disease
  - Ovarian masses
- Urologic causes:
  - Chronic urinary tract infections
  - Kidney stones
  - Interstitial cystitis
- Gastroenterologic causes:
  - Constipation
  - Irritable bowel disease
  - Lactose intolerance
  - Inflammatory bowel disease
  - Hernia
  - Chronic appendicitis
  - Abdominal migraines
- Musculoskeletal causes:
  - Trauma or old injury
  - Leg length discrepancy
  - Postural problems
  - Trigger points
- Psychosocial causes:
  - Depression/anxiety
  - School avoidance
  - Physical or sexual abuse
  - Eating disorders
  - Substance abuse

Appendix 1.15.2 Malignant ovarian masses

Germ cell tumors
Teratomas
Gonadoblastoma
Choriocarcinoma
Dysgerminoma
Embryonal carcinoma
Polyembryoma
Endodermal sinus tumor
Mixed forms

Sex cord-stromal tumors
Sertoli–Leydig cell tumor
Granulosa cell tumor
Gynandroblastoma
Lipid cell tumors

Epithelial tumors
Serous
Mucinous
Small cell
Clear cell
Endometrioid
Transitional
Brenner
Mixed malignant
Mesodermal
Undifferentiated

Metastases to ovary

Modified from the World Health Organization's International Histologic Classification of Ovarian Tumors. Reproduced with permission from Emans SJ, Laufer MR, Goldstein DP. Benign and malignant ovarian masses. In: Pediatric and Adolescent Gynecology, 2005:685–728. Lippincott Williams & Wilkins.

Appendix 1.15.3 Differential diagnosis of a unilocular cyst in the pediatric age group

- Follicular cyst
- Cystadenoma:
  - Mucinous: can get very large
  - Serous
- Paratubal (para-ovarian) cyst
- Hydrosalpinx, salpingitis, pelvic inflammatory disease
- Mesenteric cyst
- Urachal cyst
- Appendiceal abscess
- Obstructed genital lesions (imperforate hymen, noncommunicating uterine horn)

Appendix 1.15.4 Differential diagnosis of mixed echogenic adnexal masses in the adolescent age group

- Corpus luteum cyst
- Germ cell neoplasms:
  - Benign cystic teratoma: most common
  - Serous cystadenoma
  - Mucinous cysadenoma
  - Malignant ovarian germ cell tumors
- Endometrioma
- Ectopic pregnancy
- Pelvic inflammatory disease:
  - Tubo-ovarian abscess
  - Tubo-ovarian complex
  - Pyosalpinx

Appendix 2 Useful web resources for adolescents, their parents/caregivers, and clinicians

For parents

General topics

Children Now – Talking about difficult topics with 8–12 year olds
http://www.talkingwithkids.org/

Nemours teen health – General health, including the reproductive system, growth and development, puberty, nutrition, weight
http://teenshealth.org/

The American Academy of Pediatrics – Information from pediatricians
http://www.healthychildren.org

Gynecology and reproductive health

The Center for Young Women's Health (CYWH) – Information for parents of teens
http://www.youngwomenshealth.org/

Sex education

Advocates for Youth – Parent sex education center
http://www.advocatesforyouth.org/
Campaign for Our Children – Parent resource center, sexuality and communication
http://www.cfoc.org/
Society of Obstetricians and Gynecologists of Canada
www.sexualityandu.ca/parents

Obesity and eating disorders

American Academy of Pediatrics, Changing Your Role: Helping Your Overweight Adolescents
http://www.healthychildren.org/English/health-issues/conditions/obesity/pages/Your-Changing-Role-Helping-Your-Overweight-Teen.aspx

Something Fishy – Eating disorders and compulsive overeating
www.something-fishy.org

National Eating Disorders Association (NEDA)
www.nationaleatingdisorders.org

For teens

General topics

Columbia University's Health Promotion Program – Including weight, eating disorders, sexual health, relationships, nutrition, physical activity
http://www.goaskalice.columbia.edu/

Nemours teen health – General health, including the reproductive system, growth and development, puberty, nutrition, weight
http://teenshealth.org/

Gynecology and reproductive health

The Center for Young Women's Health (CYWH) – Endometriosis, PCOS, MRKH, POI
http://www.youngwomenshealth.org/

Practical Pediatric and Adolescent Gynecology, First Edition. Edited by Paula J. Adams Hillard.
© 2013 John Wiley & Sons, Ltd. Published 2013 by John Wiley & Sons, Ltd.

Sexual health and sexuality

Advocates for Youth – LGBTQ
http://www.youthresource.org

The American Social Health Association – Sexual health
http://www.iwannaknow.org

Campaign for Our Children – Teen guide
http://www.cfoc.org/

Rutgers, the State University of New Jersey – sex education by teens, for teens
http://www.sexetc.org/

MTV collaboration with Kaiser Family Foundation – Pregnancy, STDs, relationships
http://www.itsyoursexlife.com/

Planned Parenthood Teens – Am I ready for sex?, LGBTQ, sex, masturbation, relationships, birth control
http://www.teenwire.com/

California Family Health Council – Contraception, STDs, resources
http://www.teensource.org

Society of Obstetricians and Gynecologists of Canada
www.sexualityandu.ca

Contraception

The National Campaign to Prevent Teen and Unintended Pregnancy – For older teens and young adults
http://www.bedsider.org

Planned Parenthood Teens – Am I ready for sex?, pregnancy, pregnancy options, relationships, birth control
http://www.teenwire.com/

Pregnancy

Planned Parenthood Teens – Am I ready for sex?, pregnancy, pregnancy options, LGBTQ, sex, masturbation, relationships, birth control
http://www.teenwire.com/

Pregnancy Options Workbook – Abortion, adoption, childbirth, parenting
www.pregnancyoptions.info

Backline – "Unconditional and judgment-free support for the full spectrum of decisions, feelings and experiences with pregnancy, parenting, adoption and abortion"
www.yourbackline.org

Abortion Care Network – Mom, Dad I'm Pregnant
www.abortioncarenetwork.org

Faith Aloud – "Overcoming the religious stigma of abortion and sexuality"; supporting *all* pregnancy options
www.faithaloud.org/faith/faith-counseling.php

For kids

General topics

Nemours teen health – General health including puberty for 8–12 year olds
http://teenshealth.org/

For clinicians

Policy statements and guidelines on contraception, abortion, LGBTQ, STDs, eating disorders

American Academy of Pediatrics (AAP)
http://www.aap.org

American College of Obstetrics and Gynecology (ACOG)
http://www.acog.org

North American Society for Pediatric and Adolescent Gynecology (NASPAG)
http://www.naspag.org

American Academy of Family Practice (AAFP)
http://www.aafp.org

Centers for Disease Control (CDC)
http://www.cdc.gov

Gay and Lesbian Medical Association
http://www.glma.org

National Institute of Mental Health (NIMH)
http://www.nimh.nih.gov

National Eating Disorders Association (NEDA)
www.nationaleatingdisorders.org

Centers for Disease Control and Prevention, Healthy Weight – It's not a diet, it's a lifestyle!
http://www.cdc.gov/healthyweight/assessing/bmi/childrens_bmi/about_childrens_bmi.html

Index

Practical Pediatric and Adolescent Gynecology, First Edition. Edited by Paula J. Adams Hillard.
© 2013 John Wiley & Sons, Ltd. Published 2013 by John Wiley & Sons, Ltd.